Non-Interpretive Skills for Radiology

CASE REVIEW SERIES

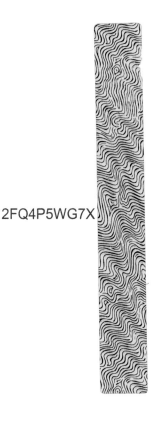

Series Editor

David M. Yousem, MD, MBA
Associate Dean of Professional Development
Director of Neuroradiology
Johns Hopkins School of Medicine
Baltimore, Maryland

Volumes in the CASE REVIEW Series

Series Foreword

I have been very gratified by the popularity and positive feedback that the authors of the Case Review series have received on the publication of their volumes. Reviews in journals and online sites as well as word-of-mouth comments have been uniformly favorable. The authors have done an outstanding job in filling the niche of an affordable, easy-to access, case-based learning tool that supplements the material in the Requisites series. I have been told by residents, fellows, and practicing radiologists that the Case Review series books are the ideal means for studying for rotations and clinical practice.

Although some students learn best in a non-interactive study book mode, others need the anxiety or excitement of being quizzed. The selected format for the Case Review series (which consists of showing a few images needed to construct a differential diagnosis and then asking a few clinical and imaging questions) was designed to simulate the board examination experience. The only difference is that the Case Review books provide the correct answer and immediate feedback. The limit and range of the reader's knowledge are tested through scaled cases ranging from relatively easy to very hard. The Case Review series also offers feedback on the answers, a brief discussion of each case, a link back to the pertinent Requisites volume, and up-to-date references from the literature. In addition, we have recently included labeled figures, figure legends, and supplemental figures in a new section at the end of the book, which provide the reader more information about the case and diagnosis.

This new title on non-interpretive skills does not follow the image-followed-by question format of the other titles in the series by necessity. I hope the chance to learn this new and challenging content is both rewarding and fun.

We have upcoming volumes yet to be published, so stay tuned for even more Case Review favorites to come. Personally, I am very excited about the future. Join us.

David M. Yousem, MD, MBA

Non-Interpretive Skills for Radiology

CASE REVIEW SERIES

David M. Yousem, MD, MBA
Associate Dean of Professional Development
Director of Neuroradiology
Johns Hopkins School of Medicine
Baltimore, Maryland

The 2015-2016 Trainees
Department of Radiology
Johns Hopkins Medical Institution
Baltimore, Maryland

ELSEVIER

ELSEVIER

1600 John F. Kennedy Blvd.
Ste 1800
Philadelphia, PA 19103-2899

NON-INTERPRETIVE SKILLS FOR RADIOLOGY: CASE REVIEW SERIES   ISBN: 978-0-323-47352-1

Notices

Knowledge and best practice in this field are constantly changing. As new research and experience broaden our understanding, changes in research methods, professional practices, or medical treatment may become necessary.

Practitioners and researchers must always rely on their own experience and knowledge in evaluating and using any information, methods, compounds, or experiments described herein. In using such information or methods they should be mindful of their own safety and the safety of others, including parties for whom they have a professional responsibility.

With respect to any drug or pharmaceutical products identified, readers are advised to check the most current information provided (i) on procedures featured or (ii) by the manufacturer of each product to be administered, to verify the recommended dose or formula, the method and duration of administration, and contraindications. It is the responsibility of practitioners, relying on their own experience and knowledge of their patients, to make diagnoses, to determine dosages and the best treatment for each individual patient, and to take all appropriate safety precautions.

To the fullest extent of the law, neither the Publisher nor the authors, contributors, or editors, assume any liability for any injury and/or damage to persons or property as a matter of products liability, negligence or otherwise, or from any use or operation of any methods, products, instructions, or ideas contained in the material herein.

Library of Congress Cataloging-in-Publication Data
Names: Yousem, David M., author.
Title: Non-interpretive skills for radiology : case review / David M. Yousem.
Other titles: Case review series.
Description: Philadelphia, PA : Elsevier, Inc., [2017] | Series: Case review
 series | Includes bibliographical references.
Identifiers: LCCN 2016029283 (print) | LCCN 2016029758 (ebook) | ISBN
 9780323473521 (pbk. : alk. paper) | ISBN 9780323473743 (E-Book)
Subjects: | MESH: Radiology | Examination Questions | Case Reports
Classification: LCC RC78.15 (print) | LCC RC78.15 (ebook) | NLM WN 18.2 | DDC
 616.07/57076–dc23
LC record available at https://lccn.loc.gov/2016029283

Executive Content Strategist: Robin R. Carter
Senior Content Development Specialist: Joan Ryan
Publishing Services Manager: Hemamalini Rajendrababu
Senior Project Manager: Beula Christopher
Senior Designer: Amy Buxton

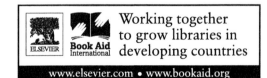

Working together
to grow libraries in
developing countries

www.elsevier.com • www.bookaid.org

NOUSHIN YAHYAVI FIROUZ ABADI, MD
Instructor of Radiology and Radiological Science
Johns Hopkins School of Medicine
Baltimore, MD

RAAG AIRAN, MD
Fellow, Department of Radiology
Johns Hopkins School of Medicine
Baltimore, MD

GULCIN ALTINOK, MD
Fellow, Department of Radiology
Johns Hopkins School of Medicine
Baltimore, MD

EMILY AMBINDER, MD
Resident, Department of Radiology
Johns Hopkins School of Medicine
Baltimore, MD

LUKASZ BABIARZ, MD
Instructor of Radiology and Radiological Science
Johns Hopkins School of Medicine
Baltimore, MD

DAVID BADGER, MD
Resident, Department of Radiology
Johns Hopkins School of Medicine
Baltimore, MD

JASON CALDWELL, MD
Fellow, Department of Radiology
Johns Hopkins School of Medicine
Baltimore, MD

AMMAR CHAUDHRY, MD
Fellow, Department of Radiology
Johns Hopkins School of Medicine
Baltimore, MD

CHRISTOPHER CHIN, MD
Fellow, Department of Radiology
Johns Hopkins School of Medicine
Baltimore, MD

RYAN CUNNINGHAM, MD
Fellow, Department of Radiology
Johns Hopkins School of Medicine
Baltimore, MD

MICHAEL DIGIANVITTORIO, MD
Fellow, Department of Radiology
Johns Hopkins School of Medicine
Baltimore, MD

PETER DUGGAN, MD
Fellow, Department of Radiology
Johns Hopkins School of Medicine
Baltimore, MD

MEHRDAD FETRAT, MD
Fellow, Department of Radiology
Johns Hopkins School of Medicine
Baltimore, MD

CHRISTOPHER FUNG, MD
Fellow, Department of Radiology
Johns Hopkins School of Medicine
Baltimore, MD

MICHAEL HAKKY, MD
Fellow, Department of Radiology
Johns Hopkins School of Medicine
Baltimore, MD

JIP INTRAPIROMKUL, MD
Fellow, Department of Radiology
Johns Hopkins School of Medicine
Baltimore, MD

JEFF JENSEN, MD
Resident, Department of Radiology
Johns Hopkins School of Medicine
Baltimore, MD

ARASH KAMALI, MD
Instructor of Radiology and Radiological Science
Johns Hopkins School of Medicine
Baltimore, MD

RIHAM EL-KHOULI, MD
Fellow, Department of Radiology
Johns Hopkins School of Medicine
Baltimore, MD

MARINOS KONTZIALIS, MD
Instructor of Radiology and Radiological Science
Johns Hopkins School of Medicine
Baltimore, MD

SALVATORE LABRUZZO, MD
Blanchfield Army Community Hospital
Fort Campbell, KY

DAVID LEE, MD
Fellow, Department of Radiology
Johns Hopkins School of Medicine
Baltimore, MD

KURT MESSER, MD
Fellow, Department of Radiology
Johns Hopkins School of Medicine
Baltimore, MD

CHARLES MITCHELL, MD
Fellow, Department of Radiology
Johns Hopkins School of Medicine
Baltimore, MD

CHIEDOZIE MKPOLULU, MD
Fellow, Department of Radiology
Johns Hopkins School of Medicine
Baltimore, MD

ANNA JEAN MORELAND, MD
Resident, Department of Radiology
Johns Hopkins School of Medicine
Baltimore, MD

Contributors

MY-LINH NGUYEN, MD
Resident, Department of Radiology
Johns Hopkins School of Medicine
Baltimore, MD

BENJAMIN NORTHCUTT, MD
Fellow, Department of Radiology
Johns Hopkins School of Medicine
Baltimore, MD

KRISTINA NOWITZKI, MD
Fellow, Department of Radiology
Johns Hopkins School of Medicine
Baltimore, MD

BERNARD O'MALLEY, MD
Associate Radiologist
Memorial Sloan-Kettering Cancer Center
New York, NY

EMANUELE ORRU, MD
Fellow, Department of Radiology
Johns Hopkins School of Medicine
Baltimore, MD

BABITA PANIGRAHI, MD
Resident, Department of Radiology
Johns Hopkins School of Medicine
Baltimore, MD

PUSKAR PATTANAYAK, MD
Resident, Department of Radiology
Johns Hopkins School of Medicine
Baltimore, MD

ELIE PORTNOY, MD
Resident, Department of Radiology
Johns Hopkins School of Medicine
Baltimore, MD

DAVID REISNER, MD
Fellow, Department of Radiology
Johns Hopkins School of Medicine
Baltimore, MD

JAMIE SCHROEDER, MD
Resident, Department of Radiology
Johns Hopkins School of Medicine
Baltimore, MD

DANIEL SEEBURG, MD
Fellow, Department of Radiology
Johns Hopkins School of Medicine
Baltimore, MD

ARCHANA SIDDALINGAPPA, MD
Fellow, Department of Radiology
Johns Hopkins School of Medicine
Baltimore, MD

PARVINDER SUJLANA, MD
Resident, Department of Radiology
Johns Hopkins School of Medicine
Baltimore, MD

CHRISTOPHER TRIMBLE, MD
Fellow, Department of Radiology
Johns Hopkins School of Medicine
Baltimore, MD

EVRIM TURKBEY, MD
Chief Resident, Department of Radiology
Johns Hopkins School of Medicine
Baltimore, MD

AJAY WADGAONKAR, MD
Fellow, Department of Radiology
Johns Hopkins School of Medicine
Baltimore, MD

JESSICA WEN, MD
Resident, Department of Radiology
Johns Hopkins School of Medicine
Baltimore, MD

ELCIN ZAN, MD
Fellow, Department of Radiology
Johns Hopkins School of Medicine
Baltimore, MD

To family, friends, colleagues, students
Thanks for sharing in the joy

NOUSHIN YAHYAVI *To Pouya, love of my life, and to Jasmine, joy of my life.*

RAAG AIRAN *To my family, for putting up with my random walks.*

GULCIN ALTINOK *To my husband, Deniz Altinok, my son, Alp Altinok, and daughter, Aylin Altinok, who love and support me all the time.*

EMILY AMBINDER *To my supportive and loving family, especially my husband, Alex.*

LUKASZ BABIARZ *To my wife, Aleksandra, and my daughter, Natalia: you put a smile on my face every day!*

DAVID BADGER *To Jana, Breyton, Evie, and Peter whose support made this important contribution to the vast expanse of non-interpretive trivia possible.*

JASON CALDWELL *To my family for all your constant love and support.*

AMMAR CHAUDHRY *To my entire family, especially my mother, Amber Mirza, without whom I could not get this far.*

CHRISTOPHER CHIN *To my parents, for their unconditional love, constant encouragement, and unwavering support in all my endeavors.*

RYAN CUNNINGHAM *To Shannon and Sabrina, for the love and laughter you bring me every day.*

MICHAEL DIGIANVITTORIO *To my wife, Michaela, whose love and support make my work possible.*

PETER DUGGAN *To my lovely wife and future daughter as well as my parents and brothers: thank you.*

MEHRDAD FETRAT *To Setareh, my staunchest support.*

CHRISTOPHER FUNG *To Daisy and my kiddos. Harold Fung, I told you your name would end up in a radiology textbook.*

MICHAEL HAKKY *To my family.*

JARUNEE INTRAPIROMKUL *To my dear husband, my family and friends, who help me through the hard times.*

JEFF JENSEN *To Ashton, Melinda, and Dan who have shared both my disappointment and success.*

ARASH KAMALI *To my wife for all the dedication and support throughout the years.*

RIHAM EL KHOULI *To my family, without whom I would never been able to succeed. You mean the world to me.*

MARINOS KONTZIALIS *To Ioanna, and Spyros.*

SALVATORE LABRUZZO *To Sally, Mason, and Gavin. I adore each of you.*

DAVID LEE *To my parents, Sara, and Olivia.*

KURT MESSER *To my dad, Ray Messer, Uncle Mike, Aunt Jenny, my great-grandparents, and the entire Messer and Liddicoatt family.*

CHARLES MITCHELL *To Jen, my wife, who goes anywhere with me and is always up for an adventure.*

CHIEDOZIE MKPOLULU *To Onyekachi Obi-Mkpolulu, the love of my life, and to Chiebuka Stefan Mkpolulu, the excellence of my youth.*

ANNA MORELAND *To Dr. Fred T. Lee, for incredible generosity in mentorship.*

MY-LINH NGUYEN *To my parents and husband. Thank you for your love and support.*

BENJAMIN NORTHCUTT *To my wife, Dania, and the rest of my family for all their support.*

KRISTINA NOWITZKI *To Ms. Schaffer, who taught me to think and write in concrete detail.*

BERNARD O'MALLEY *To my family, my friends, and all those at Johns Hopkins who supported my sabbatical process. Thank you all.*

EMANUELE ORRU' *To my parents and to my mentors around the world.*

BABITA PANIGRAHI *For all who see magic in the world. As Vonnegut said, "Science is magic that works."*

PUSKAR PATTANAYAK *Thank you to my parents, Namra and Kalidas, and my brother, Mithun, for all your love and support.*

ELIE PORTNOY *Meira, all steps forward that we take, are rooted in your incredible devotion to us and to our boys. With endless thanks ....*

DAVID REISNER *To my beautiful wife, Kendra, and our wonderful daughter, Hannah. My love grows daily.*

JAMIE SCHROEDER *With appreciation for the support of my family and the excellent teaching faculty of Hopkins Radiology.*

DANIEL SEEBURG *To my wife, Whitney, and my three children, Katia, Carsten, and Clara.*

ARCHANA SIDDALINGAPPA *To my father, Dr. Siddalingappa, who has guided me through life; my mother, Rekha, who has nurtured and showered me with love; my brother, Adarsh, who has always cared for me and protected me; and my dearest husband, Guru, who has brought so much joy into my life and made my life complete.*

PARVINDER SUJLANA *To my parents, Prithipal and Rajwant Sujlana, my sister, Sukhpreet Kaur, and my better half, Shreya Kanth.*

CHRIS TRIMBLE *To my wife, Suzette, and my children, Claire, Jack, and Max, for your unwavering love and support.*

EVRIM BENGI TURKBEY *To my husband, Baris Turkbey, my son, Uygar, and my entire family for continuous support and love.*

AJAY WADGAONKAR *To my wife, Anjuli, my limitless source of light and inspiration.*

JESSICA WEN *To my sister, Anna, for whom I wish only the very best.*

ELCIN ZAN *With love to my family and universe.*

You would think that writing on a topic like non-interpretive skills would be a pretty dull experience. I must say that the opposite was true. I offered the trainees—residents, fellows, instructors—in the diagnostic radiology and nuclear medicine fields in the Department of Radiology of the Johns Hopkins Medical Institution the opportunity to co-author this book with me, and WOW, the enthusiasm was amazing. Forty-four residents and fellows signed up to write explanatory paragraphs for 10 questions each out of the 600 questions and answers I had created. Crowd-sourcing a book! It was so much fun. Then I had to revise those paragraphs to get them in a similar "voice," fact check them, and write 150 of my own …. And voilà! It was done in 4 months! Record setting! And something I can now share with the trainee class of 2015–2016.

I want to thank all of them for their outstanding effort and for believing in the project. They are the future leaders in radiology, and they showed their mettle.

As for the readers, this book is designed to help all of the radiology trainees, the newly minted radiologists, the subspecialty certified radiologists, and the sustaining MOC-taking radiologists who fear the "nonradiology" component of the examination. While this material may not be as enthralling as the diagnostic/therapeutic procedures you must perform, it rounds you out into the consummate professional. Business principles, ethics, quality improvement guidelines, patient safety issues, occupational health provisions, federal regulations, drug regimens, and resuscitation techniques are reviewed here in a manner designed to pique your interest … and prepare you for the non-interpretive skills section of board/certification exams.

I want to thank Robin Carter for supporting the project from start to finish, Joan Ryan for guiding the production with a gentle hand, and Beula Christopher for bringing it across the finish line. But above all, thanks to all the young authors who share the dedication page for this book. We did it!

CONTENTS

QUESTIONS

1. According to a *Journal of the American College of Radiology* (*JACR*) article by Blackmore et al from 2011, clinical decision support (CDS) implementation led to reductions in lumbar spine MRI imaging for low back pain by:
   A. 0–25%
   B. 26–50%
   C. 51–75%
   D. >75%

2. According to the same *JACR* article by Blackmore et al from 2011, CDS implementation led to reductions in brain MRI imaging for headache by:
   A. 0–25%
   B. 26–50%
   C. 51–75%
   D. >75%

3. According to the same *JACR* article by Blackmore et al from 2011, CDS implementation led to reductions in sinus CT scan imaging for sinusitis by:
   A. 0–25%
   B. 26–50%
   C. 51–75%
   D. >75%

4. Decision support systems are best validated if based on:
   A. Institutional preferences
   B. Availability of modalities
   C. Subspecialty expertise
   D. Evidence-based medicine

5. According to a *Canadian Medical Association Journal* article by Jenkins et al, a meta-analysis of all means for reducing inappropriate lumbar spine imaging for low back pain found that the most effective strategy was:
   A. Clinical decision support
   B. Targeted reminders
   C. Practitioner audits
   D. Dissemination of guidelines

6. According to the same *Canadian Medical Association Journal* article by Jenkins et al, the meta-analysis showed how much of a reduction in lumbar spine imaging for low back pain resulted from implementing CDS?
   A. 0–25%
   B. 26–50%
   C. 51–75%
   D. >75%

7. According to a *Radiology Journal* article by Dunne et al in 2015, CDS in the use and yield of inpatient computed tomographic pulmonary angiography (CTPA) for acute pulmonary embolism reduced CTPA rates by an average of:
   A. 0–25%
   B. 26–50%
   C. 51–75%
   D. >75%

1. **A, 0–25%.** Blackmore et al noted that "use of imaging clinical decision support (CDS) was associated with substantial decreases in the utilization rate of lumbar MRI for low back pain, head MRI for headache, and sinus CT for sinusitis. Utilization rates for the head CT control group were not significantly changed." The rates of imaging after the intervention were 23.4% lower for low back pain lumbar MRI.

Blackmore et al developed a checklist of indications that had to occur at the EMR entry level for an outpatient study to be ordered, as an attempt to reduce the number of inappropriate advanced imaging examinations. One of the keys to this successful CDS intervention was offering alternatives such as physical therapy or a specialist consult instead of the advanced imaging. The authors collaborated with the various stakeholders such as neurologists and neurosurgeons on evidence-based guidelines for the imaging criteria to obtain "buy-in" by all parties. Blackmore was following a LEAN quality improvement model.

Reference:
Blackmore CC, et al. Effectiveness of clinical decision support in controlling inappropriate imaging. *J Am Coll Radiol*. 2011;8(1):19-25.

2. **A, 0–25%.** In the same article, there was a significant reduction in the utilization of brain MRI for headache after implementing the CDS checklist. This eliminated cases in which imaging was not indicated, such as chronic unchanged headaches without evidence of new neurologic findings. The rates of imaging after the intervention were 23.2% lower for headache-related brain MRI.

Reference:
Blackmore CC, et al. Effectiveness of clinical decision support in controlling inappropriate imaging. *J Am Coll Radiol*. 2011;8(1):19-25.

3. **B, 26–50%.** The impact of the Blackmore CDS intervention at the physician order step was most apparent in sinus CT imaging where reductions in testing amounted to 26.8%. The peak of the impact was found in year 3 after the CDS implementation began. The results were sustained for at least 3 years thereafter.

Reference:
Blackmore CC, et al. Effectiveness of clinical decision support in controlling inappropriate imaging. *J Am Coll Radiol*. 2011;8(1):19-25.

4. **D, Evidence-based medicine.** Blackmore et al developed their own evidence-based guidelines based on national standards and collaboration with their other institutional stakeholders such as neurosurgery or neurology. They stated that the "intervention was based on a set of locally derived evidence-based decision rules for when imaging is appropriate. These decision rules were developed by Virginia Mason providers from the involved specialties after review of national and international evidence-based guidelines and primary literature and were vetted extensively in the institution before implementation."

Reference:
Blackmore CC, et al. Effectiveness of clinical decision support in controlling inappropriate imaging. *J Am Coll Radiol*. 2011;8(1):19-25.

5. **A, Clinical decision support.** In a meta-analysis of seven studies, including five clustered random controlled trials and two interrupted time studies, interventions to reduce imaging for patients with lower back pain were studied within the primary care and acute hospital settings. Types of interventions utilized were grouped into four overall categories: clinical decision support and targeted reminders, audits and feedback, practitioner education, and guideline dissemination. Clinical decision support and targeted reminders produced the largest decrease in imaging studies. Clinical decision support was best exhibited in a prospective study conducted by Baker et al in 1987, evaluating the effectiveness of a special requisition form for imaging of back pain, with a limited number of clear clinical indications for imaging. This intervention decreased imaging studies by 36.8%. An additional study by Eccles et al studied the effectiveness of targeted educational reminders attached to ordered imaging studies. An imaging reduction equivalent of 22.5% was achieved. Practitioner face-to-face education sessions demonstrated a 1.4% increase in imaging compared to a control group and a decrease of 17% in radiographs and 8% in CT scans when compared to guideline dissemination. Guideline dissemination alone did not demonstrate a significant difference in imaging studies ordered compared to a control.

References:
Baker SR, Rabin A, Lantos G, et al. The effect of restricting the indications for lumbosacral radiography in patients with acute back symptoms. *AJR Am J Roentgenol*. 1987;149(3):535-538.
Eccles M, Steen N, Grimshaw J, et al. Effect of audit and feedback, and reminder messages on primary-care radiology referrals: a randomised trial. *Lancet*. 2001;357(9266):1406-1409.
Jenkins HJ, Hancock MJ, French SD, et al. Effectiveness of interventions designed to reduce the use of imaging for low-back pain: a systematic review. *Can Med Assoc J*. 2015;187(6):401-408.

6. **B, 26–50%.** Clinical decision support and targeted reminders produced the largest decrease in imaging studies. Clinical decision support was shown by Baker et al in 1987 to decrease imaging studies by 36.8% in patients with back pain. Baker employed a special requisition form that had to be completed to order imaging in patients with low back pain. This provided the evidence-based limited number of clinical indications for appropriately imaging patients with low back pain.

Reference:
Baker SR, Rabin A, Lantos G, et al. The effect of restricting the indications for lumbosacral radiography in patients with acute back symptoms. *AJR Am J Roentgenol*. 1987;149(3):535-538.

7. **A, 0–25%.** In this large-scale study of CDS for ordering CT pulmonary angiography studies, clinicians were informed of the pretest probability of pulmonary embolism for patients suspected of having a pulmonary embolism prior to the CTPA. The CDS was implemented through the computerized physician order entry system and included three stops for clinicians within the order system: (1) clinician selection of low, intermediate, or high clinical suspicion along with entry of a D-dimer value, (2) automated statement provided in the scenario of intermediate and low suspicion patients without D-dimer test performed, and (3) automated statement provided for patients in the scenario of intermediate and low clinical suspicion with a negative D-dimer value. Clinicians were advised of the pretest probability of a positive exam with automated statements at each of the three steps and given the option of cancelling the imaging order. This generated a statistically significant relative reduction of 12.3% in examinations ordered, with a small increase in the clinical yield that was not statistically significant.

Reference:
Dunne RM, Ip IK, Abbett S, et al. Effect of evidence-based clinical decision support on the use and yield of CT pulmonary angiographic imaging in hospitalized patients. *Radiology*. 2015;276(1):167-174.

8. According to that same *Radiology Journal* article by Dunne et al in 2015, the CTPA positive rates for acute pulmonary embolism went up after CDS by:
   A. 0–25%
   B. 26–50%
   C. 51–75%
   D. >75%

9. According to an article in the *American Journal of Emergency Medicine* by Ip et al in 2015, use of CDS resulted in:
   A. A reduction in utilization of CT for head trauma cases by 10–15% with a rate of missed findings on follow-up exams of 5–10%
   B. A reduction in utilization of CT for head trauma cases by 5–10% with a rate of missed findings on follow-up exams of 10–15%
   C. A reduction in utilization of CT for head trauma cases by 10–15% with a rate of missed findings on follow-up exams of 0%
   D. A reduction in utilization of CT for head trauma cases by 16–20% with a rate of missed findings on follow-up exams of <5%

10. Implementing CDS to guide appropriate head CT use in patients with mild traumatic brain injury (MTBI) can result in improved adherence to evidence-based guidelines for imaging in emergency department (ED) patients with MTBI by what percentage?
    A. 0–25%
    B. 26–50%
    C. 51–75%
    D. >75%

11. With regard to image data compression, lossless compression is considered:
    A. Mathematically reversible
    B. Mathematically irreversible
    C. Always more efficient than lossy compression
    D. Required for entry into a PACS system

8. **A, 0–25%.** Prior to the above described CDS intervention, CTPA yield was approximately 10.3%. Following intervention, yield increased to 12.1%, an equivalent of a 16.3% increase in yield. This increase, however, was not statistically significant (p = 0.65). More importantly, patients with pulmonary emboli were NOT missed by having studies discouraged after advising the ordering physicians of the probability of a positive study.

Reference:
Dunne RM, Ip IK, et al. Effect of evidence-based clinical decision support on the use and yield of CT pulmonary angiographic imaging in hospitalized patients. *Radiology.* 2015;276(1):167-174.

9. **C, A reduction in utilization of CT for head trauma cases by 10–15% with a rate of missed findings on follow-up exams of 0%.** In this study, a CDS model for patients presenting with mild traumatic brain injury (MTBI) was derived based on multi-institutional studies and guidelines, including the New Orleans Criteria, Canadian CT Head Rule, and the CT in Head Injury Patients Prediction Rule. This model was implemented through the computerized physician order entry system. The rate of head CT imaging decreased from 58.1% of MTBI ED visits to 50.3%, a relative reduction of 13.4%. Secondary outcome was defined as delayed imaging after initial ED visit within 7 days of presentation, or delayed diagnosis of significant imaging findings. The change in delayed imaging or diagnosis from 6.7% to 9.4% was not statistically significant. Delayed diagnosis of radiologically significant findings was 0% in both the control and CDS intervention groups.

Reference:
Ip IK, Raja AS, Gupta A, et al. Impact of clinical decision support on head computed tomography use in patients with mild traumatic brain injury in the ED. *Am J Emerg Med.* 2015;33(3):320-325.

10. **C, 51–75%.** Gupta et al investigated the effect of a CDS system on compliance with evidence-based practice guidelines for CT head imaging of patients with MTBI. MTBI is defined as trauma-induced disruption of brain function as indicated by loss of consciousness for no greater than 30 minutes, altered mental status, or focal neurological deficits, without GCS < 13 or amnesia for more than 24 hours. Compliance prior to CDS implementation was determined based on review of electronic health records by two attending physicians. A CDS system was created through the computerized physician order entry, which also allowed for monitoring of compliance. Preintervention compliance with clinical practice guidelines for the ordering of CT scans of the head was 49% and increased to approximately 76.5% following CDS implementation. This represented a relative increase of 56.1% (p < 0.001).

Reference:
Gupta A, Ip IK, Raja AS, et al. Effect of clinical decision support on documented guideline adherence for head CT in emergency department patients with mild traumatic brain injury. *J Am Med Inform Assoc.* 2014;21(e2):e347-e351.

11. **A, Mathematically reversible.** Compression is the processing of imaging data to create a smaller file size, which is useful in facilitating imaging data transfer and storage. Lossless compression by definition uses a mathematically reversible process, while lossy compression by definition uses a mathematically irreversible process. Lossless compression is less efficient than lossy compression because it uses lower compression ratios and therefore results in larger file sizes. Compression is not a prerequisite for image data entry into a PACS system (Fig 1-1).

Reference:
Morgan P, Frankish C. Image quality, compression and segmentation in medicine. *J Audiov Media Med.* 2002;25(4):149-154. PMID: 12554293.

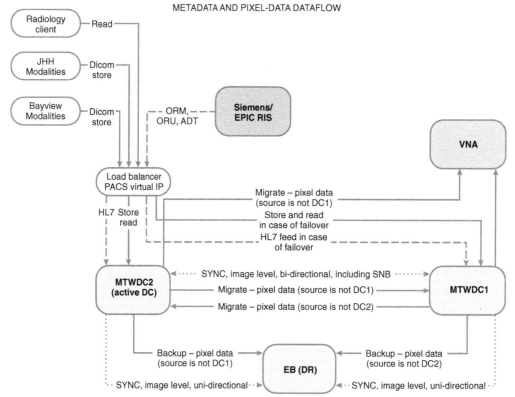

Figure 1-1 PACS system.

12. Diagnostically acceptable irreversible compression (DAIC) refers to mathematically irreversible compression that:
    A. Is lossless
    B. Does not affect a particular diagnostic task
    C. Cannot be converted to hard media
    D. All of the above

13. For compression, the DICOM standard allows compression using:
    A. JPEG
    B. MPEG
    C. Both JPEG and MPEG
    D. Neither JPEG nor MPEG

14. U.S. Food and Drug Administration (FDA) requires that when an image is displayed, it must be labeled with:
    A. Whether irreversible compression has been applied
    B. The compression ratio utilized
    C. The compression scheme used
    D. All of the above

15. In what scenario does the FDA NOT allow irreversible compression to be applied?
    A. PET scans
    B. Mammograms
    C. Digital subtraction angiograms
    D. DEXA scans

16. Recommended minimum graphic bit depth for diagnostic workstations is:
    A. 8 or more bit depth
    B. 10 or more bit depth
    C. 12 or more bit depth
    D. No bit depth specified

17. American College of Radiology (ACR) recommendations specify that images be displayed as:
    A. At least 256×256 pixel values
    B. At least 512×512 pixel values
    C. At least 1024×1024 pixel values
    D. No matrix is specified

18. To reduce eye fatigue, room lighting should be at:
    A. Complete darkness
    B. Standard fluorescent room lighting at 120 lux
    C. 60-80 lux
    D. None of the above

12. **B, Does not affect a particular diagnostic task.** Diagnostically acceptable irreversible compression is defined as an irreversible compression ratio that results in differences in postprocessing images that do not affect diagnostic performance. The permissible ratio varies by the compression algorithm used, the amount of data in the original image file, and the diagnostic task. DAIC is by definition irreversible (a). Lossless compression is reversible. Lossy compression is irreversible. Compression, in fact, facilitates image data transfer to storage on hard media (c).

Reference:
European Society of Radiology (ESR). Usability of irreversible image compression in radiological imaging. A position paper by the European Society of Radiology (ESR). *Insights Imaging.* 2011;2(2):103-115. doi: 10.1007/s13244-011-0071-x; PMCID: PMC3259360.

13. **C, Both JPEG and MPEG.** JPEG and MPEG are both compression algorithms compliant with the DICOM standard. JPEG, JPEG-LS, and JPEG-2000 are algorithms used for still imaging data. These algorithms may be either reversible or irreversible. Compression algorithms for video data, among which MPEG is an example, are typically irreversible.

Reference:
European Society of Radiology (ESR). Usability of irreversible image compression in radiological imaging. A position paper by the European Society of Radiology (ESR). *Insights Imaging.* 2011;2(2):103-115. doi: 10.1007/s13244-011-0071-x; PMCID: PMC3259360.

14. **D, All of the above.** The most recent guidelines from the FDA specify labeling guidelines for the display of medical images processed with a compression algorithm. The FDA requires that an image label must state the compression scheme (ie, JPEG, MPEG) and the compression ratio (ie, 1:3, 1:5) utilized. If irreversible compression has been applied, a message accompanying the image must indicate this (a).

Reference:
Center for Devices and Radiological Health. *Guidance for the submission of premarket notifications for medical image management devices.* Rockville, MD: U.S. Department of Health and Human Services; 2000.

15. **B, Mammograms.** The only imaging study type for which the FDA does not permit the use of irreversible compression (in transmission, storage, or interpretation) is mammography. Oddly enough, mammography has actually been shown to tolerate very high compression ratios (compared to brain CT, eg) while maintaining diagnostic performance. For all other study types, irreversible compression is permitted. However, the interpreting physician is ultimately responsible for ensuring that irreversibly compressed images are DAIC-compliant.

References:
Center for Devices and Radiological Health. *Guidance for the submission of premarket notifications for medical image management devices.* Rockville, MD: U.S. Department of Health and Human Services; 2000.
European Society of Radiology (ESR). Usability of irreversible image compression in radiological imaging. A position paper by the European Society of Radiology (ESR). *Insights Imaging.* 2011;2(2):103-115. doi: 10.1007/s13244-011-0071-x; PMCID: PMC3259360.

16. **A, 8 or more bit depth.** The minimum graphic bit depth required by the FDA for diagnostic workstations is 8 bits (conferring $2^8 = 256$ output levels per R/G/B color

channel). In clinical practice, the contemporary standard bit depth for diagnostic workstations is at least 12 bits ($2^{12} = 4096$ output levels). Even at bit depths of 12 bits, there is truncation of available Hounsfield units (HU) output values during imaging of metal density objects, which contributes to artifact during CT examinations involving orthopedic hardware, for example. New data suggest that higher bit depths (ie, 14 bit) may extend the available output range to a diagnostically useful extent in such scenarios, with increased available HU outputs minimizing artifact interference.

Reference:
Glide-Hurst C, Chen D, Zhong H, et al. Changes realized from extending bit-depth and metal artifact reduction in CT. *Med Phys.* 2013;40(6):061711. PMID: 23718590.

17. **D, No matrix is specified.** ACR recommendations do not specify a minimum matrix display for diagnostic workstations. The FDA, however, recommends that images be labeled with the matrix display when it has been reduced through processing as compared to the original image data. The ACR's rule of thumb for matrix display is that it should be selected according to the modality. Modalities with high matrix input (ie, computed radiography, digital radiography, digitized film, and digital mammography) should be interpreted using a high matrix, and modalities with low matrix input (ie, CT, MR, US, NM, digital fluorography, digital subtraction imaging) may be interpreted using a low matrix.

References:
Center for Devices and Radiological Health. *Guidance for the submission of premarket notifications for medical image management devices.* Rockville, MD: U.S. Department of Health and Human Services; 2000.
Norweck JT, Seibert JA, Andriole KP, et al. ACR-AAPM-SIIM technical standard for electronic practice of medical imaging. *J Digit Imaging.* 2013;26(1):38-52. PMID: 22992866.
Indrajit I, Verma B. Monitor displays in radiology: Part 1. *Indian J Radiol Imaging.* 2009;19(1):24-28. doi: 10.4103/0971-3026.45341; PMCID: PMC 2747408.

18. **D, None of the above.** Ambient lighting in the recommended range corresponds to the light emitted by the diagnostic monitor plus some additional ambient lighting. When subject to typical office lighting ($\approx$100–480 lux) or just the light of the monitor ($\approx$7 lux), radiologists demonstrate worse diagnostic performance. Overly bright light interferes with diagnostic performance by decreasing contrast ratios, which occurs when luminance reflecting off the monitor registers in areas of the image that ought to be dark. On the other hand, too-low levels of ambient lighting are hypothesized to detract from diagnostic performance by causing eye fatigue—in addition to posing a general safety hazard (ie, risk for injury while moving about a dark room). Viewing conditions should be optimized to minimize eye fatigue. Reading room lighting should prevent reflections on the monitor. In general, although not specified or required by any governing body, 20 to 40 lux is recommended in the work space environment.

Reference:
Brennan PC, McEntee M, Evanoff M, et al. Ambient lighting: effect of illumination on soft copy viewing of radiographs of the wrist. *AJR Am J Roentgenol.* 2007;188(2):W177-W180. PMID: 17242225.

19. Which of the following is a correct definition?
    A. Ambient luminance (L_{amb}): Brightness even when the monitor is turned off
    B. Minimum luminance (L_{min}): The luminance of the lowest gray value that can still be detected by the human eye
    C. Maximum luminance (L_{max}): The brightest pixel on the monitor
    D. All of the above

20. JPEG refers to:
    A. Joint Picture Electronic Graphic
    B. Joint Photographic Electronic Group
    C. Joint Photographic Experts Group
    D. Just Picture Electronic Graphic

21. The difference between de-identified data and anonymized data is:
    A. De-identified data could be linked by a code back to the original data but fully anonymized data are not relinkable to the original data
    B. Anonymized data could be linked by a code back to the original data but de-identified data are not relinkable to the original data
    C. Anonymized data are HIPAA compliant but de-identified are not
    D. De-identified data are HIPAA compliant but anonymized data are not

22. Which of the following are acceptable means for authentication prior to access to patient data?
    A. Signing of a HIPAA compliance document
    B. Permission by the patient
    C. Retinal scans
    D. All of the above

23. Authentication is to login as authorization is to:
    A. Logoff
    B. Login
    C. Security
    D. Access

24. To prevent data from getting into the wrong hands, most security experts recommend use of:
    A. Data compression and encryption
    B. Restriction of access and data encryption
    C. Passwords and biometric (fingerprint/retinal scan/voice recognition) hard stops
    D. Data encryption and data sequestration

25. Nonrepudiation is a system that confirms:
    A. Senders and receivers of data/messages
    B. "Garbage in garbage out"
    C. Access denial to encrypted data
    D. Fail-safe methods to prevent authentication cyberattacks

19. **D, All of the above.** According to the following reference:

Ambient luminance (L_{amb}): Brightness due to diffusely reflected room lighting. Ambient luminance should be less than one-fourth of the luminance of the darkest gray level.

Minimum luminance (L_{min}): luminance of the lowest gray value, $L'_{min} = L_{min} + L_{amb}$, should be at least 1.0 cd/m² for diagnostic interpretation and 0.8 cd/m² for other uses

Maximum luminance (L_{max}): the luminance for the maximum gray value

Luminance ratio (LR): the ratio of L_{max} (the luminance for the maximum gray value) to L_{min}

Of note, all of these values vary with the level of ambient lighting. The accepted criterion for minimum L_{max} is 170 cd/m². A high LR is required for adequate image contrast, with an LR of at least 420 cd/m² recommended for mammography, and an LR of at least 350 cd/m² being appropriate for all other applications. Furthermore, luminance must demonstrate uniformity across the faceplate of a monitor, varying by no more than 30% based on test patterns provided by and nonuniformity coefficients described by the AAPM.

References:
Norweck JT, Seibert JA, Andriole KP, et al. ACR-AAPM-SIIM technical standard for electronic practice of medical imaging. *J Digit Imaging*. 2013;26(1):38-52. PMID: 22992866.

Samei E, Badano A, Chakraborty D, et al. Assessment of display performance for medical imaging systems: executive summary of AAPM TG18 report. *Med Phys*. 2005;32(4):1205-1225.

20. **C, Joint Photographic Experts Group.** Compressing image files allows for decreased storage requirement as well as easier data transmission. Images can be compressed in two ways: lossless or lossy. Lossless compression is reversible but is only able to achieve a small amount of data compression. Lossy compression algorithms are irreversible but allow a much greater potential for data compression and thus use much less storage space. A common example of a lossy algorithm is the Joint Photographic Experts Group standard, otherwise known as JPEG.

Reference:
Goldberg MA. Image data compression. *J Digit Imaging*. 1997;10(suppl 1):9-11. doi: 10.1007/BF03168640.

21. **A, De-identified data could be linked by a code back to the original data, but fully anonymized data are not relinkable to the original data.** Anonymized data have been severed from the patient irreversibly and cannot be relinked to the supplying patient, even by the study organizer. On the other hand, de-identified data have been severed from the patient in a reversible manner, and thus the data can be relinked to the supplying patient in some cases. Thus, health information that has been anonymized is more secure than data that have been de-identified. De-identification can be accomplished by the Safe Harbor Method, which details 18 data features that must be removed, in conjunction with the Statistical or Expert Determination Method, requiring a statistician to verify that it is unlikely the data could be traced back to a particular patient, even if the data were shared with a trusted researcher.

References:
ACR-AAPM-SIIM practice parameter for electronic medical information privacy and security. <http://www.acr.org/~/media/419A8512DBDB4FDE99EC75B3C68B01CF.pdf>; 2014.

Godard B, Schmidtke J, Cassiman JJ, et al. Data storage and DNA banking for biomedical research: informed consent, confidentiality, quality issues, ownership, return of benefits. A professional perspective. *Eur J Hum Genet*. 2003;11(suppl 2):S88-S122. doi: 10.1038/sj.ejhg.5201114.

Fullerton SM, Anderson NR, Guzauskas G, et al. Meeting the governance challenges of next-generation biorepository research. *Sci Transl Med*. 2010;2(15):15cm3. doi: 10.1126/scitranslmed.3000361.

22. **C, Retinal scans.** Authentication refers to the verification of a user's identity in the computer system. The system can authenticate a particular user via a specific user name and password or security questions. Likewise, it may use biometric data such as retina scanning or fingerprints. Signing of a HIPAA compliance document or patient permission are not sufficient to authenticate a user prior to accessing patient data.

Reference:
ACR-AAPM-SIIM practice parameter for electronic medical information privacy and security. <http://www.bu.edu/tech/about/security-resources/bestpractice/auth/>; 2014.

23. **D, Access.** Authentication refers to the verification of a user's identity in the computer system. It uses varying methods for determining each user's unique identity such as individualized passwords, digital certificates, smart cards, and biometrics. Once authenticated, a person will be able to log in to the system. However, authentication only verifies one's identity; it does not delineate one's rights to access patient information. Authorization, on the other hand, refers to defining and limiting what information and processes a particular individual can access. Thus, authentication verifies "who you are," and authorization defines "what you can do" in the system.

Reference:
ACR-AAPM-SIIM practice parameter for electronic medical information privacy and security. <http://www.bu.edu/tech/about/security-resources/bestpractice/auth/>; 2014.

24. **B, Restriction of access and data encryption.** There are two methods for ensuring data remain confidential. The first is restricting access. The fewer users who have access to data, the less likely it is to fall into the wrong hands. The second method of data protection is encryption. Encrypted data are more difficult to access even if they were to be stolen, and this is thus a recommended component of data security. Encrypted data may have a private key, in which individuals enter their own passcodes to decode or encode information, or a public key in which there is a passcode shared by multiple users.

References:
ACR-AAPM-SIIM practice parameter for electronic medical information privacy and security. <http://www.acr.org/~/media/419A8512DBDB4FDE99EC75B3C68B01CF.pdf>; 2014.

What Is Encryption? Surveillance Self-Defense Project. Electronic Frontier Foundation website. <https://ssd.eff.org/en/module/what-encryption>. Accessed 3 November 2014.

25. **A, Senders and receivers of data/messages.** Nonrepudiation refers to the method of ensuring that individuals cannot deny having sent or received a particular encrypted electronic message. It can be accomplished by verifying the send/receive data by cross-checking them with the private or public key encryption data to ensure a particular user was the sender/recipient of the message. Alternatively, user activity may be audited and logged following authentication of a particular user. Either method can accomplish the goal of uniquely identifying the parties involved in a particular message.

References:
ACR-AAPM-SIIM practice parameter for electronic medical information privacy and security. <http://www.acr.org/~/media/419A8512DBDB4FDE99EC75B3C68B01CF.pdf>; 2014.

McCullagh A. Non-repudiation in the digital environment. *First Monday (online)*. 2000;5(8):7. Articles.

26. With regard to decision support physician order entry software interventions, what two studies are most often cited as being inappropriately ordered (low utility)?
    A. Brain CT and MRI
    B. Spine CT and MRI
    C. Abdominal CT and US
    D. None of the above

27. The greatest percentage of low utility (not appropriate to be ordered) studies ordered on outpatients are:
    A. Spine CT and MRI
    B. Nuclear cardiology
    C. Obstetrical ultrasound
    D. Cardiac CTA

28. According to the 2006 study on decision support by Rosenthal et al, in what percentage of the studies that were graded as low utility by decision support does the ordering physician override the system and still order the study?
    A. 0-25%
    B. 26-50%
    C. 51-75%
    D. >75%

29. After the use of decision support for CT and MR at the Massachusetts General Hospital:
    A. CT volume decreased
    B. MR volume decreased
    C. US volume increased
    D. All of the above

30. After the use of decision support for CT and MR at the Massachusetts General Hospital:
    A. CT volume growth rate decreased
    B. MR volume growth rate decreased
    C. US volume growth rate decreased
    D. All of the above

31. Which is not true of the educational effect of decision support software programs compared to the gatekeeper effect?
    A. It is longer lasting
    B. It can cross modalities even when the rationale for ordering the test is not required
    C. It affects US more than CT
    D. It is learned behavior

26. **B, Spine CT and MRI.** Among the answer choices, the studies that were consistently graded the lowest utility were the combined spinal MRI and CT examinations. Spinal CT was found to be of low clinical utility in 20% of cases and spinal MRI in 12% of cases. They comprised 53% of all low utility studies (among 22,208 total studies) evaluated in one recent publication.

    Chest MRI was another low utility clinical study (approximately 18% of cases). However, in contrast to spinal studies, which were quite common, chest MRIs comprised only a small fraction of the total study number (and only roughly 2% of all low utility studies).

    Reference:
    Rosenthal DI, Weilburg JB, Schultz T, et al. Radiology order entry with decision support: initial clinical experience. *J Am Coll Radiol.* 2006;3(10):799-806.

27. **B, Nuclear cardiology.** The greatest percentage of low utility scores (examinations with utility scores of 1 to 3 on a scale of 1-9 with 9 being most appropriate and 1 being least appropriate) occurred with nuclear cardiac imaging. While the percentage was low at 6%, it compared with MRI at 5% and CT at 1%. Nonetheless, because nuclear cardiology only accounted for 4% of total orders (n = 2801) versus 61% for CT (n = 43,995) and 35% for MR (n = 25,200), it had a minor impact. The largest absolute number of inappropriate low utility studies were from MR at 1260, compared to 439 CTs and 168 nuclear cardiology studies. As a percentage, nuclear cardiology was the biggest contributor, but in absolute numbers, MRI was the biggest contributor.

    Reference:
    Rosenthal DI, Weilburg JB, Schultz T, et al. Radiology order entry with decision support: initial clinical experience. *J Am Coll Radiol.* 2006;3(10):799-806.

28. **D, >75%.** In 91% of cases that received low utility scores, the users overrode the CDS recommendation and proceeded to schedule the examinations. Several reasons were cited by the requesting physicians for proceeding to order the low utility examinations. Among them were a recommendation by a specialist (55%), disagreement with guidelines (25%), patient demand (9%), and other imaging was tried and unhelpful (6%). Physicians frequently overrode the warning and proceeded with the study despite the soft barrier placed by the programming tool.

    Reference:
    Rosenthal DI, Weilburg JB, Schultz T, et al. Radiology order entry with decision support: initial clinical experience. *J Am Coll Radiol.* 2006;3(10):799-806.

29. **A, CT volume decreased.** CT volumes demonstrated the most significant decline with the implementation of decision support at MGH. All other examinations, including MRI and US, demonstrated a nonsignificant trend toward decline as well, without definitive evidence of change in either direction.

    The CT findings were hypothesized to have occurred on the basis of two independent factors. One was the "gatekeeper effect" in which the extra steps needed to process a study when decision support is in use may have dissuaded a certain degree of exam volume from being ordered. The second element discussed was the "educational effect" in which ordering physicians learned new indications (or lack thereof) for various studies, through which their ordering patterns shifted over the course of time, even if not entirely persuasive initially. No clear reasoning could be suggested for the specific change in CT over other modalities; however, the reference below cited several hypotheses.

    Reference:
    Sistrom CL, Dang PA, Weilburg JB, et al. Effect of computerized order entry with integrated decision support on the growth of outpatient procedure volumes: seven-year time series analysis. *Radiology.* 2009;251(1):147-155.

30. **D, All of the above (but ultrasound was not included in decision support).** Although one might have hoped for marked reductions in actual rates of utilization after the implementation of decision support at MGH, in fact what was slowed was just the rate of growth of the modalities over a 7-year period. This is like saying that health care costs have not gone down in the United States but the rate of rise in health care costs has been slowing—not very satisfying. One would hope for a true decrease. Sistrom found a significant decrease in CT volume growth by 2.75% per quarter, a decrease in MR growth rate by 1.2% without a significant reduction in quarterly volume growth. The growth rate of US at 1.3% decreased after order entry implementation even though it was not included in the decision support program.

    Reference:
    Sistrom CL, Dang PA, Weilburg JB, et al. Effect of computerized order entry with integrated decision support on the growth of outpatient procedure volumes: seven-year time series analysis. *Radiology.* 2009;251(1):147-155.

31. **B, It can cross modalities even when the rationale for ordering the test is not required.** Part of the rationale for use of decision support software is that it will educate physicians. For example, while directing an emergency physician to order ultrasound for children suspected of having appendicitis, it teaches that ED doctor that US is an excellent substitute for a radiation-heavy procedure such as CT. This may have benefits down the road for suggesting appropriateness of evaluating neck masses in children, or adults, with ultrasound, even if that is not a test that is currently directed via decision support. These are examples of the educational effect. Learned behavior is longer lasting than a pure gatekeeper effect that prevents a physician from ordering the wrong study without a rationalization. On the other hand, one can put up a "stop sign" for any modality with any study using the gatekeeper function. Thus CT and MR scans of the head can be prevented in neonates by applying a gatekeeper hard stop function such that the ordering physician is required to speak to a radiologist to gain approval for overriding use of neonatal head ultrasound.

    Reference:
    Sistrom CL, Dang PA, Weilburg JB, et al. Effect of computerized order entry with integrated decision support on the growth of outpatient procedure volumes: seven-year time series analysis. *Radiology.* 2009;251(1):147-155.

32. Implementation of CDS is encouraged by the ACR as a reaction to:
    A. Electronic medical record utilization
    B. Meaningful use requirements
    C. Radiology benefit management
    D. Fee for service down regulation

33. Positive results occur in what percentage of appropriate studies versus inappropriate studies according to Lehnert et al?
    A. 61% of inappropriate and 37% of appropriate tests ordered
    B. 58% of appropriate and 24% of inappropriate tests ordered
    C. 43% of appropriate and 21% of inappropriate tests ordered
    D. 21% of appropriate and 14% of inappropriate tests ordered

34. Which of the following tests accounts for the smallest percentage of inappropriate tests ordered?
    A. MR abdomen
    B. MR knee
    C. MR pelvis
    D. MR shoulder

35. Use of decision support guidelines for an incidental lung nodule (found on abdominal CT) workup resulted in what factor of improvement in ordering the appropriate follow-up?
    A. 5×
    B. 4×
    C. 3×
    D. 2×

36. The Radiology Reporting Initiative:
    A. Standardizes the order of indication, technique, comparison, recommendations, and impression in reports
    B. Aims to standardize language in radiology reports to an eighth-grade level as required by Congress
    C. Is part of meaningful use legislation
    D. Creates clear and concise report templates

32. **C, Radiology benefit management.** The CDS emphasis is a reaction to the unpleasant experience of having to go through multiple layers of preauthorization by insurers or through radiology benefits management (RBM). The RBMs serve as middle men in screening for inappropriate or redundant services but can be heavy-handed in their hard stop approach that some physicians feel disempowers them and interferes with the doctor-patient relationship.

The same legislation that fixed the sustainable growth rate dilemma in Medicare payment also has kick-started the use of physician order entry. The law mandates that physicians ordering CT, MRI, nuclear medicine, and PET must use clinical decision support gatekeeper software to access government-approved, evidence-based appropriate-use criteria. Payment for these services will be made only to those groups documenting that the referring physicians employed appropriateness criteria in the ordering of those studies. Documentation as to whether the order followed or did not follow the appropriateness guideline will be required down the road with data supplied to CMS (whether the exam ordered adhered or did not adhere to an acceptable CDS rating).

Reference:
Keen CD. The clinical decision-support mandate: Now what? *Radiol Bus.* 2014;<http://www.radiologybusiness.com/topics/policy/clinical-decision-support-mandate-now-what>.

33. **B, 58% of appropriate and 24% of inappropriate tests ordered.** In Lehnert et al's study, appropriateness criteria developed by a radiology benefit management company were used to determine the rate at which referring physicians ordered the "correct" high RVU procedures. Based on their analysis, 26% were not considered appropriate. When an appropriate study was ordered, the rate of positive results was 58%. When inappropriate studies were ordered, only 13% were positive and/or affected management of the patient.

Inappropriate low yield studies can be reduced by requiring a physician, not just his or her support staff, to order the study if that test failed to comply with appropriateness criteria recommendations built into the CDS. This was exemplified by a study by Vartanians et al that showed a reduction in low yield studies ordered from 5.43% of all studies ordered to 1.92% after implementation of a rule that studies with low yield decision support scores could not be scheduled if placed by nonclinician support staff. To override the CDS "block," the referring clinician had to log in to complete the process.

References:
Lehnert BE, Bree RL. Analysis of appropriateness of outpatient CT and MRI referred from primary care clinics at an academic medical center: how critical is the need for improved decision support? *J Am Coll Radiol.* 2010;7(3):192-197.
Vartanians VM, Sistrom CL, Weilburg JB, et al. Increasing the appropriateness of outpatient imaging: effects of a barrier to ordering low-yield examinations. *Radiology.* 2010;255(3):842-849. doi: 10.1148/radiol.10091228.

34. **A, MR abdomen.** Inappropriate MRs of the abdomen account for just 7% of all inappropriate studies ordered. MRs of the knee come in at 14%, followed by MRs of the pelvis (20%) and MRs of the shoulder at 37% inappropriate.

Lehnert and Bree's data were flawed in part by small numbers collected and that the studies were limited to outpatient primary care clinics, but what they found was:

Study Percentage Inappropriate by RBM HealthHelp Criteria	
CT head/brain	62%
CT maxillofacial	36%
CT spine	53%
MR shoulder	37%
MR spine	35%
CT chest/abd/pelvis	30%
CT/CTA	21%
MR pelvis	20%
MR knee	14%
MR brain and orbits	13%
MR abdomen	7%

Reference:
Lehnert BE, Bree RL. Analysis of appropriateness of outpatient CT and MRI referred from primary care clinics at an academic medical center: how critical is the need for improved decision support? *J Am Coll Radiol.* 2010;7(3):192-197.

35. **D, 2×.** Prior to CDS guideline implementation 50% of solitary noncalcified pulmonary nodules seen on abdominal CT were worked up inappropriately. After the CDS program was implemented, 95% of pulmonary nodules followed guidelines for workup. During the same period, if the guideline software was not utilized (but concurrent with those cases directed by the guidelines), only 45% of the pulmonary nodules were triaged for workup appropriately. This shows the strength and value of using CDS appropriateness criteria in directing the workup of such incidental findings commonly seen on imaging.

The factor that most determines whether or not pulmonary nodules are worked up according to Fleischner Society rules is the size of the nodule. Adherence is highest in the 4- to 6-mm nodule group but diminishes both for smaller and bigger nodules.

Reference:
Lu MT, Rosman DA, Wu CC, et al. Radiologist point-of-care clinical decision support and adherence to guidelines for incidental lung nodules. *J Am Coll Radiol.* 2016;13(2):156-162. [Epub 2015 Nov 11].

36. **D, Creates clear and concise report templates.** The Radiology Reporting Initiative is "a library of clear and consistent report templates." They are created by twelve subcommittees of subspecialty experts, with the goal of creating uniformity and improving communication with referring providers.

Although these templates are not part of Medicare meaningful use of EHRs, they are part of other CMS pay-for-performance incentives.

The templates are not limited to the order of sections within a report, and they also include specific information fields for data that referring physicians would be interested in, depending on the indication of the exam.

Although the AMA previously estimated health literacy of the U.S. general public at around the eighth-grade level, Congress has not mandated an eighth-grade reading level for radiology reports.

References:
Radiological Society of North America. Radiology reporting initiative. <www.rsna.org/Reporting_Initiative.aspx>.
Weis BD. *Health literacy: a manual for clinicians.* Chicago, IL: American Medical Association and American Medical Foundation; 2003.
Kahn CE, Langlotz CP, Burnside ES, et al. Towards best practices in radiology reporting. *Radiology.* 2009;252(3):852-856.

37. The Radiology Reporting Initiative:
    A. Is an initiative by the AMA
    B. Is being organized through the Radiological Society of North America (RSNA)
    C. Is managed by subspecialty societies
    D. Is a mandate of The Joint Commission

38. What is the most widely used radiology lexicon?
    A. BI-RADS
    B. Urban Dictionary
    C. *Merriam-Webster's*
    D. RadPeer

39. Radlex is one attempt at:
    A. Standardizing report formats
    B. Creating structured reports
    C. Getting all reports to a single page in length
    D. Defining the terms radiologists use

40. LI-RADS refers to:
    A. Liver reporting
    B. Limb MSK reporting
    C. Breast reporting, lateral views
    D. There is no such thing currently

41. Regarding structured reports:
    A. When presented with the option of receiving narrative versus structured reports, clinicians overwhelmingly preferred structured reports
    B. When presented with the option of receiving narrative versus structured reports, clinicians overwhelmingly preferred narrative reports
    C. When presented with the option of creating narrative versus structured reports, radiologists overwhelmingly preferred structured reports
    D. None of the above

42. Which is true about radiologists' attitudes about structured reports (as of 2009)?
    A. Structured reports are more accurate than narrative reports
    B. Structured reports are felt to be overly constraining with regard to report content and time-consuming to use
    C Radiologists prefer structured reports
    D. Structured reports are more complete than narrative reports

43. Image Gently is to pediatric CT scanning as Step Lightly is to pediatric:
    A. Gastrointestinal procedures
    B. Genitourinary procedures
    C. Neuroradiology
    D. Interventional radiology

37. **B, Is being organized through the RSNA.** The Radiology Reporting Initiative was organized by the RSNA to create "a library of clear and consistent report templates." The AMA was not involved in the initiative. Although there are subcommittees composed of subspecialty experts who create the various specialty templates, the subspecialty societies are not directly involved.

The templates that have been created by the Radiology Reporting Initiative are not mandated by the Joint Commission or any health care payers, but they may be incorporated into other CMS pay-for-performance incentives.

Reference:
Kahn CE, Langlotz CP, Burnside ES, et al. Towards best practices in radiology reporting. *Radiology.* 2009;252(3):852-856. <https://www.rsna.org/Reporting_Initiative.aspx>.

38. **A, BI-RADS.** The Breast Imaging Reporting and Data System (BI-RADS) is a lexicon (controlled vocabulary) developed in 1993 by the American College of Radiology to standardize mammographic reporting and reduce confusion regarding mammographic findings. Use of this lexicon was codified into law by the Mammography Quality Standards Act (MQSA) of 1997, which required that all mammograms in the United States include the BI-RADS terminology and categories of assessment.

Urban Dictionary is a commercial website that describes itself as "a veritable cornucopia of streetwise lingo, posted and defined by its readers." Merriam-Webster, Inc. is an American company that publishes reference books, especially dictionaries. RadPeer is a web-based program to perform cross-institution peer review. Organized by the ACR, RadPeer "allows peer review to be performed during the routine interpretation of current images."

References:
Liberman L, Menell JH. Breast imaging reporting and data system (BI-RADS). *Radiol Clin North Am.* 2002;40(3):409-430.
MQSA final rule. *Fed Regist.* 62(208):55988. <http://www.acr.org/Quality-Safety/RADPEER>.

39. **D, Defining the terms radiologists use.** Radlex, a portmanteau term for radiology lexicon, is "a unified language of radiology terms for standardized indexing and retrieval of radiology information." The purpose of such a lexicon is to have a single set of terms with agreed upon meaning and minimal ambiguity that all radiologists can use.

Standardizing reporting formats and creating structured reports is a purpose of the RSNA Radiology Reporting Initiative, which makes templates for reports created by subspecialty committees freely available to radiologists. There is no word or page limit to radiology reports endorsed by ACR or RSNA.

References:
Radiological Society of North America website. <https://www.rsna.org/RadLex.aspx>.
American College of Radiology website. <http://www.acr.org/News-Publications/News/News-Articles/2013/ACR-Bulletin/201311-Setting-the-Standard>.
Langlotz CP. RadLex: a new method for indexing online educational materials. *Radiographics.* 2006;26(6):1595-1597.

40. **A, Liver reporting.** The Liver Imaging Reporting and Data System (LI-RADS) was created in 2008 by an ACR-appointed committee, consisting of diagnostic radiologists with expertise in hepatic CT and MR imaging, interventional radiologists with expertise in HCC therapy, transplant hepatologists, liver transplant surgeons, and health informatics experts. ACR released the first draft of the guidelines in 2011 and updates in 2013 and 2014 fashioned after the successful implementation of BI-RADS.

BI-RADS is the breast radiology reporting scheme after which the LI-RADS system was modeled, and it includes data from all breast imaging views. There currently is no standard system or scale for limb reporting.

References:
Tang A, Cruite I, Sirlin CB. Toward a standardized system for hepatocellular carcinoma diagnosis using computed tomography and MRI. *Expert Rev Gastroenterol Hepatol.* 2013;7(3):269-279.
American College of Radiology. Liver Imaging Reporting and Data System version 2014. From <http://www.acr.org/Quality-Safety/Resources/LIRADS>. Accessed November 2015.

41. **A, When presented with the option of receiving narrative versus structured reports, clinicians overwhelmingly preferred structured reports.** Structured reporting is composed of three tiers. First, reports are divided into sections such as "Indication," "Findings," and "Impression." Second, the "Findings" section is further divided into smaller categories—for example, into organs and organ systems. In the third tier, standardized language is required, such as BI-RADS. In a July 2011 *Radiology* article, referring clinicians overwhelmingly preferred structured reports to narrative (free form) reports.

References:
Cramer JA, Eisenmenger LB, Pierson NS, et al. Structured and templated reporting: an overview. *Appl Radiol.* 2014.
Schwartz LH, Panicek DM, Berk AR, et al. Improving communication of diagnostic radiology findings through structured reporting. *Radiology.* 2011;260(1):174-181. doi: 10.1148/radiol.11101913; [Epub 2011 Apr 25]; PubMed PMID: 21518775.

42. **B, Structured reports are felt to be overly constraining with regard to report content and time-consuming to use.** An October 2009 *Radiology* article evaluated the quality of radiology reports by residents using a structured reporting system compared to a free-text dictation. There was no difference in accuracy between reports. On a post-study opinion survey, the majority of residents agreed that a structured reporting system has benefits but felt that the software was overly constraining and inefficient. This continues to be the attitude of many practicing radiologists, which accounts for the poor dissemination of structured reports in private and academic practice.

Reference:
Johnson AJ, Chen MY, Swan JS, et al. Cohort study of structured reporting compared with conventional dictation. *Radiology.* 2009;253(1):74-80. doi: 10.1148/radiol.2531090138; [Epub 2009 Aug 25]; PubMed PMID: 19709993.

43. **D, Interventional radiology.** Due to increased utilization of diagnostic imaging procedures and potential risk of radiation from these procedures, especially in the pediatric population, the Society of Pediatric Radiology (SPR) formed the Alliance for Radiation Safety in Pediatric Imaging and started the Image Gently campaign. Their main objectives included increased awareness of the risk associated with radiation exposure and the need to modify radiation dose to limit overall radiation exposure during diagnostic procedures. In 2009, SPR expanded its efforts to limit radiation exposure by initiating the Step Lightly campaign to increase awareness and decrease radiation exposure during interventional pediatric radiology procedures.

References:
Goske MJ, Applegate KE, Boylan J, et al. The Image Gently campaign: working together to change practice. *AJR Am J Roentgenol.* 2008;190(2):273-274.
Goske MJ, Applegate KE, Boylan J, et al. Image Gently™: a national education and communication campaign in radiology using the science of social marketing. *J Am Coll Radiol.* 2008;5(12):1200-1205.
Sidhu M, Goske MJ, Connolly B, et al. Image Gently, Step Lightly: promoting radiation safety in pediatric interventional radiology. *AJR Am J Roentgenol.* 2010;105(4):W299-W301.

44. The best solution for "Image gently" is to:
    A. Substitute ultrasonography
    B. Decrease maS
    C. Decrease kvP
    D. Decrease DLP

45. The best solution for "Image wisely" is to:
    A. Substitute ultrasonography
    B. Decrease maS
    C. Decrease kvP
    D. Decrease DLP

46. A useful application of "Image wisely" is:
    A. Radiology benefits managers
    B. Iterative reconstruction of CT studies
    C. Decision support software
    D. Computer-assisted diagnosis (CAD)

47. When revenue is reported on the income statement in the period in which the payment for x-ray studies is received from customers it is called:
    A. Cash basis of accounting
    B. Revenue basis of accounting
    C. Accrual basis of accounting
    D. All of the above

48. When expenses are paid out by check on the income statement in the period in which the payment for contrast dye is provided to one's suppliers it is called:
    A. Cash basis of accounting
    B. Expense basis of accounting
    C. Accrual basis of accounting
    D. All of the above

49. When revenue is listed on the income statement at the time that a particular service is billed to a patient it is called:
    A. Cash basis of accounting
    B. Expense basis of accounting
    C. Accrual basis of accounting
    D. All of the above

50. The matching principle states that:
    A. Every revenue entry must be offset by an expense entry
    B. All expenses must be matched in the same accounting period to the revenues they helped to earn
    C. Every number in the income statement must match that in the balance statement
    D. None of the above

44. A, Substitute ultrasonography. Computed tomography (CT) plays a key role in patient evaluation, especially in emergency situations where acquisition of CT reduces mortality, morbidity and incidence of exploratory laparotomy. However, there is ample evidence in the literature to support the use of alternative radiation-free modalities (namely, ultrasound and magnetic resonance imaging), as part of the Imaging Gently campaign to reduce radiation exposure without compromising patient care. Ultrasound is readily available, does not use radiation, and can provide sufficient diagnostic information to allow for optimal patient care. Therefore, the SPR recommends use of these radiation-free modalities when applicable.

References:
Strauss KJ, Goske MJ, Kaste SC, et al. Image Gently: ten steps you can take to optimize image quality and lower CT dose for pediatric patient. *AJR Am J Roentgenol.* 2010;194(4):868-873.
Goske MJ, Applegate KE, Bell C, et al. Image Gently: providing practical educational tools and advocacy to accelerate radiation protection for children worldwide. *Semin Ultrasound CT MR.* 2010;31(1):57-63.

45. A, Substitute ultrasonography. Although every effort should be made to minimize CT radiation dose in cases where CT is the imaging modality of choice, it is important to remember that ultrasound is the imaging modality of choice for a variety pediatric of pelvic, abdominal, and cardiovascular indications. Because ultrasound does not expose the patient to ionizing radiation, its application in pregnant patients and women of childbearing age is particularly important. Some examples of indications for which ultrasound is the imaging modality of choice include pelvic pain, evaluation of pelvic masses, right upper quadrant pain, acute pancreatitis, assessment for free fluid in the setting of blunt abdominal trauma, abdominal aortic aneurysm, extremity deep vein thrombosis, and assessment of extracranial carotid artery patency.

Reference:
Image Wisely website. <http://www.imagewisely.org/imaging-modalities/computed-tomography/imaging-physicians/articles/use-of-ultrasound-as-an-alternative-to-ct>.

46. C, Decision support software. Nonionizing imaging options are always preferable to any test with ionizing radiation, particularly in the pregnant patient. Ordering physicians may not have access to the patients' imaging or radiation dose history and/or may lack or be unaware of recommended criteria to guide their decisions, thereby potentially exposing patients to unnecessary radiation. Promotion of alternative nonionizing imaging modalities and providing ordering clinicians with information to help better inform their image-ordering decision-making process can be accomplished with decision support software.

References:
Image Wisely website. <http://www.imagewisely.org/imaging-modalities/computed-tomography/medical-physicists/articles/the-pregnant-patient>.
White paper. Initiative to reduce unnecessary radiation exposure from medical imaging. <http://www.fda.gov/Radiation-EmittingProducts/RadiationSafety/RadiationDoseReduction/ucm199994.htm>.

47. A, Cash basis of accounting. If you wait until you actually receive payment for a service you have provided, it is considered cash basis accounting. This means that you may have expenses for a service in one time period but the payment listed for that service in a different time period. If you are selling an item in a store, cash basis of accounting makes more sense than when you are providing a service that gets billed for later. How can you convert your service-based practice into a cash basis enterprise? Some family practitioners notify patients that "Payment is due on the date of service." Patients pay that day for the physical examination in whole. The physician then has patients submit their insurance claims for repayment to the patient. The physician gets the money that day as cash. Patients have to deal with the insurance carrier.

References:
Patriot Software website. <https://www.patriotsoftware.com/accounting/training/blog/cash-basis-vs-accrual-comparing-accounting-methods/>.
Accounting Coach website. <http://www.accountingcoach.com/blog/cash-basis-accrual-basis-of-accounting>.

48. A, Cash basis of accounting. If you are spending money for contrast that you will eventually use, and you list that as a current expense even though you have not used that contrast, it is cash basis accounting. Paying by check does not hit your account until that check is cashed. However when you write the check, not when it is cashed or clears the bank, is the point of entry for cash basis accounting. If you have to pay the electricity bill for December on February 1, it is listed in February as an expense on the cash basis of accounting even though the expense was "earned" in December's electricity.

Reference:
Accounting Coach website. <http://www.accountingcoach.com/blog/cash-basis-accrual-basis-of-accounting>.

49. C, Accrual basis of accounting. When the bill is sent to the patient you haven't actually "realized" that income. That is, you do not have cash in hand that you can spend for your expenses or use as salary. Yes, you have provided a service that has value, but, no, you do not actually have payment. What if the patient does not pay? What if the patient dies on the way home? What if you never actually "see" that money? Your time is gone. The contrast dye has been used. The technician's salary has been paid. But you have nothing in hand. You sent a bill.

To list the amount charged on your income statement probably does not make sense but is the concept of the accrual basis of accounting. The payment you will receive is listed as if it was in the bank to offset the expense of that service. Hence accounts receivables are consider a current asset/income in the accrual basis of accounting.

In a similar fashion, if you charge the contrast dye on your visa in January and you do not receive it until February, it is listed in January for cash basis and in February for accrual basis accounting.

Reference:
Accounting Coach website. <http://www.accountingcoach.com/blog/cash-basis-accrual-basis-of-accounting>.

50. B, All expenses must be matched in the same accounting period as the revenues they helped to earn. The matching principle states that all expenses on an income statement must be reported in the same accounting period as the revenues they helped to earn. This allows the most accurate assessment of profitability for that period. This is why the balance sheet is truly balanced and why the income statement is able to account for all of the moneys in a practice. Recognizing an expense earlier than is appropriate lowers net income by not countering it with that income just as citing an expense later than appropriate raises net income. Reporting revenues for a period without reporting all the expenses that brought them could result in overstated profits.

Reference:
E-conomic website. What is the matching principle? <https://www.e-conomic.com/accountingsoftware/accounting-words/matching>.

51. A radiology group's balance sheet is:
    A. A snapshot of a company's financial condition
    B. The only statement that applies to a single point in time
    C. Provided at least once a year
    C. All of the above

52. The radiology group's income statement does not show:
    A. A company's earnings for a given period
    B. A company's holdings on a specific date
    C. Profitability over a given interval
    D. All of the money a company spent

53. The concept of commoditization of radiology supports the notion of:
    A. Image wisely
    B. Contracts go to the lowest bidder
    C. Incorporation will protect the specialty
    D. Radiologists as consultants

54. Teleradiology after-hours service is an example of:
    A. Consultants' agreements
    B. Market forces
    C. Commoditization risk
    D. Professional laziness

55. An accountant CPA group owns an imaging center with MR and CT outside their professional office. They employ radiologists to interpret the images at the freestanding imaging center. This is an example of:
    A. Business opportunity
    B. Commoditization
    C. Stark law violation
    D. Self-referral

51. **D, All of the above.** The balance sheet is a statement that provides all the assets and liabilities at a specific point in time for a company. The current (one year) and long term (more than one year) assets and liabilities are listed for the financial document. The bottom line of a balance sheet lists the net worth/shareholder equity for which a company has "invested in itself." Within shareholder equity lies retained earnings that may be reduced by declaring dividends to the shareholders. The assets are any item of value. In radiology these are usually the accounts receivables of bills for studies that have been performed but for which the money has not been received. There is cash from receipts. The other big assets are the value of the imaging machinery that the group owns. By the same token, the greatest liabilities are the salaries paid to operate the business and the debt on the, for example, 12 MRI scanners, 6 CT scanners and 3 PET scanners in the practice. The loans and leases for such equipment and the buildings account for liabilities.

Useful data points are:

Debt-to-Equity Ratio = Total Liabilities / Shareholders' Equity
P/E Ratio = Price per share / Earnings per share
Operating Margin = Income from Operations / Net Revenues

Reference:
U.S. Securities and Exchange Commission website. Beginners' guide to financial statements. <http://www.sec.gov/investor/pubs/begfinstmtguide.htm>.

52. **B, A company's holdings on a specific date.** An income statement is analogous to a profit/loss statement that is assessed over a period of time, usually quarterly. A balance statement is the financial statement that "takes stock" of one's position at a point in time. "Income from operations" (one of the few bottom lines of an income statement) is derived from subtracting the operating expenses from the gross profit. This is called earnings before interest, taxes and depreciation and amortization (EBITDA) and is sometimes referred to as a company's operating profitability. However, most income statements then proceed to deduct from the income from operations the interest expense and the depreciation/amortization expenses. This leaves earnings before taxes (EBT). Finally taxes are removed for the net profit/income/earning after EBITDA.

If you divide the total net earnings by the number of shares in the company, you get earnings per share, or EPS.

Reference:
U.S. Securities and Exchange Commission website. Beginners' guide to financial statements. <http://www.sec.gov/investor/pubs/begfinstmtguide.htm>.

53. **B, Contracts go to the lowest bidder.** Commoditization (or commodification) is defined as "the transformation of goods and services into a commodity." Many centers now bundle services into disease- or treatment-based products (eg, pain, cancer, fertility, easier surgery). Such "commodities" are widely advertised and promoted to both the public and primary care physicians. Restructuring the specialty of radiology as a product will result in its commoditization. Technology, after-hours imaging and teleradiology services, financial incentives, reimbursement policies, radiologists themselves, imaging growth and requirements for expertise, and patients are drivers of radiology commoditization. These drivers share the commonality of interpretation only, with a dissociation of the other integrated components of an imaging examination, including necessity and appropriateness, performance quality, and consultation with a referring physician. Commoditization implies a nonexistent low value relationship with the clinicians whom radiologists serve. It is a bad thing. For interpretation-only services, hospitals and payers seek to maximize profit margins by brokering radiologists' fees at less than full value.

References:
Borgstede JP. Radiology: commodity or specialty. *Radiology.* 2008;247(3):613-616.
Krestin GP. Commoditization in radiology: threat or opportunity? *Radiology.* 2010;256(2):338-342.

54. **C, Commoditization risk.** Drivers toward commoditization of radiology are technology, after-hours imaging and teleradiology services, financial incentives, reimbursement policies, radiologists themselves, imaging growth and requirements for expertise, and patients. After-hours imaging and teleradiology services are commoditization drivers because they offer nonintegrated interpretation-only services. They do not foster long term relationships between radiologists and their (day-time) clinical colleagues. The implication is that you can buy an interpretation from anyone, and the benefits of collegiality and long term relationships are minimal.

Reference:
Borgstede JP. Radiology: commodity or specialty. *Radiology.* 2008;247(3):613-616.

55. **A, Business opportunity.** Radiology has become a very complex business. Business opportunity involves the offer of a product that will enable the purchaser to begin a business. In this scenario, the accountants are not self-referring, so there is no Stark Law violation. They view the ability to use their space for a lucrative purpose as a business opportunity. It is not commoditization because the radiologists may build relationships with referring clinicians independent of who owns the building or the equipment. It may be true that the radiologists who are employed by the CPAs would not otherwise be able to purchase the equipment themselves and may not otherwise be employed.

References:
Business opportunity. <http://www.entrepreneur.com/encyclopedia/business-opportunity>. Accessed December 16, 2015.
Yousem DM, Beauchamp NJ. *Radiology Business Practice: How to Succeed.* 1st ed. Philadelphia, PA: Elsevier; 2008.

QUESTIONS

1. The ACR practice parameter for communication states that the impression of a report should include all of the following except:
   A. The radiation dosage of studies where radiation was used
   B. A specific diagnosis when possible
   C. A differential diagnosis when appropriate
   D. Follow-up or additional diagnostic studies to clarify or confirm the impression when appropriate

2. If a report is modified from preliminary result to the final result in a manner that could affect patient care:
   A. It should be labeled as a critical finding
   B. It should document communication of the discrepancy
   C. It should be returned to the medical record unscathed
   D. The final report should be signed off by the person who provided the initial reading

3. In the case of a critical finding where the referring physician or his or her designee cannot be contacted, the radiologist is obligated to contact:
   A. The emergency department personnel in charge
   B. The chief of that service
   C. The patient
   D. The radiology administrator on duty

4. Non-routine communications include all of the following except:
   A. Findings that suggest a need for immediate or urgent intervention
   B. Findings that disagree with a preceding interpretation of the same examination and where failure to act may adversely affect patient health
   C. Findings where the referring physician's opinion and what he or she suspects disagree with what the radiologist believes to be the source of the patient's symptoms
   D. Findings that the radiologist reasonably believes may be seriously adverse to the patient's health and may not require immediate attention but, if not acted on, may worsen over time and possibly result in an adverse patient outcome

5. Documentation of nonroutine communication must occur in:
   A. The medical record only
   B. A departmental log only
   C. A personal journal only
   D. The medical record or a departmental log or a personal journal

6. The optimal means of communication of critical findings is:
   A. Verbal
   B. Texting
   C. Email
   D. Via the medical record

7. As for "curbside consultations" by radiologists, the ACR's suggestion for this is:
   A. Don't do them
   B. Document the interpretation somewhere
   C. Require formal readings
   D. Provide compassionate, collegial care in the spirit of the Good Samaritan rule

8. In the case of a self-referred patient, the obligation is to communicate the result with:
   A. The patient's primary care physician
   B. The patient's referring physician for the study
   C. The patient
   D. None of the above

9. Patient identifiable data may be transmitted without a patient's authorization under which of the following circumstances?
   A. Payment activities
   B. Quality assurance programs
   C. Fraud claims
   D. All of the above

1. **A, The radiation dosage of studies where radiation was used.** Unless a report is brief, each report should contain an "impression" or "conclusion." The impression should include:
   - A specific diagnosis when possible
   - A differential diagnosis when appropriate
   - Follow-up or additional diagnostic studies to clarify or confirm the impression when appropriate
   - Any significant patient reaction

   The impression need not include radiation dose of studies where radiation was used.

   Reference:
   <http://www.acr.org/~/media/C5D1443C9EA4424AA12477D1AD1D927D.pdf>.

2. **B, It should be labeled as a critical finding.** According to the *ACR Practice Parameter for Communication of Diagnostic Imaging Findings,* if a report is modified from preliminary result to the final result in a manner that could affect patient care this discrepancy must be communicated appropriately, and the final result should include documentation of the discrepancy and communication.

   Reference:
   <http://www.acr.org/~/media/C5D1443C9EA4424AA12477D1AD1D927D.pdf>.

3. **C, The patient.** According to the *ACR Practice Parameter for Communication of Diagnostic Imaging Findings,* in the case of a critical finding where the referring physician or his or her designee cannot be contacted, the radiologist is obligated to contact the patient.

   Reference:
   <http://www.acr.org/~/media/C5D1443C9EA4424AA12477D1AD1D927D.pdf>.

4. **C, Findings where the referring physician's opinion and what he or she suspects disagree with what the radiologist believes to be the source of the patient's symptoms.**

   In emergent or other nonroutine clinical situations, the interpreting physician should expedite delivery of the diagnostic imaging report to ensure timely receipt of the findings. Such nonroutine communications include:
   - Findings that suggest a need for immediate or urgent intervention
   - Findings that are discrepant with a preceding interpretation of the same examination and where failure to act may adversely affect patient health
   - Findings that the interpreting physician reasonably believes may be seriously adverse to the patient's health and may not require immediate attention but, if not acted on, may worsen over time and possibly result in an adverse patient outcome

   According to the *ACR Practice Parameter for Communication of Diagnostic Imaging Findings,* findings where the clinician's opinion and what he or she suspects are discrepant with what the radiologist believes to be the source of the patient's symptoms do not require nonroutine communication.

   Reference:
   <http://www.acr.org/~/media/C5D1443C9EA4424AA12477D1AD1D927D.pdf>.

5. **D, The medical record or a departmental log or a personal journal.** According to the *ACR Practice Parameter for Communication of Diagnostic Imaging Findings,* interpreting physicians should document all nonroutine communications. Documentation is optimally placed in the patient's radiology report or medical record but may be entered into a departmental log or personal journal. Documentation should include the time, method of communication, and the name of the person to whom the communication was delivered.

   Reference:
   <http://www.acr.org/~/media/C5D1443C9EA4424AA12477D1AD1D927D.pdf>.

6. **A, Verbal. According to the *ACR Practice Parameter for Communication of Diagnostic Imaging Findings,* the optimal means of communication of critical findings is verbal, either in person or via telephone.** Verbal communication ensures timely receipt of the critical information. Other methods of communication, including texting, facsimile, instant messaging, and email may not guarantee the receipt of the information in a timely fashion and are therefore not preferred.

   Reference:
   <http://www.acr.org/~/media/C5D1443C9EA4424AA12477D1AD1D927D.pdf>.

7. **B, Document the interpretation somewhere.** On occasion, an interpreting physician may be asked to provide an interpretation that does not result in a formal report but that may be used to guide treatment decisions. Such "curbside consultations" or "wet readings" may not allow for immediate documentation and may occur under less than ideal viewing conditions or without relevant prior imaging available for comparison. Such interpretations carry inherent risk, and interpreting physicians providing consultation of this kind are strongly encouraged to formally document the interpretation, limitations that may have affected interpretation, and any associated communication.

   Reference:
   <http://www.acr.org/~/media/C5D1443C9EA4424AA12477D1AD1D927D.pdf>.

8. **C, The patient.** Most patients undergoing imaging procedures have been referred by health care professionals. Some patients, however, may be self-referred (often breast imaging or cosmetic interventional radiology procedures). Interpreting physicians should recognize that providing interpretive services for self-referred patients establishes a doctor-patient relationship that includes an obligation for communicating the results directly to the patient and arranging any appropriate follow-up.

   Reference:
   <http://www.acr.org/~/media/C5D1443C9EA4424AA12477D1AD1D927D.pdf>.

9. **D, All of the above.** A covered entity is permitted to use and disclose protected health information, without an individual's authorization, for the following purposes or situations:
   1. To the individual
   2. Treatment, payment, and health care operations: A covered entity may use and disclose protected health information for its own treatment, payment, and health care operations activities. A covered entity also may disclose protected health information for the treatment activities of any health care provider, the payment activities of another covered entity and of any health care provider, or the health care operations of another covered entity involving either quality or competency assurance activities or fraud and abuse detection and compliance activities, if both covered entities have or had a relationship with the individual and the protected health information pertains to the relationship.
   3. Opportunity to agree or object
   4. Incident to an otherwise permitted use and disclosure
   5. Public interest and benefit activities
   6. Limited data set for the purposes of research, public health or health care operations

   Covered entities may rely on professional ethics and best judgments in deciding which of these permissive uses and disclosures to make.

   Reference:
   <http://www.hhs.gov/ocr/privacy/hipaa/understanding/summary/>.

10. Patient identifiable data may be transmitted without a patient's authorization under which of the following circumstances?
    A. During domestic violence investigations
    B. During claims of tuberculosis exposure
    C. During claims of implicit bias
    D. All of the above

11. Which is the ACR's philosophy about communication?
    A. Patient confidentiality trumps timeliness for critical findings.
    B. Timeliness should not negate appropriate methods of information delivery.
    C. Timely receipt of information outweighs issues of the means in which the report is delivered.
    D. A written communication is more valuable than a verbal communication.

12. Which of the following is a critical test?
    A. Tension pneumothorax
    B. CTA for pulmonary embolus
    C. 3-mm subdural hematoma
    D. NCCT for change in mental status

13. The Joint Commission has specified that accredited facilities must define:
    A. Critical tests
    B. Critical results
    C. Both critical tests and critical results
    D. None of the above

14. Which of the following best describes The Joint Commission requirements for communicating critical results?
    A. The Joint Commission requires communication of critical results directly to a physician.
    B. The Joint Commission categorizes radiologic actionable findings as either "critical," "urgent," or "significant."
    C. The Joint Commission requires institutions to monitor their performance on reporting critical findings.
    D. The Joint Commission categorizes radiologic actionable findings as either "red," "orange," or "yellow."

15. According to ACR Actionable Reporting Work Group recommendations, communication of a Category 1 finding that could lead to death or significant morbidity if not promptly recognized, communicated, and acted upon, should be done within:
    A. Minutes
    B. Hours
    C. Days
    D. None of the above

10. **A, During domestic violence investigations.** There are 12 national priority purposes for which the Privacy Rule permits use and disclosure of protected health information without an individual's authorization or permission. Limitations apply to each public interest purpose, balancing privacy of an individual with the benefit of the public good. These purposes are:

1. Required by law
2. Public health activities
3. Victims of abuse, neglect, or domestic violence
4. Health oversight activities
5. Judicial and administrative proceedings
6. Law enforcement purposes
7. Decedents
8. Cadaveric organ, eye, or tissue donation
9. Research
10. Serious threat to health or safety
11. Essential government functions
12. Workers' compensation

Reference:
<http://www.hhs.gov/ocr/privacy/hipaa/understanding/summary/>.

11. **C, Timely receipt of information outweighs issues of the means by which the report is delivered.** As detailed in the ACR's Practice Parameter for Communication of Diagnostic Imaging Findings, the timely receipt of the report is more important than the method of report delivery. This paper stresses the importance of effective communication as a critical component of radiology. The characteristics of effective communication are those that promote optimal patient care, are timely, and limit the risk of miscommunication. There is a responsibility of the ordering provider to provide relevant clinical information, a working diagnosis, and pertinent signs/symptoms that prompt the need for imaging.

Reference:
Revised 2014 (Resolution 11)* ACR practice parameter for communication of diagnostic imaging findings. <http://www.acr.org/~/media/ACR/Documents/PGTS/guidelines/Comm_Diag_Imaging.pdf>.

12. **B, CTA for pulmonary embolus.** The second national 2015 patient safety goal of The Joint Commission is to improve the effectiveness of communication among caregivers. The standards implemented as part of this goal include requiring health care organizations to identify critical tests and critical results/values. A critical test is an examination that if positive for its primary indication would yield a critical result. A critical result is one that is significantly outside the normal range and may indicate a life-threatening situation. Further, this life-threatening situation may be averted with proper and prompt care, potentiated by effective communication. CTA for pulmonary embolus meets these criteria. A tension pneumothorax and 3 mm subdural hematoma are critical **findings** not critical **tests**.

Reference:
<http://www.jointcommission.org/assets/1/6/2015_NPSG_HAP.pdf>.

13. **C, Both critical tests and critical results.** TJC specified that accredited facilities define both critical tests and critical results as a standard aimed to improve effective communication among caregivers. A critical test (CTA for pulmonary embolus) is an examination that if positive for its primary indication would yield a critical result (tension pneumothorax). A critical result is one that is significantly outside the normal range and may indicate a life-threatening situation. Further, this life-threatening situation may be averted with proper and prompt care, potentiated by effective communication.

Reference:
<http://www.jointcommission.org/assets/1/6/2015_NPSG_HAP.pdf>.

14. **C, The Joint Commission requires institutions to monitor their performance on reporting critical findings.** TJC allows institutions leeway to define and categorize their own critical results, requiring only that staff "get important test results to the right person on time" and "regularly measure and assess documentation and communication processes as part of an established quality assurance program." They define a critical result as "any result or finding that may be considered life threatening or that could result in severe morbidity and require urgent or emergent clinical attention."

References:
Larson PA, Berland LL, Griffith B, et al. Actionable findings and the role of IT support: report of the ACR Actionable Reporting Work Group. *J Am Coll Radiol.* 2014;11(6):552-558.
Anthony SG, Prevedello LM, Damiano MM, et al. Impact of a 4-year quality improvement initiative to improve communication of critical imaging test results. *Radiology.* 2011;259(3):802-807. doi:10.1148/radiol.11101396; [Epub 2011 Apr 5].
Joint Commission NPSGs. <http://www.jointcommission.org/assets/1/6/2015_NPSG_HAP.pdf>. Accessed December 4, 2015.
ACR Practice Guideline for Communication of Diagnostic Imaging Findings. <http://www.acr.org/~/media/C5D1443C9EA4424AA12477D1AD1D927D.pdf>. Accessed December 4, 2015.

15. **A, Minutes.** Neither TJC nor ACR has developed a standard list for critical results or tests and each facility is given the leeway to define and categorize its own critical tests and results and timeline for communication. This is entirely a local decision. However, their recommendation for Category 1 (Category 1: Communication Within Minutes. Category 1 findings are those that could lead to death or significant morbidity if not promptly recognized, communicated and acted upon. Direct verbal communication to the ordering clinician is generally required as promptly as possible) is verbal communication "within minutes." Such items as intracranial hemorrhage, severe spinal cord compression, and tension pneumothorax fall into this category.

The ACR referred to the Massachusetts Coalition for the Prevention of Medical Errors (MCPME), which developed a list of actionable findings. The MCPME used numeric categories 1, 2, and 3 to categorize common findings and their urgency. Category 1 is defined above. Category 2 are findings that are clinically significant, explain a patient's acute presentation, and require specific medical or surgical treatment and should be communicated in hours. Category 3 findings do not require any immediate treatment or other action, but could still be significant and should be communicated directly within days. Brigham and Women's has employed a color coded scheme that includes red alerts that require "interruptive notification" of the referring physicians within 60 minutes of discovery of the critical findings, for scenarios such as ischemic bowel or intracerebral hemorrhage.

References:
Larson PA, Berland LL, Griffith B, et al. Actionable findings and the role of IT support: report of the ACR Actionable Reporting Work Group. *J Am Coll Radiol.* 2014;11(6):552-558.
Anthony SG1, Prevedello LM, Damiano MM, et al. Impact of a 4-year quality improvement initiative to improve communication of critical imaging test results. *Radiology.* 2011;259(3):802-807. doi:10.1148/radiol.11101396; [Epub 2011 Apr 5].

16. Category 2 findings are defined by the ACR Actionable Reporting Work Group as clinically significant observations that generally explain a patient's acute presentation and require specific medical or surgical treatment but are not as urgent as Category 1, life threatening findings. These should be communicated within:
    A. Minutes
    B. Hours
    C. Days
    D. None of the above

17. Which of the following qualifies as a Category 2 (orange alert) finding?
    A. Tension pneumocephalus
    B. An obstructing ureteral stone
    C. Thyroid nodule
    D. All of the above

18. Which of the following is NOT considered a Category 2 (orange alert) finding?
    A. Abdominal abscess
    B. Impending pathologic hip fracture
    C. Open displaced skull fracture without intracranial hemorrhage
    D. Leaking aortic aneurysm

19. Which of the following is a good example of a Category 3 (yellow alert) communication result?
    A. Solid 2.5-cm renal mass
    B. 10-mm subdural hematoma
    C. Femoral neck fracture
    D. Pneumothorax

20. The ACR Practice Guideline for Communication of Diagnostic Imaging Findings suggests including what elements of documentation when communicating actionable findings?
    A. Date, time of communication, who reported the findings, who received the findings, means of communication (ie, call, fax, email)
    B. Date, time of communication, who reported the findings, who received the findings, when the finding was observed
    C. Date, time of communication, who made the phone call of the findings, who received the findings
    D. Date, time of communication, who reported the findings, who received the findings, means of communication (ie, call, fax, email), date and time the finding was discovered

21. Dr. Jones revises a resident's preliminary report in the electronic medical record (EMR). He signs the report and it goes from preliminary designation to finalized designation in the EMR. He then notices an additional finding. He wants to add that finding to the report. Which of the following is the best way to revise the report?
    A. Have the report he originally finalized sent back to his queue to correct it, and sign it.
    B. Have the original resident's report sent back to his queue to correct and sign.
    C. Write an addendum to his finalized report.
    D. None of the above

22. In the case above, which of the reports needs to be retrievable for an audit?
    A. The resident's report
    B. The initial signed report by Dr. Jones
    C. The final revised/addended signed report by Dr. Jones
    D. All of the above

23. In what instance would Dr. Jones have to call the referring physician to notify that doctor about the addendum he made?
    A. In all cases
    B. If it was anything but a typographical error
    C. If the new finding was not previously reported
    D. If the information in the addendum changes the diagnosis

16. **B, Hours.** The ACR Actionable Reporting Work Group recognized that some findings are important but immediacy is not as critical as far as communication. To this they ascribe category 2. The radiologist must document such communication and ensure that it has been received and, in some case, it has been acted on appropriately.

The analogy in the Brigham and Women's policy would be an orange alert. These are findings that could result in mortality or significant morbidity if not appropriately treated within 2 to 3 days, such as an intraabdominal abscess or impending pathologic hip fracture. Nonetheless, they set the orange alert bar at notification within 3 hours of discovery of findings.

References:
The Joint Commission National Patient Safety Goals Effective January 1, 2014. <http://www.jointcommission.org/assets/1/6/2014_HAP_NPSG_E.pdf> Accessed 8.16.2014.
Anthony SG1, Prevedello LM, Damiano MM, et al. Impact of a 4-year quality improvement initiative to improve communication of critical imaging test results. *Radiology.* 2011;259(3):802-807. doi:10.1148/radiol.11101396; [Epub 2011 Apr 5].
Singh H, Vij MS. Eight recommendations for policies for communicating abnormal test results. *Jt Comm J Qual Patient Saf.* 2010;36(5):226-232.
ACR Practice Parameter for Communication of Diagnostic Imaging Findings (rev 2014). <http://www.acr.org/~/media/ACR/Documents/PGTS/guidelines/Comm_Diag_Imaging.pdf> Accessed 9/20/2014.
Larson PA, Berland L, Griffith B, et al. Actionable findings and the role of information. *J Am Coll Radiol.* 2014;11(6):552-558.

17. **B, An obstructing ureteral stone.** Tension pneumocephalus, because it can cause life-threatening herniation of brain tissue, stroke, and increased intracranial pressure, would be considered a category 1 finding. By the same token, a thyroid nodule does not have to be communicated within hours. The thyroid nodule can be worked up at a more leisurely pace that does not require such urgency. An obstructing ureteral stone does not have the immediacy of a tension pneumothorax or pneumocephalus but should be addressed in a prompt fashion. Hence it has been listed as a category 2 finding.

References:
The Joint Commission National Patient Safety Goals Effective January 1, 2014. <http://www.jointcommission.org/assets/1/6/2014_HAP_NPSG_E.pdf> Accessed August 16, 2014.
Rossi LP, Leblanc MM, Miguel K, et al. The Joint Commission, national patient safety goals, and radiology. In: Abujudeh HH, Bruno MA, eds. *Quality and Safety in Radiology.* New York: Oxford University Press; 2012:80-92.
Singh H, Vij MS. Eight recommendations for policies for communicating abnormal test results. *Jt Comm J Qual Patient Saf.* 2010;36(5):226-232.
ACR Practice Parameter for Communication of Diagnostic Imaging Findings (rev 2014). <http://www.acr.org/~/media/ACR/Documents/PGTS/guidelines/Comm_Diag_Imaging.pdf> Accessed September 20, 2014.
Larson PA, Berland L, Griffith B, et al. Actionable findings and the role of information. *J Am Coll Radiol.* 2014;11(6):552-558.

18. **D, Leaking aortic aneurysm.** A leaking aortic aneurysm is a medical emergency that would classify as a critical finding, category 1, or red alert. As such, it should be addressed immediately with communication within minutes after discovery.

References:
Anthony SG1, Prevedello LM, Damiano MM, et al. Impact of a 4-year quality improvement initiative to improve communication of critical imaging test results. *Radiology.* 2011;259(3):802-807.
Larson PA, Berland L, Griffith B, et al. Actionable findings and the role of information. *Radiology.* 2011;259(3):802-807. doi:10.1148/radiol.11101396; [Epub 2011 Apr 5].
ACR Practice Parameter for Communication of Diagnostic Imaging Findings (rev 2014). <http://www.acr.org/~/media/ACR/Documents/PGTS/guidelines/Comm_Diag_Imaging.pdf>. Accessed September 20, 2014.

19. **A, Solid 2.5 cm renal mass.** The Brigham and Women's classification for a renal mass and a lung nodule is yellow alert. They specify that this demands notification within 3 days of discovery. This is a finding that must be addressed but does not have the same level of urgency as abscesses

and tension pneumothoraces. The analogous classification for the ACR workgroup is category 3. The items in Category 3 include definitive diagnoses of new malignancies to questionable masses that may be more likely benign than malignant.

References:
Larson PA, Berland LL, Griffith B, et al. Actionable findings and the role of IT support: report of the ACR Actionable Reporting Work Group. *J Am Coll Radiol.* 2014;11(6):552-558.
Anthony SG1, Prevedello LM, Damiano MM, et al. Impact of a 4-year quality improvement initiative to improve communication of critical imaging test results. *Radiology.* 2011;259(3):802-807. doi:10.1148/radiol.11101396; [Epub 2011 Apr 5].

20. **B, Date, time of communication, who reported the findings, who received the findings, when the finding was observed.** The ACR Practice Guideline for Communication of Diagnostic Imaging Findings section II.C.2.b suggests including "the time, method of communication, and the name of the person to whom the communication was delivered" any time an actionable finding is reported.

Reference:
ACR Practice Guideline for Communication of Diagnostic Imaging Findings. <http://www.acr.org/~/media/C5D1443C9EA4424AA12477D1AD1D927D.pdf>. Accessed December 4, 2015.

21. **C, Write an addendum to his finalized report.** Communication of information is only as effective as the system that conveys the information. A copy of the final report should be archived by the imaging facility as part of the patient's medical record and be retrievable for future reference. Situations that may warrant nonroutine communication include "findings that are discrepant with a preceding interpretation of the same examination and where failure to act may adversely affect patient health." These cases may occur when the final interpretation is discrepant with a preliminary report or when significant discrepancies are encountered upon subsequent review of a study after a final report has been submitted.

Reference:
ACR Practice Parameter for Communication of Diagnostic Imaging Findings. <http://www.acr.org/~/media/ACR/Documents/PGTS/guidelines/Comm_Diag_Imaging.pdf>. Accessed December 13, 2015.

22. **D, All of the above.** Preliminary communications should be reproduced into a permanent format as soon as practical and appropriately labeled as a preliminary report, distinct from the final report, and archived because clinical decisions may have been based on the preliminary report. A copy of the final report should be archived by the imaging facility as part of the patient's medical record and be retrievable for future reference. Retention and distribution of these records must be in accordance with state and federal regulations and facility policies. Interpreting physicians should document all nonroutine communications. Documentation is best placed in the radiology report or the patient's medical record.

Reference:
ACR Practice Parameter for Communication of Diagnostic Imaging Findings. <http://www.acr.org/~/media/ACR/Documents/PGTS/guidelines/Comm_Diag_Imaging.pdf>. Accessed December 13, 2015.

23. **D, If the information in the addendum changes the diagnosis.** As soon as possible, a significant variation in findings and/or conclusions between the preliminary and final interpretations should be reported in a manner that reliably ensures receipt by the ordering or treating physician/health care provider, particularly when such changes may affect patient care.

Reference:
ACR Practice Parameter for Communication of Diagnostic Imaging Findings. <http://www.acr.org/~/media/ACR/Documents/PGTS/guidelines/Comm_Diag_Imaging.pdf>. Accessed December 13, 2015.

24. Electronic signature is appropriate for radiology reports:
    A. In all situations
    B. In finalized reports only
    C. In preliminary reports only
    D. If signing for another person

25. What does CMS require for a signature to be valid?
    A. Services that are provided or ordered must be authenticated by the ordering practitioner
    B. Signatures are handwritten, electronic, or stamped (stamped signatures are only permitted in the case of an author with a physical disability who can provide proof to a CMS contractor of an inability to sign due to a disability)
    C. Signatures are legible
    D. All of the above

26. If a signature is not legible, what is the recourse for Center for Medicare and Medicaid Services (CMS) orders?
    A. Use a signature log submitted to CMS to support the identity of the illegible signature
    B. Convert to a verbal order co-signed by a nurse
    C. Co-sign the order by someone else
    D. None of the above

27. A radiologist's signature on an order for diphenhydramine is undated in the medical record. What is a valid way to establish the date of an order?
    A. Use the date before the order
    B. Use the date after the order
    C. If the date before and after the order is the same, use that date
    D. None of the above

28. Digital Imaging and Communications in Medicine (DICOM) standards improved upon the ACR-NEMA Standard by:
    A. Improving speed
    B. Implementing networking capability by TCP/IP protocols
    C. Interfacing with radiology PACS
    D. Allowing nonradiologists to use the PACS

29. Digital Imaging and Communications in Medicine (DICOM) standards added what additional guidelines to the ACR-NEMA Standard?
    A. Established offline media standards as in CDs
    B. Created methodology for rapid offline 3D postprocessing
    C. Set standards for jump-drive duplication of radiology data
    D. Created rules for nonradiologists to use an RIS for their images

30. The DICOM standard does not specify:
    A. The implementation details of any features of the standard on a device claiming conformance
    B. The overall set of features and functions to be expected from a system implemented by integrating a group of devices each claiming DICOM conformance
    C. A testing/validation procedure to assess an implementation's conformance to the standard
    D. All of the above

31. Health Level Seven (HL7) refers to:
    A. A level of emergency that requires all hospital employees to "remain in place" in the event of a disaster
    B. A DICOM code that refers to transfer of imaging data between modalities
    C. The "language" used to transfer clinical and administrative data within the health care environment
    D. The seven key performance measures (KPMs) that The Joint Commission uses to accredit hospitals

24. **A, In all situations.** The final report should be completed in accordance with appropriate state and federal requirements. Electronic or rubber-stamp signature devices, instead of a written signature, are acceptable unless contrary to state law, if access to such devices is secure.

Reference:
ACR Practice Parameter for Communication of Diagnostic Imaging Findings. <http://www.acr.org/~/media/ACR/Documents/PGTS/guidelines/Comm_Diag_Imaging.pdf>. Accessed December 13, 2015.

25. **D, All of the above.** For a signature to be valid the criteria to be met include:
    - Services that are provided or ordered must be authenticated by the ordering practitioner.
    - Signatures are handwritten, electronic, or stamped.*
    - Signatures are legible.
    - One may not add late signatures to medical records (beyond the short delay that occurs during the transcription process).
    - Systems and software products must include protections against modification, and one should apply administrative safeguards that correspond to standards and laws.
    - Stamped signatures are only permitted in the case of an author with a physical disability who can provide proof to a CMS contractor of an inability to sign due to a disability.

References:
Department of Health and Human Services. Complying with Medicare signature requirements. <https://www.cms.gov/Outreach-and-Education/Medicare-Learning-Network-MLN/MLNProducts/downloads/Signature_Requirements_Fact_Sheet_ICN905364.pdf>. Accessed December 3, 2015.

26. **A, Use a signature log submitted to CMS to support the identity of the illegible signature.** You may submit a signature log or attestation statement to support the identity of the illegible signature. If the original record contains a printed signature below the illegible signature, this may be accepted.

    Providers will sometimes include a signature log in the documentation they submit that lists the typed or printed name of the author associated with initials or illegible signature. The signature log might be included on the actual page where the initials or illegible signature are used or might be a separate document. Alternatively, providers will sometimes include an attestation statement in the documentation they submit. To be considered valid for Medicare medical review purposes, an attestation statement must be signed and dated by the author of the medical record entry and must contain sufficient information to identify the beneficiary.

References:
Department of Health and Human Services, Complying with Medicare Signature Requirements. <https://www.cms.gov/Outreach-and-Education/Medicare-Learning-Network-MLN/MLNProducts/downloads/Signature_Requirements_Fact_Sheet_ICN905364.pdf>. Accessed December 3, 2015.
Centers for Medicaid and Medicare Services. Medicare program integrity manual (Pub. 100-08), Chapter 3, Section 3.3.2.4.A. <https://www.cms.gov/Regulations-and-Guidance/Guidance/Manuals/downloads/pim83c03.pdf>.

27. **C, If the date before and after the order is the same, use that date.** Medicare Administrative Contractors, Comprehensive Error Rate Testing auditors, and Zone Program Integrity contractors shall ensure that the documentation contains enough information for the reviewer to determine the date on which the service was performed/ordered. If the date before and after an order is the same, use that date.

Reference:
Centers for Medicaid and Medicare Services. Medicare program integrity manual (Pub. 100-08), Chapter 3, Section 3.3.2.4.A. <https://www.cms.gov/Regulations-and-Guidance/Guidance/Manuals/downloads/pim83c03.pdf>.

28. **B, Implementing networking capability by TCP/IP protocols.** The ACR and National Electrical Manufacturers Association (NEMA) formed a joint committee in 1983 to develop a standard way of transferring images between various manufacturers and digital formats to allow for interoperability among a variety of devices. ACR-NEMA standards were published and eventually upgraded and developed into the DICOM standard, which exhibits several improvements on prior versions. These include application of the standard to a network environment with networking protocols as well as application to offline media. The DICOM standard also has expanded on previous equipment specifications to allow for multiple levels of device conformance to the standard. The DICOM does allow for interfacing with PACS systems; however, this was already available in prior ACR-NEMA standards.

Reference:
ACR IT reference guide for the practicing radiologist. <http://dicom.nema.org/standard.html>.

29. **A, Established offline media standards as in CDs.** Multiple improvements on the ACR-NEMA standards were made in the creation of the DICOM standard. These include applicability to a networked environment with standard networking protocol, as well as application to offline media. Industry standard offline file systems and media, including CDs, are also supported by the DICOM standard. Remote jump-drive technology is not designated in the DICOM, nor is specification of who is eligible to use the PACS system.

Reference:
ACR IT reference guide for the practicing radiologist. <http://dicom.nema.org/standard.html>.

30. **D, All of the above.** To allow for interoperability among a large variety of imaging devices, the DICOM standard designates device specifications; to conform to this standard, medical imaging equipment must follow a set of protocols for network communications, as well as a specific syntax for commands and information exchange. Media must also be stored within specific formats and services.

    Although the DICOM standard designates these specifications, it does not provide details for implementation or ways of assessing conformance, nor does it specify a set of expected features and functions on a particular device.

Reference:
ACR IT reference guide for the practicing radiologist. <http://dicom.nema.org/standard.html>.

31. **C, The "language" used to transfer clinical and administrative data within the health care environment.** Health Level Seven International is a nonprofit organization accredited by the American National Standards Institute. Founded in 1987, its mission is to provide standards for the exchange of electronic health care information. The number 7 in the organization's name refers to seventh layer of the International Standards Communications model, Application. HL7 is a standard created by the organization that provides a framework and format to facilitate the transfer of health care information and data.

Reference:
<http://www.hl7.org/implement/standards/>.
<http://www.cdc.gov/ehrmeaningfuluse/docs/introduction_to_hl7_03022011_anderson_cleared.pptx>.

32. According to the HL7 Clinical Document Architecture, which of the following characteristics is required for a clinical document?
    A. Subjectivity
    B. Assessments
    C. Patient information data
    D. Readability

33. According to the HL7 Clinical Document Architecture standard, which of the following additional characteristics are required for a clinical document?
    A. Persistence
    B. Stewardship
    C. Wholeness
    D. All of the above

34. The Systemized Nomenclature of Medicine Clinical Terms is used as the basis of terms used in:
    A. PACS
    B. RIS
    C. EHR
    D. DICOM

35. The American Medical Association Code of Medical Ethics states that when a patient suffers significant medical complications that may have resulted from the physician's mistake or judgment, the physician is ethically required to:
    A. Say "I'm sorry"
    B. Disclose to the patient all the facts necessary to ensure understanding of what has occurred
    C. Identify all members of the medical team participating in the patient's care
    D. None of the above

36. Expressions of sympathy following an accident or error are:
    A. Recommended by the AMA
    B. Inadmissible in civil court to prove liability in most states
    C. Admissible in civil court in most states
    D. Termed *qui tam* laws

37. The most widely used definition of patient-centered care is:
    A. Care that honors and responds to patients' preferences, needs, values, and goals
    B. Care that treats patients as they would like to be treated
    C. Safe and effective care that does no harm
    D. All of the above

32. **D, Readability.** HL7's purpose is to allow access and use of health care data and informatics with the ease of interoperability. HL7 provides standards for the creation of clinical documents so that they may easily be interpreted and exchanged between clinicians and patients. Examples of a clinical document include a history and physical, progress note, discharge summary, or imaging report. The six characteristics of a clinical document include:
1. Persistence
2. Stewardship
3. Potential for authentication
4. Context
5. Wholeness
6. Human readability

   Human readability allows both clinicians and patients to understand the content of the clinical document. Subjectivity, assessments, and patient information data are not necessarily part of a clinical document.

References:
<http://www.hl7.org/implement/standards/>.
<https://en.wikipedia.org/wiki/Health_Level_Seven_International>.
Dolin RH, Alschuler L, Beebe C, et al. The HL7 Clinical Document Architecture. *JAMIA.* 2001;8(6):552-569.

33. **D, All of the above.** As described in the previous question, the six characteristics of a clinical document as defined by HL7 include persistence, stewardship, potential for authentication, context, wholeness, and human readability. All of the listed choices are required characteristics of a health care document. Persistence implies that a clinical document will exist in its unaltered state for a specified period of time. Stewardship implies that an individual or organization is entrusted with maintaining the document. Wholeness implies that the entire clinical document is liable for authentication, rather than selected portions of the document out of context.

References:
<http://www.hl7.org/implement/standards/>.
Dolin RH, Alschuler L, Beebe C, et al. The HL7 Clinical Document Architecture. *JAMIA.* 2001;8(6):552-569.

34. **C, EHR.** EHR stands for electronic health record, the digital form of health records for individuals or populations, and may be used in a wide variety of medical settings. It is important that the terminology used in these records is consistent, and therefore systemized medical nomenclature is used. PACS stands for picture archiving and communication system, the imaging storage system used to access images of multiple modalities. RIS stands for radiology information system and is a database used to schedule, track, and report the results of patient imaging to facilitate efficient workflow. DICOM stands for digital imaging and communications in medicine and is the standard format of medical imaging and related information.

Reference:
Geeslin MG, Gaskin CM. Electronic health record-driven workflow for diagnostic radiologists. *J Am Coll Radiol.* 2016 Jan;13(1):45-53. [Epub 2015 Oct 22].

35. **B, Disclose to the patient all the facts necessary to ensure understanding of what has occurred.** As opposed to admissions of sympathy, empathy, or guilt, physicians are obligated to disclose to patients and their attorneys all the information needed to pursue a claim against the health care providers. All records and notes on a case must be provided without exception if requested. Many physicians opine that good disclosure strengthens the patient-physician relationship and is part and parcel of patient-centered care. Although 90% of physicians say that errors that are discovered should be reported, in practice only 30% actually do so. In a study looking at breast cancer misses, less than 15% of radiologists surveyed said that they would disclose the miss to their patients.

Reference:
Leonard B. To disclose or not to disclose radiologic errors: should "patient-first" supersede radiologist self-interest? *Radiology.* 2013;268(1):4-7.

36. **B, Inadmissible in civil court to prove liability in most states.** Most states have addressed the issue as to whether saying "I'm sorry" to a patient is admissible as an acknowledgement of guilt or is incriminating. They have followed the state of Massachusetts, which does not allow a statement of regret or sympathy to a patient or family to be an admission of liability in a civil action. Such apology-immunity statutes have been passed in 36 states, but some of these do not cover expressions of guilt. A statement of fault to a patient, the family, or to colleagues may therefore be admissible even in states with "I'm Sorry" laws.

   Qui tam laws are a type of civil lawsuit in which "insiders" blow the whistle on wrongdoers (and often reap monetary reward). This is the term used when a person in a billing operation turns in the business manager of a practice for fraudulently billing for studies that were not performed or inappropriate. The False Claims Act encourages such *qui tam* whistleblowers by providing up to 25% of the money recovered to the whistleblower if the government intervenes and as high as 30% if the whistleblower team secures the monetary reward through a negotiation or trial.

Reference:
Leonard B. Will saying "I'm sorry" prevent a malpractice lawsuit? *Am J Roentgenol.* 2006;187(1):10-15. <http://www.ajronline.org/doi/abs/10.2214/AJR.06.0110>.

37. **A, Care that honors and responds to patients' preferences, needs, values, and goals.** According to the Institute of Medicine, patient-centered care is "Providing care that is respectful of and responsive to individual patient preferences, needs, and values, and ensuring that patient values guide all clinical decisions." Such care informs and involves the patients in all of their care decisions, encourages self-management, coordinates the patient's care, provides psychosocial support, and respects the patient's core values about health. In this vein, complementary and alternative medicine plays a larger role in patients' care, especially if a track record of success with homeopathic medications has shown success. More emphasis is placed on diet, meditation, physical activity, and nutritional supplements as the patient wishes. Patient-centered care places the patient and the physician in a partnership for the healing process. The result of this new approach has been improved outcomes and patient satisfaction and reduced utilization of care.

Reference:
Crossing the quality chasm: a new health system for the 21st century. IOM, March 2001. <http://www.nap.edu/books/0309072808/html>.

38. The average indemnity payment for primary errors in communication by radiologists is:
    A. Five times as high as when appropriate communication occurs
    B. Four times as high as when appropriate communication occurs
    C. Three times as high as when appropriate communication occurs
    D. Two times as high as when appropriate communication occurs

39. The types of communication errors that can occur in radiology do not typically include:
    A. Errors of documentation
    B. Errors of commission
    C. Communication of inaccurate or incomplete information
    D. Failures in the communication loop

40. When a radiologist does not have clinical information available at the time of her reading of a study, what type of communication error has occurred?
    A. Error of documentation
    B. Inaccurate or incomplete information
    C. No communication error has occurred
    D. All of the above

41. When a radiologist fails to inform a radiology nurse that a patient is allergic to contrast dye prior to a study, what type of communication error has occurred?
    A. Error of documentation
    B. Failure in the communication loop
    C. No communication error has occurred
    D. All of the above

42. Dr. Stein gets a call from Mr. Woods asking her to send him a report of the postreduction x-ray of his 19-year-old son. Dr. Stein should:
    A. Send the report after obtaining patient information confirming the son's identity
    B. Ask for permission from the son on the phone via a conference call
    C. Obtain a HIPAA release form from the son before providing the report
    D. Call risk management

43. Dr. Stein gets a call from Mr. Woods' son's lawyer asking her to send him a report of the postreduction x-ray. Dr. Stein should:
    A. Send the report after obtaining patient information confirming the son's identity
    B. Ask for permission from the son on the phone via a conference call
    C. Obtain a HIPAA release form from the patient before providing the report
    D. Call risk management

38. **D, Two times as high as when appropriate communication occurs.** The average indemnity payment when a radiologist did not communicate positive findings was $231K whereas if effective communication occurred, the average indemnity payment was less than $105K. In the article cited they refer to four types of communication errors:

- Type A: Radiologist failed to directly communicate with both the treating physician and the patient
- Type B: Radiologist communicated with treating physician but the information did not reach the patient
- Type C: Radiologist failed to directly communicate with the treating physician but did communicate with the patient
- Type D: Radiologist communicated to the treating physician and the patient

The average payout for Type A ($375K), Type B ($262K), Type C ($143K), and Type D ($0K) on behalf of the radiologist for asymptomatic patients with breast cancer tracked directly with the degree of communication provided.

The bottom line, the authors opined, is "The most defensible form of communication … is direct communication, because this approach ensures that the information reaches the intended party."

Reference:
Brenner RJ1, Bartholomew L. Communication errors in radiology: a liability cost analysis. *J Am Coll Radiol*. 2005 May;2(5):428-431.

39. **B, Errors of commission.** The three types of communication errors that Brook et al describe are errors of documentation, communication of inaccurate or incomplete information, and failures in the communication loop. These errors may have the radiologist as the "perpetrator" or the "recipient" of the error. The lack of documentation may be when a clinician fails to note an unconscious patient's previous reaction to a contrast dye in the electronic medical record or the radiologist fails to document the administration of diphenhydramine for hives in a drowsy patient returning to an outpatient clinic in an altered state. Incomplete information is often the result of inadequate clinical history as in the site of pain for a patient being evaluated for a lower extremity fracture. It may also be when a radiologist fails to recommend the proper next step in the workup of a patient for inferior vena cava venous thrombosis who has a negative Doppler ultrasound of the calf. Failures in the communication loop refer to the passage of information from one health care employee to the next to ensure no mistakes are made.

References:
<http://pubs.rsna.org/doi/full/10.1148/rg.305105013>.
Brook OR, O'Connell AM, Thornton E, et al. Quality initiatives: anatomy and pathophysiology of errors occurring in clinical radiology practice. *Radiographics*. 2010;30(5):1401-1410.

40. **B, Inaccurate or incomplete information.** The absence of clinical information has been shown to decrease the accuracy of radiology reports. In a 2004 meta-analysis, no studies were identified that suggested a blinded read, without clinical information, produces a more accurate interpretation of that study. Thus, the rate of true positive interpretations increases when there is good clinical history.

Reference:
Loy CT, Irwig L. Accuracy of diagnostic tests read with and without clinical information, a systematic review. *JAMA*. 2004;292(13):1602-1609.

41. **B, Failure in the communication loop.** The communication loop refers to the transfer of information from the schedulers to the office staff to the transporter to the technologist to the nurse to the radiologist to the transcriptionist to the referring physician. All along the loop there may be breakdowns in communication. Thus, even though the scheduler may ask a patient if she has an iodine allergy, the transmission of that information all around the loop is fraught with potential errors. Does that information get to the nurse administering the contrast agent? Does the doctor know in advance so that ready access to potential resuscitative medications is available? Does the radiologist comment on this in his report so that future "events" are avoided? Does the referring physician list that as an allergy in the electronic medical record so that the patient receives appropriate prophylaxis for the next study? Typically when such mistakes are made, there are numerous points of failure all along the way in the communication loop. Multiple digital safeguards that ask pertinent questions (Is the patient allergic to iodine? Did the patient receive appropriate prophylaxis? Is iodine allergy listed in the known allergy section of the HER?) before proceeding may reduce such errors.

Reference:
Brook OR, O'Connell AM, Thornton E, et al. Quality initiatives: anatomy and pathophysiology of errors occurring in clinical radiology practice. *Radiographics*. 2010;30(5):1401-1410.

42. **C, Obtain a HIPAA release form from the son before providing the report.** Under the HIPAA privacy rule, adolescents who legally are adults and emancipated minors can exercise the rights of individuals. HIPAA defers to state law to determine the age of majority and the rights of parents to act for a child in making health care decisions, and thus, the ability of the parent to act as the personal representative of the child for HIPAA purposes (45 CFR 164.502(g)). The age of majority is 18 in most states. Therefore, in this case, Mr. Woods' son is a legal adult and considered the "individual." A covered entity must obtain the individual's written authorization for any use or disclosure of protected health information that is not for treatment, payment, or health care operations or otherwise permitted or required by the privacy rule (45 CFR § 164.512(j)).

References:
<http://www.ecfr.gov/cgi-bin/text-idx?SID=938e08839465e82e2c30c3bd4a359ce2&node=pt45.1.164&rgn=div5%23se45.1.164_1402-se45.1.164_1502>.
<http://www.hhs.gov/hipaa/for-professionals/privacy/laws-regulations/index.html>.

43. **C, Obtain a HIPAA release form from the patient before providing the report.** Under the privacy rule, a covered entity may not use or disclose an individual's protected health information (PHI) for purposes unrelated to treatment, payment, health care operations, or certain defined exceptions without first obtaining the individual's prior written authorization. A covered entity can disclose PHI without an individual's written authorization in specific circumstances: when complying with a court order, subpoena, or summons; when responding to an administrative subpoena, investigative demand, or other administrative request; for a proceeding before a health oversight agency; and for law enforcement purposes. A litigant can discover PHI by three methods: (1) A litigant can seek a signed individual authorization for access to the information; (2) there is a court order allowing access to specific medical information; or (3) a litigant can procure a subpoena, discovery request, or other lawful process and either give notice of the request to the individual or enter into a HIPAA-approved protective order.

Reference:
<https://www.law.uh.edu/healthlaw/perspectives/LDHIPAAAuthorizations.pdf>.
<http://www.americanbar.org/publications/gp_solo/2011/september/navigating_hipaa_claims_litigation.html>.

44. Dr. Stein gets a call from Mr. Woods' 19 year old son asking her to send him a report of his own postreduction x-ray. Dr. Stein should:
    A. Send the report after obtaining patient information confirming the son's identity
    B. Ask for permission from the son on the phone
    C. Obtain a HIPAA release form from the son before providing the report
    D. Call risk management

45. Dr. Stein gets a call from Mr. Woods asking her to send him a report of the postreduction x-ray of his 17-year-old son. Dr. Stein should:
    A. Send the report after obtaining patient information confirming the son's identity
    B. Ask for permission from the son on the phone
    C. Obtain a HIPAA release form from the son before providing the report
    D. Call risk management

46. Dr. Stein gets a call from Mr. Woods' 17-year-old lawyer asking her to send him a report of the postreduction x-ray of his 17-year-old son from 17 days earlier. Dr. Stein should:
    A. Send the report after obtaining patient information confirming the son's identity
    B. Ask for permission from the son on the phone
    C. Obtain a HIPAA release form before providing the report
    D. Call risk management

47. What is the best definition for *full disclosure*?
    A. All the information available about a recommended treatment
    B. All the information a patient requests from a health care provider
    C. All the information the physician decides to share with the patient
    D. All the information a patient needs to make an informed treatment choice

48. Of those radiologists listed, which specialist plays the largest role in communicating directly with patients and recommending care to patient-centric teams, multidisciplinary tumor boards, and care teams?
    A. Abdominal radiologists
    B. Interventional radiologists
    C. Neuroradiologists
    D. Musculoskeletal radiologists

49. What steps are most viable for diagnostic radiologists toward increasing visibility and adding real value as an integral member of a health care team?
    A. Actively engaging clinicians through involvement in multidisciplinary conferences
    B. Providing clinician- and patient-targeted imaging education
    C. Being accessible any day, any time for consultations
    D. All of the above

50. Radiologist participation in tumor-board conferences has been shown to produce major changes in what percent of cases?
    A. 17%
    B. 27%
    C. 37%
    D. 47%

44. **A, Send the report after obtaining patient information confirming the son's identity.** A covered entity is permitted, but not required, to use and disclose protected health information, without an individual's authorization, for the following purposes or situations: (1) to the individual who is the subject of the information; (2) treatment, payment, and health care operations; (3) opportunity to agree or object; (4) incident to an otherwise permitted use and disclosure; (5) public interest and benefit activities; and (6) limited data set for the purposes of research, public health, or health care operations.

Reference:
<http://www.hhs.gov/hipaa/for-professionals/privacy/laws-regulations/index.html>.

45. **A, Send the report after obtaining patient information confirming the son's identity.** In most cases under the privacy rule, a parent, guardian, or other person acting in loco parentis is the personal representative of the minor child and can exercise the minor's rights with respect to protected health information. Therefore, in most cases, parents can exercise individual rights, such as access to the medical record, on behalf of their minor children. In certain exceptional cases, the parent is not considered the personal representative. In these situations, the privacy rule defers to state and other law to determine the rights of parents to access and control the protected health information of their minor children. If state and other law is silent concerning parental access to the minor's protected health information, a covered entity has discretion to provide or deny a parent access to the minor's health information, provided the decision is made by a licensed health care professional in the exercise of professional judgment.

References:
<http://www.hhs.gov/hipaa/for-professionals/privacy/laws-regulations/index.html>.
<http://www.hhs.gov/hipaa/for-professionals/privacy/guidance/personal-representatives/index.html>.

46. **D, Call risk management.** Something is clearly amiss when you have a 17-year-old lawyer. That the 17-year-old lawyer is representing a 17-year-old client smells like a rat. At this point, Dr. Stein needs to inform risk management that something unusual is occurring and there is concern that an illegal access request is being made.

References:
<http://www.hhs.gov/hipaa/for-professionals/privacy/laws-regulations/index.html>.
<http://www.hhs.gov/hipaa/for-professionals/privacy/guidance/personal-representatives/index.html>.

47. **D, All the information a patient needs to make an informed treatment choice.** Physicians must disclose enough information for the patient to make an informed decision. This information includes (1) condition being treated; (2) nature and character of the proposed treatment or surgical procedure; (3) anticipated results; (4) recognized possible alternative forms of treatment; and (5) recognized serious possible risks, complications, and anticipated benefits involved in the treatment or surgical procedure, as well as the recognized possible alternative forms of treatment, including nontreatment. Physicians must also disclose information that a reasonable person in the patient's position would find important and explain any benefits or risks that may be significant to the particular patient.

Reference:
Murray B. Informed consent: what must a physician disclose to a patient? *AMA J Ethics*. 2012;14(7):563-566. <http://journalofethics.ama-assn.org/2012/07/hlaw1-1207.html>.

48. **B, Interventional radiologists.** Interventional radiologists (IRs) frequently work in the context of collaborative, patient-centric teams as well as being integral members of multidisciplinary tumor boards and vascular care teams. They frequently communicate directly with patients regarding treatment options after consulting team members in patient care. Communication has long been a critical role for IRs both with other caregivers and with patients and their families. IR practice models can provide effective strategies for more visible participation in value-based health care systems.

Reference:
Charalel RA, McGinty F, Brant-Zawadzki M, et al. Interventional radiology delivers high-value health care and is an Imaging 3.0 vanguard. *J Am Coll Radiol*. 2015;12(5):504.

49. **D, All of the above.** Radiologist participation in tumor-board conferences, as one example, has demonstrated improvements in higher quality, more timely, and more cost-effective imaging services. Engaging and educating patients and routinely delivering prompt exam results improve patients' understanding, respect, and involvement. Overall results are a significant effect on cost efficiencies and levels of patient satisfaction and increased professional satisfaction for radiologists. Being accessible in the modern era of mobile phones and 24/7 availability is part of service-oriented and value-added radiology.

Reference:
Charalel RA, McGinty G, Brant-Zawadzki M, et al. Interventional radiology delivers high-value health care and is an Imaging 3.0 vanguard. *J Am Coll Radiol*. 2015;12(5):504.

50. **C, 37%.** In a study on cancer patient management it was found that radiologist participation on tumor-board conferences produced *major* changes in 37% of the cases and *minor* changes in 15% of oncologic patient care management. They defined major changes in this way:

> *A major change in treatment was defined as that which dramatically changed patient management, e.g., change from curative to palliative treatment, change of chemotherapeutic protocol due to insufficient response, etc. Significant information was defined as not only information that caused a major change in treatment (eg, a bone lesion thought to be a malignant lytic lesion reinterpreted as a benign osteoporotic lesion; a lung nodule reinterpreted as a blood vessel; increase in tumor size reread as no change in size of lesion) but also information not directly associated with the primary disease, such as complications of therapy and unrelated diseases.*

Reference:
Brook OR, Hakmon T, Brook A, et al. The effect of a Radiology Conference consultation on cancer patients management. *Ann Oncol*. 2011;22(5):1204-1208.

QUESTIONS

1. Which of the following is not one of the six core competencies of maintenance of certification (MOC)?
   A. Medical knowledge
   B. Ethical behavior
   C. Professionalism
   D. Practice-based learning and improvement

2. When Dr. Smith is able to signal a respiratory arrest alert, drawing upon different practitioners in various departments (anesthesiology, cardiology, pulmonary) to coordinate the care of a patient having an anaphylactic reaction in the radiology suite, he is demonstrating his proficiency in which core competency?
   A. Patient care
   B. Interpersonal and communication skills
   C. Systems-based practice
   D. Practice-based learning and improvement

3. Which is not true for the Milestones concept for Training Programs in Core Competencies?
   A. They substitute for medical knowledge testing
   B. They provide explicit and transparent expectations of performance
   C. They guide curriculum development
   D. They provide public accountability

4. For radiology, the Milestones for training were developed by representatives of:
   A. ABR, ACR, ABMS
   B. ACGME, ABMS, ABR
   C. ACGME, ACR, ABR
   D. ACGME, ABMS, AMA

5. Which level is not correct for radiology?
   A. "Level 1: The resident demonstrates milestones expected of one who has had some education in diagnostic radiology."
   B. "Level 2: The resident is advancing and demonstrating additional milestones."
   C. "Level 3: The resident continues to advance and demonstrate additional milestones; the resident consistently demonstrates the majority of milestones targeted for residency."
   D. "Level 4: The resident has advanced beyond performance targets set for residency and is demonstrating "aspirational" goals which might describe the performance of someone who has been in practice for several years."

1. **B, Ethical behavior.** These are the six core competencies of MOC:
   1. Patient Care—Provide care that is compassionate, appropriate, and effective treatment for health problems and to promote health.
   2. Medical Knowledge—Demonstrate knowledge about established and evolving biomedical, clinical, and cognate sciences and their application in patient care.
   3. Interpersonal and Communication Skills—Demonstrate skills that result in effective information exchange and teaming with patients, their families, and professional associates (eg, fostering a therapeutic relationship that is ethically sound and uses effective listening skills with nonverbal and verbal communication; working as both a team member and at times as a leader).
   4. Professionalism—Demonstrate a commitment to carrying out professional responsibilities, adherence to ethical principles, and sensitivity to diverse patient populations.
   5. Systems-based Practice—Demonstrate awareness of and responsibility to larger context and systems of health care. Be able to call on system resources to provide optimal care (eg, coordinating care across sites or serving as the primary case manager when care involves multiple specialties, professions, or sites).
   6. Practice-based Learning and Improvement—Able to investigate and evaluate patient care practices, appraise and assimilate scientific evidence, and improve the practice of medicine.

   Ethical behavior falls under Professionalism but is not a separate core competency.

   Reference:
   Relyea-Chew A, Talner LB. A dedicated general competencies curriculum for radiology residents development and implementation. *Acad Radiol.* 2011;18(5):650-654.

2. **C, Systems-based practice.** Dr. Smith is demonstrated the core competency of Systems-based Practice—Demonstrate awareness of and responsibility to larger context and systems of health care. Be able to call on system resources to provide optimal care (eg, coordinating care across sites or serving as the primary case manager when care involves multiple specialties, professions, or sites).

   Reference:
   Relyea-Chew A, Talner LB. A dedicated general competencies curriculum for radiology residents development and implementation. *Acad Radiol.* 2011;18(5):650-654.

3. **A, They substitute for medical knowledge testing.** Specifically stated on the ACGME website, milestones fulfill the following:
   - Provide public accountability—report at a national level on aggregate competency outcomes by specialty
   - Guide curriculum development
   - Provide more explicit and transparent expectations of performance

   In addition, "Milestones provide a framework for the assessment of the development of the resident or fellow physician in key dimensions of the elements of physician competency in a specialty or subspecialty. They neither represent the entirety of the dimensions of the six domains of physician competency, nor are they designed to be relevant in any other context."

   Milestones therefore only provide a framework but do not substitute for or represent the entirety of the six domains of physician competency. The six domains of core competencies are:
   1. Medical Knowledge
   2. Patient Care and Technical Skills
   3. Professionalism
   4. Interpersonal and Communication Skills
   5. Practice-based Learning and Improvement
   6. Systems-based Practice

   References:
   Milestones. Accreditation Council for Graduate Medical Education. Web. 29 Dec. 2015. <http://www.acgme.org/acgmeweb/tabid/430/ProgramandInstitutionalAccreditation/NextAccreditationSystem/Milestones.aspx>.
   The Next Accreditation System: A Resident Perspective. Accreditation Council for Graduate Medical Education, 2013. Web. 29 Dec. 2015. <http://www.acgme.org/acgmeweb/Portals/0/PDFs/Resident-Services/9NASResidentsMay2014.pdf.

4. **B, ACGME, ABMS, ABR.** The Diagnostic Radiology Milestone Project, published in July 2015, was a joint initiative by the Accreditation Council for Graduate Medical Education (ACGME) and the American Board of Radiology (ABR).

   In addition, as stated on the ACGME website, "Each specialty's Milestones Working Group was co-convened by the ACGME and relevant American Board of Medical Specialties (ABMS) specialty board(s), and was composed of ABMS specialty board representatives, program director association members, specialty college members, ACGME Review Committee members, residents, fellows, and others."

   References:
   The Diagnostic Radiology Milestone Project. A Joint Initiative of The Accreditation Council for Graduate Medical Education and The American Board of Radiology. Accreditation Council for Graduate Medical Education, July 2015. Web. 29 Dec. 2015. <http://www.acgme.org/acgmeweb/tabid/430/ProgramandInstitutionalAccreditation/NextAccreditationSystem/Milestones.aspx>.
   Milestones. Accreditation Council for Graduate Medical Education. Web. 29 Dec. 2015. <http://www.acgme.org/acgmeweb/tabid/430/ProgramandInstitutionalAccreditation/NextAccreditationSystem/Milestones.aspx>.

5. **D, "Level 4: The resident has advanced beyond performance targets set for residency and is demonstrating "aspirational" goals which might describe the performance of someone who has been in practice for several years."** According to the Accreditation Council for Graduate Medical Education (AGCME) milestones, "**Level 4:** The resident has advanced so that he or she now substantially demonstrates the milestones targeted for residency. This level is designed as the graduation target."

   Answer D describes the **Level 5 milestone:** "The resident has advanced beyond performance targets set for residency and is demonstrating "aspirational" goals which might describe the performance of someone who has been in practice for several years. It is expected that only a few exceptional residents will reach this level."

   Reference:
   The Diagnostic Radiology Milestone Project. A joint initiative of The Accreditation Council for Graduate Medical Education and The American Board of Radiology. Accreditation Council for Graduate Medical Education, July 2015. Web. 29 Dec. 2015. <http://www.acgme.org/acgmeweb/tabid/430/ProgramandInstitutionalAccreditation/NextAccreditationSystem/Milestones.aspx>.

6. The level that is the target for graduation from a residency program in radiology is:
   A. Level 2
   B. Level 3
   C. Level 4
   D. Level 5

7. "Able to teach procedures to junior-level residents and competently performs complex procedures, modifies procedures as needed, and anticipates and manages complications of complex procedures." This is an example of what level competency?
   A. Level 2
   B. Level 3
   C. Level 4
   D. Level 5

8. "Uses established evidence-based imaging guidelines such as American College of Radiology (ACR) Appropriateness Criteria" is an example of what level achieved?
   A. Level 1
   B. Level 2
   C. Level 3
   D. Level 4

9. "Selects appropriate protocols and contrast agent/dose for advanced imaging as defined by the residency program" is an example of what level achieved?
   A. Level 1
   B. Level 2
   C. Level 3
   D. Level 4

10. "Completes a systems-based practice project as required by the ACGME Review Committee" is an example of what level achieved?
    A. Level 1
    B. Level 2
    C. Level 3
    D. Level 4

11. "States relative costs of common procedures" is an example of what level core competency achieved?
    A. Level 1
    B. Level 2
    C. Level 3
    D. Level 4

12. "Communicates, under indirect* supervision, in challenging circumstances (eg, cognitive impairment, cultural differences, language barriers, low health literacy)" is an example of what level core competency achieved?
    A. Level 2
    B. Level 3
    C. Level 4
    D. Level 5

13. "Efficiently generates clear and concise reports that do not require substantive correction on routine cases" is an example of what level core competency achieved?
    A. Level 2
    B. Level 3
    C. Level 4
    D. Level 5

14. "Applies principles of Image Gently and Image Wisely" is an example of what level core competency achieved?
    A. Level 2
    B. Level 3
    C. Level 4
    D. Level 5

15. "Recognizes and manages contrast reactions" is an example of what level core competency achieved?
    A. Level 1
    B. Level 2
    C. Level 3
    D. Level 4

16. "Participates in local and national organizations to advance professionalism in radiology" is an example of what level core competency achieved?
    A. Level 2
    B. Level 3
    C. Level 4
    D. Level 5

6. **C, Level 4.** According to the Accreditation Council for Graduate Medical Education (AGCME) milestones, level 4 is the target for graduation. "**Level 4:** The resident has advanced so that he or she now substantially demonstrates the milestones targeted for residency. This level is designed as the graduation target." Additionally, the ACGME milestones state, "Level 4 is designed as the graduation *target* but does *not* represent a graduation *requirement*. Making decisions about readiness for graduation is the purview of the residency program director."

Reference:
The Diagnostic Radiology Milestone Project. A joint initiative of The Accreditation Council for Graduate Medical Education and The American Board of Radiology. Accreditation Council for Graduate Medical Education, July 2015. Web. 29 Dec. 2015. <http://www.acgme.org/acgmeweb/tabid/430/ProgramandInstitutionalAccreditation/NextAccreditationSystem/Milestones.aspx>.

7. **D, Level 5.** According to the Diagnostic Radiology Milestone Project (patient care and technical skills section), the ability to teach procedures to junior-level residents and competently performing complex procedures, modifying procedures as needed and anticipating and managing complication of complex procedures are definitions of level 5 core competency.

Reference:
The Diagnostic Radiology Milestone Project. A joint initiative of Accreditation Council For Graduate Medical Education and American Board of Radiology, July 2015. <https://www.acgme.org/acgmeweb/Portals/0/PDFs/Milestones/DiagnosticRadiologyMilestones.pdf>.

8. **A, Level 1.** According to the Diagnostic Radiology Milestone Project (patient care and technical skills section), using established evidence-based guidelines such as American College of Radiology appropriateness criteria and appropriately using the electronic health record to obtain relevant clinical information are definitions of level 1 core competency.

Reference:
The Diagnostic Radiology Milestone Project. A joint initiative of Accreditation Council For Graduate Medical Education and American Board of Radiology, July 2015. <https://www.acgme.org/acgmeweb/Portals/0/PDFs/Milestones/DiagnosticRadiologyMilestones.pdf>.

9. **C, Level 3.** According to the Diagnostic Radiology Milestone Project (medical knowledge), selection of appropriate protocols and contrast agent/dose for advanced imaging as defined by the residency program and demonstrating knowledge of physical principles to optimize image quality are definitions of level 3 core competency.

Reference:
The Diagnostic Radiology Milestone Project. A joint initiative of Accreditation Council For Graduate Medical Education and American Board of Radiology, July 2015. <https://www.acgme.org/acgmeweb/Portals/0/PDFs/Milestones/DiagnosticRadiologyMilestones.pdf>.

10. **D, Level 4.** According to the Diagnostic Radiology Milestone Project (systems-based practice section), the ability to complete a systems-based practice project as required by the ACGME Review Committee and the ability to describe national radiology quality programs (eg, National Radiology Data Registry, accreditation, peer-review) are definitions of level 4 core competency.

Reference:
The Diagnostic Radiology Milestone Project. A joint initiative of Accreditation Council For Graduate Medical Education and American Board of Radiology, July 2015. <https://www.acgme.org/acgmeweb/Portals/0/PDFs/Milestones/DiagnosticRadiologyMilestones.pdf>.

11. **B, Level 2.** According to the Diagnostic Radiology Milestone Project (systems-based practice section), the ability to state the relative cost of common procedures is the definition of level 2 core competency.

Reference:
The Diagnostic Radiology Milestone Project. A joint initiative of Accreditation Council for Graduate Medical Education and American Board of Radiology, July 2015. <https://www.acgme.org/acgmeweb/Portals/0/PDFs/Milestones/DiagnosticRadiologyMilestones.pdf>.

12. **B, Level 3.** According to the Diagnostic Radiology Milestone Project (interpersonal and communication skills section), the ability to communicate under indirect supervision, in challenging circumstances (eg, cognitive impairment, cultural differences, language barriers, low health literacy) is an example of level 3 core competency.

Reference:
The Diagnostic Radiology Milestone Project. A joint initiative of Accreditation Council For Graduate Medical Education and American Board of Radiology, July 2015. <https://www.acgme.org/acgmeweb/Portals/0/PDFs/Milestones/DiagnosticRadiologyMilestones.pdf>.

13. **A, Level 2.** According to the Diagnostic Radiology Milestone Project (interpersonal and communication skills), the ability to efficiently generate clear and concise written/electronic reports that do not require substantive faculty member correction on routine cases is an example of level 2 core competency. In addition, the ability to verbally communicate the findings and recommendations in a clear and concise manner is another definition of level 2 competency.

Reference:
The Diagnostic Radiology Milestone Project. A joint initiative of Accreditation Council For Graduate Medical Education and American Board of Radiology, July 2015. <https://www.acgme.org/acgmeweb/Portals/0/PDFs/Milestones/DiagnosticRadiologyMilestones.pdf>.

14. **C, Level 4.** According to the Diagnostic Radiology Milestone Project (practice-based learning and improvement section), applying principles of Image Gently and Image Wisely is an example of level 4 core competency.

Reference:
The Diagnostic Radiology Milestone Project. A joint initiative of Accreditation Council For Graduate Medical Education and American Board of Radiology, July 2015. <https://www.acgme.org/acgmeweb/Portals/0/PDFs/Milestones/DiagnosticRadiologyMilestones.pdf>.

15. **A, Level 1.** According to the Diagnostic Radiology Milestone Project (practice-based learning and improvement section), recognizing and managing contrast reactions is an example of level 1 core competency. In addition, the ability to describe the mechanisms of radiation injury, the ALARA ("as low as reasonably achievable") concept, and describing the risks associated with MRI are other examples of level 1 core competency in this section.

Reference:
The Diagnostic Radiology Milestone Project. A joint initiative of accreditation council for graduate medical education and American Board of Radiology, July 2015. <https://www.acgme.org/acgmeweb/Portals/0/PDFs/Milestones/DiagnosticRadiologyMilestones.pdf>.

16. **D, Level 5.** According to the Diagnostic Radiology Milestone Project (professionalism section), participating in local and national organizations to advance professionalism in radiology and mentoring others regarding professionalism and ethics are examples of level 5 core competency.

Reference:
The Diagnostic Radiology Milestone Project. A joint initiative of Accreditation Council For Graduate Medical Education and American Board of Radiology, July 2015. <https://www.acgme.org/acgmeweb/Portals/0/PDFs/Milestones/DiagnosticRadiologyMilestones.pdf>.

17. The ABR promotes professionalism through:
    A. Appropriateness criteria publications
    B. RADPEER
    C. MOC
    D. All of the above

18. Which of the following is NOT a part of the modern translation of the Hippocratic Oath?
    A. I will respect the hard-won scientific gains of those physicians in whose steps I walk, and gladly share such knowledge as is mine with those who are to follow.
    B. First do no harm.
    C. I will apply, for the benefit of the sick, all measures which are required, avoiding those twin traps of over-treatment and therapeutic nihilism.
    D. I will prevent disease whenever I can, for prevention is preferable to cure.

19. Which of the following supports the "do no harm" treatise of the Hippocratic Oath?
    A. Nor shall any man's entreaty prevail upon me to administer poison to anyone; neither will I counsel any man to do so. Moreover, I will give no sort of medicine to any pregnant woman, with a view to destroy the child.
    B. With regard to healing the sick, I will devise and order for them the best diet, according to my judgment and means; and I will take care that they suffer no hurt or damage.
    C. I will not cut for the stone, but will commit that affair entirely to the surgeons.
    D. Whatever, in the course of my practice, I may see or hear (even when not invited), whatever I may happen to obtain knowledge of, if it be not proper to repeat it, I will keep sacred and secret within my own breast.

20. Which of the following from the Hippocratic Oath supports the implementation of HIPAA?
    A. Nor shall any man's entreaty prevail upon me to administer poison to anyone; neither will I counsel any man to do so. Moreover, I will give no sort of medicine to any pregnant woman, with a view to destroy the child.
    B. With regard to healing the sick, I will devise and order for them the best diet, according to my judgment and means; and I will take care that they suffer no hurt or damage.
    C. I will not cut for the stone, but will commit that affair entirely to the surgeons.
    D. Whatever, in the course of my practice, I may see or hear (even when not invited), whatever I may happen to obtain knowledge of, if it be not proper to repeat it, I will keep sacred and secret within my own breast.

21. The U.S. Preventive Services Task Force (USPSTF) has suggested a grading system for medical research. Which of the following is one of their grades?
    A. Level I: Evidence obtained from at least one properly designed randomized controlled trial
    B. Level II: Evidence from case reports
    C. Level III: Opinions from journal editors
    D. All of the above

17. **D, All of the above.** Medical professionalism can be broadly defined as "a set of core beliefs and values that guide the daily work of physicians" caring for patients. The American College of Radiology Code of Ethics emphasizes the importance of quality assurance, technology assessment, and utilization review as core radiologist responsibilities.

RADPEER is a simple process that allows peer review to be performed during the routine interpretation of current images for quality assurance. The ACR Appropriateness Criteria are evidence-based guidelines to assist referring physicians and other providers in making the most appropriate imaging or treatment decision for a specific clinical condition.

Maintenance of professionalism throughout a decades-long career in radiology requires practitioners to be actively engaged in continuous learning and self-improvement.

References:
Leung AN. Professionalism in radiology. *J Thorac Imaging.* 2014;29(5): 284-286.
ACR Quality and safety. <http://www.acr.org/Quality-Safety>. Accessed December 9, 2015.

18. **B, "First do no harm."** The modern translation of the Hippocratic Oath was written in 1964 by Louis Lasagna:

I swear to fulfill, to the best of my ability and judgment, this covenant:

I will respect the hard-won scientific gains of those physicians in whose steps I walk, and gladly share such knowledge as is mine with those who are to follow.

I will apply, for the benefit of the sick, all measures which are required, avoiding those twin traps of over-treatment and therapeutic nihilism.

I will remember that there is art to medicine as well as science, and that warmth, sympathy, and understanding may outweigh the surgeon's knife or the chemist's drug.

I will not be ashamed to say "I know not," nor will I fail to call in my colleagues when the skills of another are needed for a patient's recovery.

I will respect the privacy of my patients, for their problems are not disclosed to me that the world may know. Most especially must I tread with care in matters of life and death. If it is given me to save a life, all thanks. But it may also be within my power to take a life; this awesome responsibility must be faced with great humbleness and awareness of my own frailty. Above all, I must not play at God.

I will remember that I do not treat a fever chart, a cancerous growth, but a sick human being, whose illness may affect the person's family and economic stability. My responsibility includes these related problems, if I am to care adequately for the sick.

I will prevent disease whenever I can, for prevention is preferable to cure.

I will remember that I remain a member of society, with special obligations to all my fellow human beings, those sound of mind and body as well as the infirm.

If I do not violate this oath, may I enjoy life and art, respected while I live and remembered with affection thereafter. May I always act so as to preserve the finest traditions of my calling and may I long experience the joy of healing those who seek my help.

Reference:
Modern translation of the Hippocratic Oath. <http://guides.library.jhu.edu/c.php?g=202502&p=1335759>. Accessed December 9, 2015.

19. **B, "With regard to healing the sick, I will devise and order for them the best diet, according to my judgment and means; and I will take care that they suffer no hurt or damage."** "First do no harm" is a well-known phrase in medicine. Contrary to popular belief the phrase does not appear in the Hippocratic Oath. The oath does contain "With regard to healing the sick, I will devise and order for them the best diet, according to my judgment and means; and I will take care that they suffer no hurt or damage." A more accurate formulation can be "first do no net harm."

References:
Pavur, Claude. The Hippocratic Oath in Latin with English Translation. <http://www.academia.edu/2638728/The_Hippocratic_Oath_in_Latin_with_English_translation>. Accessed December 9, 2015.
Sokol DK. "First do no harm" revisited. *BMJ.* 2013;347:f6426.

20. **D, "Whatever, in the course of my practice, I may see or hear (even when not invited), whatever I may happen to obtain knowledge of, if it be not proper to repeat it, I will keep sacred and secret within my own breast."** Obligations of physicians about the patient's privacy and confidentiality are part of the Hippocratic Oath. The pertinent provision of the Oath reads as follows: "What I may see or hear in the course of the treatment or even outside of the treatment in regard to the life of men, which on no account must be spread abroad, I will keep to myself, holding such things shameful to be spoken about." This part of the Oath is commonly accepted to provide the ethical foundation for the physician's duty of confidentiality. The Oath expressly declares that a physician's obligation of confidentiality applies beyond matters of medical care.

Reference:
Mark A. Rothstein. The Hippocratic Bargain and Health Information Technology. *J Law Med Ethics.* 2010;38(1):7-13.

21. **A, Level I: Evidence obtained from at least one properly designed randomized controlled trial.** The U.S. Preventive Services Task Force suggested the following grading system for "hierarchy of research design":

I: Properly powered and conducted randomized controlled trial (RCT); well-conducted systematic review or meta-analysis of homogeneous RCTs
II-1: Well-designed controlled trial without randomization
II-2: Well-designed cohort or case-control analytic study
II-3: Multiple time series with or without the intervention; dramatic results from uncontrolled experiments
III: Opinions of respected authorities, based on clinical experience; descriptive studies or case reports; reports of expert committees

Reference:
The US Preventive Services Task Force Procedure Manual-Section 4. <http://www.uspreventiveservicestaskforce.org/Page/Name/procedure-manual-section-4>. Accessed December 11, 2015.

22. Which of the following is NOT level II evidence according to the USPSTF?
    A. Level II-1: Evidence obtained from well-designed controlled trials without randomization
    B. Level II-2: Evidence obtained from well-designed cohort or case-control analytic studies, preferably from more than one center or research group
    C. Level II-3: Evidence obtained from multiple time series designs with or without the intervention. Dramatic results in uncontrolled trials might also be regarded as this type of evidence.
    D. Level II-4: Evidence obtained from double blinded randomized case and non-case–controlled trial with appropriate placebo and duplicative data

23. The USPSTF also uses levels for the quality of data for an assessment of risk versus benefit. Which of these are currently in use?
    A. Level A: Good scientific evidence suggests that the benefits of the clinical service substantially outweigh the potential risks. Clinicians should discuss the service with eligible patients.
    B. Level B: At least fair scientific evidence suggests that the benefits of the clinical service outweigh the potential risks. Clinicians should discuss the service with eligible patients.
    C. Level C: At least fair scientific evidence suggests that there are benefits provided by the clinical service, but the balance between benefits and risks is too close for making general recommendations. Clinicians need not offer it unless there are individual considerations.
    D. All of the above

24. The USPSTF also uses levels for the quality of data for an assessment of risk versus benefit. Which of these are currently in use?
    A. Level G: At least fair scientific evidence suggests that the risks of the clinical service outweigh potential benefits. Clinicians should routinely offer the service to asymptomatic patients.
    B. Level H: Scientific evidence is lacking, of poor quality, or conflicting, such that the risk outweighs benefit. Do not use this test.
    C. Level I: Scientific evidence is lacking, of poor quality, or conflicting, such that the risk versus benefit balance cannot be assessed. Clinicians should help patients understand the uncertainty surrounding the clinical service.
    D. All of the above

22. **D, Level II-4: Evidence obtained from double blinded randomized case and non-case–controlled trial with appropriate placebo and duplicative data.** Level 2 evidence according to USPSTF only has 3 subtypes which are:

    II-1: Well-designed controlled trial without randomization
    II-2: Well-designed cohort or case-control analytic study
    II-3: Multiple time series with or without the intervention; dramatic results from uncontrolled experiments

Reference:
The US Preventive Services Task Force Procedure Manual-Section 4. <http://www.uspreventiveservicestaskforce.org/Page/Name/procedure-manual-section-4>. Accessed December 11, 2015.

23. **D, All of the above.** The U.S. Preventive Services Task Force (USPSTF) assigns one of five letter grades (A, B, C, D, or I) to describe the strength of recommendation to assess risk versus benefit in practice:

Grade	Definition	Suggestions for Practice
A	The USPSTF recommends the service. There is high certainty that the net benefit is substantial.	Offer or provide this service.
B	The USPSTF recommends the service. There is high certainty that the net benefit is moderate or there is moderate certainty that the net benefit is moderate to substantial.	Offer or provide this service.
C	The USPSTF recommends selectively offering or providing this service to individual patients based on professional judgment and patient preferences. There is at least moderate certainty that the net benefit is small.	Offer or provide this service for selected patients depending on individual circumstances.
D	The USPSTF recommends against the service. There is moderate or high certainty that the service has no net benefit or that the harms outweigh the benefits.	Discourage the use of this service.

Grade	Definition	Suggestions for Practice
I Statement	The USPSTF concludes that the current evidence is insufficient to assess the balance of benefits and harms of the service. Evidence is lacking, of poor quality, or conflicting, and the balance of benefits and harms cannot be determined.	Read the clinical considerations section of the USPSTF Recommendation Statement. If the service is offered, patients should understand the uncertainty about the balance of benefits and harms.

Reference:
The US Preventive Services Task Force Grade Definitions after July 2012. <http://www.uspreventiveservicestaskforce.org/Page/Name/grade-definitions>. Accessed December 11, 2015.

24. **C, Level I: Scientific evidence is lacking, of poor quality, or conflicting, such that the risk versus benefit balance cannot be assessed.** Clinicians should help patients understand the uncertainty surrounding the clinical service. The United States Preventive Services Task Force (USPSTF) is an independent panel of primary care physicians and epidemiologists who systemically review evidence of effectiveness and develop recommendations for clinical preventive services.

    The USPSTF assigns one of five letter grades (A, B, C, D, or I) to each recommendation.

Grade	Result	Meaning
A	Recommended	There is high certainty that the net benefit is substantial.
B	Recommended	There is high certainty that the net benefit is moderate or there is moderate certainty that the net benefit is moderate to substantial.
C	No recommendation	Clinicians may provide the service to selected patients depending on individual circumstances. However, for most individuals without signs or symptoms there is likely to be only a small benefit.
D	Recommended against	There is moderate or high certainty that the service has no net benefit or that the harms outweigh the benefits.
I statement	Insufficient evidence	The current evidence is insufficient to assess the balance of benefits and harms of the service.

Reference:
Grade Definitions. U.S. Preventive Services Task Force. October 2014. <http://www.uspreventiveservicestaskforce.org/page/name/grade-defintions>.

25. Your partner Dr. Perry is away on a week-long vacation. She has several overdue unsigned reports that have not been released to the clinicians. Which of the following are you compelled to do?
    A. Sign the reports
    B. Sign the reports with the proviso, "signed in Dr. Perry's absence"
    C. Hold the reports until Dr. Perry returns
    D. Use Dr. Perry's login and password to sign the reports

26. What is the next best, most expedient option for getting the overdue reports to the clinicians?
    A. Have Dr. Perry's secretary fax the reports to Dr. Perry for her approval.
    B. Reread the studies with your name as soon as possible.
    C. Send the clinicians the preliminary reports and tell them that Dr. Perry will contact them when she returns if there are changes.
    D. Have the business administrator, with the approval of legal council, release the reports under Dr. Perry's name.

27. According to the ACR bylaws, "The decision to render a service by a diagnostic radiologist, radiation oncologist, interventional radiologist, nuclear medicine physician, or medical physicist is a matter of individual physician and patient choice governed by the best interest of the _____:
    A. Profession
    B. Patient
    C. Physician
    D. Nation's electorate

28. Under which circumstance can a radiologist refuse to do an exam on a patient?
    A. Based on the sex of the patient
    B. Based on the sexual orientation of a patient
    C. As the sole proprietor, the physician's belief that the exam is not medically indicated
    D. None of the above

25. **C, Hold the reports until Dr. Perry returns.** The Centers for Medicare and Medicaid Services (CMS) requires that all radiology reports must be signed by the radiologist/practitioner who performs and/or interprets radiology services.

Although the ACR requested that if an interpreting physician is unavailable for signature that a colleague be allowed to authenticate the report, CMS did not accept that request. CMS did not accept the ACR's recommendations. CMS requires that radiologists sign their own reports. Although the CMS rule may slow the report delivery to the referring physician, the ACR urges its members to comply with it.

Reference:
Code of Federal Regulations (CFR), Title 42, section 482.26, Condition of Participation, Radiologic Services. <https://www.gpo.gov/fdsys/pkg/CFR-2011-title42-vol5/pdf/CFR-2011-title42-vol5-sec482-26.pdf>.

26. **B, Reread the studies with your name as soon as possible.** The Centers for Medicare and Medicaid Services (CMS) requires that all radiology reports must be signed by the radiologist/practitioner who performs and/or interprets radiology services (see answer 25 above).

Reference:
Code of Federal Regulations (CFR), Title 42, section 482.26, Condition of Participation, Radiologic Services. <https://www.gpo.gov/fdsys/pkg/CFR-2011-title42-vol5/pdf/CFR-2011-title42-vol5-sec482-26.pdf>.

27. **B, Patient.** The Code of Ethics of the American College of Radiology is intended to aid radiologists and radiation oncologists, individually and collectively in maintaining a high level of ethical conduct. It is not a set of laws but rather a framework. The first part of the Code of Ethics is called Principles of Ethics, which serve as goals of exemplary professional conduct. There are nine listed principles including the one quoted in this question. This states:
   1. The principal objective of the medical profession is to render service to people with full respect for human dignity and in the best interest of the patient.
   2. Members should merit the confidence of patients entrusted to their care, rendering to each a full measure of service and commitment.
   3. Members should strive continually to improve their medical knowledge and skill and make these improvements available to their patients and colleagues.
   4. Members should at all times be aware of their limitations and be willing to seek consultations in clinical situations where appropriate. These limitations should be appropriately disclosed to patients and referring physicians.
   5. The medical profession should safeguard the public and itself against physicians deficient in moral character or professional competence by reporting, to the appropriate body, without hesitation, perceived illegal or unethical conduct of members of the medical profession.
   6. Members should uphold all laws, uphold the dignity and honor of the medical profession, and accept its self-imposed discipline and deal honestly and fairly with patients and colleagues. The honored ideals of the medical profession imply that responsibilities of members extend to society in general as well as their patients. These responsibilities include the interest and participation of members in activities that improve the health and well-being of the individual and the community.
   7. Members may not reveal confidences entrusted to them in the course of medical attendance, or deficiencies they may observe in the character of patients, unless they are required to do so by law, or unless it becomes necessary to protect the welfare of the individual or of the community.
   8. A physician who has not personally interpreted the images obtained in a radiological examination should not sign a report or take attribution of an interpretation of that examination rendered by another physician in a manner that causes the reader of a report to believe that the signing radiologist was the interpreter.
   9. The decision to render a service by a diagnostic radiologist, radiation oncologist, interventional radiologist, nuclear medicine physician, or medical physicist is a matter of individual physician and patient choice governed by the best interest of the patient. The traditional bond among diagnostic radiologists, radiation oncologists, interventional radiologists, nuclear medicine physicians, and medical physicists, particularly in their professional relationships with each other, is a powerful aid in the service of patients and should not be used for personal advantage.

   The second part of the Code of Ethics is called Rules of Ethics. This list includes sixteen rules that are mandatory and directive of specific minimal standards of professional conduct.

Reference:
2015–2016 ACR Code of Ethics. <http://www.acr.org/~/media/ACR/Documents/PDF/Membership/Governance/2015_2016Code of Ethics.pdf>.

28. **C, As the sole proprietor, the physician's belief that the exam is not medically indicated.** A radiologist can refuse to do an exam if it is known to be scientifically invalid, has no medical indication, and offers no possible benefit to the patient.

   The AMA code of ethics says:
   1. Physicians should respond to the best of their ability in cases of medical emergency
   2. Physicians cannot refuse to care for patients based on race, gender, sexual orientation, or any other criteria that would constitute invidious discrimination, nor can they discriminate against patients with infectious diseases
   3. Physicians may not refuse to care for patients when operating under a contractual arrangement that requires them to treat. Exceptions to this requirement may exist when patient care is ultimately compromised by the contractual arrangement.

Reference:
American Medical Association Code of Medical Ethics. Potential Patients. <http://www.ama-assn.org/ama/pub/physician-resources/medical-ethics/code-medical-ethics/opinion1005.page?> Accessed on December 5, 2015.

29. Dr. Jones does not believe in the value of ultrasound elastography. However, his employer, Kaiser Permanente, has a contract with a health club that they will offer US elastography. Dr. Jones:
    A. Must perform the US elastography
    B. Need not perform it, based on his belief that the exam is not medically indicated
    C. Should consider leaving his place of employment
    D. Should tell the health club it should not contract with Kaiser

30. Which of the following is not considered a component of professionalism?
    A. Punctuality
    B. Accurate charting
    C. Concern for patient rights
    D. None of the above

31. Of the core competencies, which one evaluates departmental quality improvement (QI) initiatives, root cause analyses, and RVU-based measures of productivity?
    A. Professionalism
    B. Systems-based practice
    C. Practice-based learning
    D. Medical knowledge

32. Of the core competencies, which one looks at out-of-hospital care, modifying factors, legal/professional issues, diagnostic studies, consultation and disposition, prevention and education, multitasking, and team management?
    A. Professionalism
    B. Systems-based practice
    C. Practice-based learning
    D. Medical knowledge

29. **A, Must perform the US elastography.** Despite his personal beliefs, Dr. Jones is operating under a contractual arrangement with Kaiser Permanente that requires him to perform ultrasound elastography. As stated in the previous answer, the AMA code of ethics says "Physicians may not refuse to care for patients when operating under a contractual arrangement that requires them to treat." Other tenets of the AMA include that it may be ethically permissible for physicians to decline a potential patient when:
    1. The treatment request is beyond the physician's current competence.
    2. The treatment request is known to be scientifically invalid, has no medical indication, and offers no possible benefit to the patient.
    3. A specific treatment sought by an individual is incompatible with the physician's personal, religious, or moral beliefs.
    4. Physicians, as professionals and members of society, should work to assure access to adequate health care (and provide charity care but not to the degree that would seriously compromise the care provided to existing patients. When deciding whether to take on a new patient, physicians should consider the individual's need for medical service along with the needs of their current patients. Greater medical necessity of a service engenders a stronger obligation to treat.

Reference:
American Medical Association Code of Medical Ethics. Potential Patients. <http://www.ama-assn.org/ama/pub/physician-resources/medical-ethics/code-medical-ethics/opinion1005.page?> Accessed December 5, 2015.

30. **D, None of the above.** Professionalism encompasses the virtues of honesty, altruism, service, commitment, commitment to excellence, and accountability. Applied to radiology and the milestone project, behaviors that demonstrate patient advocacy, truthfulness, self-improvement, and maintenance of the boundaries of the doctor-patient relationship are considered representative of professionalism. Dealing with ethical issues of medical research by advocating for full disclosure about consent or social justice issues such as the value of opening electronic health records to patients may be other ways of demonstrating this core competency. Some specialty societies have established professionalism codes of conduct that further define the goals of this core competency.

References:
Larkin GLL, Binder L, Houry D, et al. Defining and evaluating professionalism: a core competency for graduate emergency medicine education. *Acad Emerg Med.* 2002;9(11). <https://www.acgme.org/acgmeweb/Portals/0/PDFs/Milestones/DiagnosticRadiologyMilestones.pdf>.

31. **B, Systems-based practice.** Systems-based practice is exemplified in the following milestone listed under diagnostic radiology core competencies (Table 3-1):
    • Describes departmental QI initiatives
    • Describes the departmental incident/occurrence reporting system

• Incorporates QI into clinical practice
• Participates in the departmental incident/occurrence reporting system
• Identifies and begins a systems-based practice project incorporating QI methodology
• Completes a systems-based practice project
• Describes national radiology quality programs (eg, National Radiology Data Registry, accreditation, peer review)
• Routinely participates in root cause analysis

The means for evaluating the core competency are listed as:
• End-of-rotation global assessment
• 360-degree evaluation/multi-rater/peer
• Direct observation and feedback
• Self-assessment and reflections/portfolio
• Semi-annual evaluation with program director
• Written feedback on project (with mentor)
• Project presentation feedback (faculty, peers, others in system)
• Critical incidents reporting and feedback

References:
Dyne PL1, Strauss RW, Rinnert S. Systems-based practice: the sixth core competency. *Acad Emerg Med.* 2002;9(11):1270-1277. <http://www.ncbi.nlm.nih.gov/pubmed/12414481>.
<https://www.acgme.org/acgmeweb/Portals/0/PDFs/Milestones/DiagnosticRadiologyMilestones.pdf>.

32. **B, Systems-based practice.** The ACGME defines systems-based practice as (1) understanding how the components of the local and national health care system function interdependently and how changes to improve the system involve group and individual efforts, (2) optimizing coordination of patient care both within one's own practice and within the health care system, (3) consulting with other health care professionals, and (4) educating health care consumers, regarding the most appropriate utilization of resources. In that regard, the activities described (out-of-hospital care, modifying factors, legal/professional issues, diagnostic studies, consultation and disposition, prevention and education, multitasking, and team management) are in that bailiwick of actions that demonstrate an awareness of and responsiveness to the larger context and system of health care and the ability to effectively call on system resources to provide high value optimal care. Getting involved in state or national radiological societies would also be relevant to this core competency. Fighting against Stark Law exemptions, for example, could demonstrate fulfillment of systems-based practice requirements.

Reference:
Dyne PL1, Strauss RW, Rinnert S. Systems-based practice: the sixth core competency. *Acad Emerg Med.* 2002;9(11):1270-1277.
<http://www.ncbi.nlm.nih.gov/pubmed/12414481>.

Table 3-1 SYSTEMS-BASED PRACTICE (SBP1)

SBP1: QUALITY IMPROVEMENT (QI)					
Has Not Achieved Level 1	**Level 1**	**Level 2**	**Level 3**	**Level 4**	**Level 5**
	Describes departmental QI initiatives Describes the departmental incident/occurrence reporting system	Incorporates QI into clinical practice Participates in the departmental incident/occurrence reporting system	Identifies and begins a systems-based practice project incorporating QI methodology	Completes a systems-based practice project as required by the ACGME Review Committee Describes national radiology quality programs (eg, National Radiology Data Registry, accreditation, peer-review)	Leads a team in the design and implementation of a QI project Routinely participates in root cause analysis
Comments					

33. Of the core competencies, which looks at improvement in clinical projects, quality improvement tools, and plan-do-study-act cycle worksheets?
    A. Professionalism
    B. Systems-based practice
    C. Practice-based learning
    D. Medical knowledge

34. Mona Mohamed is from a conservative Bedouin family. She requests to have a chaperone during her pelvic obstetric ultrasound examination performed by Dr. John Silver.
    A. An authorized health professional chaperone should be provided.
    B. If the facility has a policy that chaperones are not provided, then Mrs. Mohamed should not expect a chaperone.
    C. A chaperone should be provided by Mrs. Mohamed's family.
    D. None of the above

35. If Dr. Silver is going to explain his findings to Mrs. Mohamed:
    A. The chaperone should not be present.
    B. The chaperone must be present.
    C. The chaperone should only be present if Mrs. Mohamed requests her to stay.
    D. None of the above

36. With regard to the questioning of Mrs. Mohamed about her obstetric history prior to the performance of the pelvic ultrasound:
    A. The chaperone should not be present.
    B. The chaperone must be present.
    C. The chaperone should be one that Mrs. Mohamed chooses.
    D. None of the above

37. According to Title IX sexual harassment regulations, if a student or his or her parent does not want to file a complaint or does not request that the school take any action on the student's behalf, if a school knows or reasonably should know about possible sexual harassment or sexual violence:
    A. It cannot launch an investigation.
    B. It must obtain the student's permission before filing an investigation.
    C. It must launch an investigation but cannot take steps to resolve the situation without permission.
    D. It must launch an investigation and must take steps to resolve the situation.

38. A criminal investigation into allegations of sexual harassment or sexual violence:
    A. Does not relieve the school of its duty under Title IX to resolve complaints promptly and equitably.
    B. Relieves the school of its duty under Title IX to resolve complaints promptly and equitably.
    C. Cannot be brought to bear unless the victim agrees to bring formal charges against the perpetrator.
    D. Must coincide with the school's investigation into wrongdoing

39. For sexual harassment cases to be successfully tried against a defendant:
    A. The evidence must be beyond a shadow of a doubt.
    B. The decision must require a supermajority (>66.7%) of the jury to find guilt.
    C. One juror's vote may prevent a judgment against someone.
    D. There must be a preponderance of evidence in favor of the plaintiff.

40. The Clery Act, which applies to postsecondary institutions, requires that:
    A. Both parties be informed of the outcome, including sanction information, of any institutional proceeding alleging a sex offense.
    B. Colleges and universities may require a complainant to abide by a nondisclosure agreement, in writing or otherwise.
    C. A school is NOT obligated to inform every complainant in a case of the outcome of the complaint.
    D. Institutions need not disclose crime statistics for incidents that are reported to campus security authorities (CSA) and local law enforcement as having occurred on or near the campus.

41. A trainee comes to you with a report that she has been sexually assaulted by a superior but does not wish to have the episode disclosed.
    A. To effectively respond to a report of sexual violence, the institution's security team may not be required to keep a reporter's identity or other information about the alleged assault confidential.
    B. When responding to a report of sexual violence, the institution's security team must publicly disclose the reporter's identity and other information about the alleged assault.
    C. When responding to a report of sexual violence, the institution's security team must keep a reporter's identity or other information about the alleged assault confidential until formal charges are brought against the perpetrator.
    D. To effectively respond to a report of sexual violence, the institution's security team must keep a reporter's identity or other information about the alleged assault confidential.

33. **C, Practice-based learning.** According to the ACGME, the definition of practice-based learning and improvement is: "Participation in the evaluation of one's personal practice utilizing scientific evidence, practice guidelines and standards as metrics, and self-assessment programs in order to optimize patient care through lifelong learning." Practice-based learning therefore includes such activities as quality improvement projects, root cause analysis evaluations, lean Sigma and six Sigma operations, and plan-do-study-act skill sets. Morbidity and mortality and safety conferences are also included under this heading. In the end, some element of self-assessment is encouraged.

Reference:
Coleman MT1, Nasraty S, Ostapchuk M, et al. Introducing practice-based learning and improvement ACGME core competencies into a family medicine residency curriculum. *Jt Comm J Qual Saf.* 2003;29(5):238-247. Available from: <http://www.ncbi.nlm.nih.gov/pubmed/12751304>.

34. **A, An authorized health professional chaperone should be provided.** Physicians have to make every effort to create a comfortable and considerate environment for patients, especially in the setting of an intimate examination. A chaperone, preferably a nurse or medical assistant, always should be available regardless of the physician and patient sex. This should be communicated to the patient before an encounter or procedure.

References:
American Medical Association Code of Medical Ethics. Use of chaperones during physical exams. <http://www.ama-assn.org/ama/pub/physician-resources/medical-ethics/code-medical-ethics/opinion821.page?> Accessed on December 5, 2015.
Committee on Practice and Ambulatory Medicine. Use of chaperones during the physical examination of the pediatric patient. *Pediatrics.* 2011;127(5):991-993.

35. **C, The chaperone should only be present if Mrs. Mohamed requests her to stay.** Respecting the patient's privacy and confidentiality is of paramount importance. Therefore, if a chaperone is present for the ultrasound examination, there should be a separate opportunity for a private conversation between the physician and the patient to discuss the findings. The chaperone should be present in this private discussion only if the patient requests it.

Reference:
American Medical Association Code of Medical Ethics. Use of chaperones during physical exams. <http://www.ama-assn.org/ama/pub/physician-resources/medical-ethics/code-medical-ethics/opinion821.page?> Accessed on December 5, 2015.

36. **A, The chaperone should not be present.** History-taking and inquiries, especially those of sensitive nature, should be kept to a minimum during a chaperoned examination to respect the patient's privacy and confidentiality. The obstetrical history of the patient should be obtained over a private discussion prior to the ultrasound examination.

Reference:
American Medical Association Code of Medical Ethics. Use of chaperones during physical exams. <http://www.ama-assn.org/ama/pub/physician-resources/medical-ethics/code-medical-ethics/opinion821.page?> Accessed on December 5, 2015.

37. **D, It must launch an investigation and must take steps to resolve the situation.** Title IX refers to federal laws that prohibit discrimination on the basis of sex in any federally funded education program or activity. The provisions of Title IX cover such topics as sexual harassment, the failure to provide equal opportunity in athletics between women and men, and discrimination based on pregnancy. Title IX regulations are enforced by the U.S. Department of Education's Office for Civil Rights. If a school becomes aware of incidents of sexual harassment or sexual violence, the schools are required to launch an investigation, even if the victim does not want to pursue litigation or press criminal charges. This puts the onus on the school to remedy the situation.

Reference:
<http://www2.ed.gov/about/offices/list/ocr/docs/title-ix-rights-201104.pdf>.

38. **A, Does not relieve the school of its duty under Title IX to resolve complaints promptly and equitably.** A criminal investigation into allegations of sexual harassment or sexual violence does not relieve the school of its duty under Title IX to resolve complaints promptly and equitably. If a school knows or reasonably should know about sexual harassment or sexual violence it must investigate immediately and act promptly. Even if a student or his or her parent does not want to file a complaint or does not request that the school take any action on the student's behalf, if a school knows or reasonably should know about possible sexual harassment or sexual violence, it must promptly investigate to determine what occurred and then take appropriate steps to resolve the situation.

Reference:
<http://www2.ed.gov/about/offices/list/ocr/docs/title-ix-rights-201104.pdf>.

39. **D, There must be a preponderance of evidence in favor of the plaintiff.** Large numbers of cities and states have established civil rights actions for sexual assault survivors in the employment, education, housing, and public benefits context. There are differences between the standards of proof in criminal and civil cases. Criminal cases require "proof beyond a reasonable doubt" while civil cases require only a "preponderance of the evidence."

References:
<http://www.vawnet.org/applied-research-papers/print-document.php?doc_id=2150>.
Manley H. Civil compensation for the victim of rape. *Cooley Law Rev.* 1990;7:193-211.

40. **A, Both parties be informed of the outcome, including sanction information, of any institutional proceeding alleging a sex offense.** Title IX requires that every school have and make known procedures for students to file complaints of sex discrimination. It mentions:
The Clery Act only applies to postsecondary institutions that receive federal funds. The Clery act states that both parties in a case of sexual harassment and sexual violence must be informed of the outcome and sanctions applied. Therefore non-disclosure agreements may not be valid.

Reference:
<http://www2.ed.gov/about/offices/list/ocr/docs/title-ix-rights-201104.html>.

41. **A, To effectively respond to a report of sexual violence, the institution's security team may not be required to keep a reporter's identity or other information about the alleged assault confidential.** The Office of Civil Rights strongly supports the student's request for confidentiality in sexual assault cases because disregarding these requests may discourage other students from reporting sexual violence. There are only limited situations in which the school must override the student's request for confidentiality to meet its Title IX obligations. In these cases, the information should only be securely shared with individuals who are responsible for handling the school's response to incidents of sexual harassment, offense, and violence.

Reference:
<http://www2.ed.gov/about/offices/list/ocr/docs/qa-201404-title-ix.pdf>.

42. Which communications about a sexual assault are considered confidential and cannot be disclosed?
    A. Between the investigator and the plaintiff
    B. Between a professional mentor and mentee
    C. Between a teacher and a student
    D. Between a licensed psychologist and a client

43. In which situation is there no issue with a consensual relationship?
    A. Between faculty and trainees
    B. Between residents in the same year of training (neither are chief residents)
    C. Between chief residents and junior residents
    D. Between department directors and faculty over 21 years of age

44. A physician may have a romantic relationship with a patient:
    A. As long as both are consenting adults
    B. As long as it has been disclosed to the ethics board
    C. As long as that relationship predated the physician-patient relationship
    D. After an appropriate time has elapsed following dissolution of the doctor-patient relationship

42. **D, Between a licensed psychologist and a client.** In 1994, Congress passed the Violent Crime Control and Law Enforcement Act, Pub. L. 103-322, 8 40153, which protects confidentiality of communications between sexual assault or domestic violence victims and their counselors. "Counselor" refers to the different types of individuals who may provide counseling or immediate assistance to sexual assault victims or domestic violence victims after an attack. Counselors may include social workers, physicians, psychiatrists, psychotherapists, psychologists, volunteers, advocates, or other workers employed at a rape crisis center or battered women's shelter.

Reference:
<https://www.ncjrs.gov/pdffiles1/nij/grants/169588.pdf>.

43. **B, Between residents in the same year of training.** Romantic consensual relationships are one of the most sensitive areas of employee relationships. Difficult problems arise when people are not at the same level of training or stature in a department and a power play becomes intrinsic to the relationship. Examples include relationships between a faculty and a trainee, between a chief resident who writes the schedule and a junior resident, and a department director and its faculty.

Reference:
Yousem DM, Beauchamp NJ. *Radiology Business Practice: How to Succeed.* St. Louis: Elsevier; 2007:490.

44. **D, After an appropriate time has elapsed following dissolution of the doctor-patient relationship.** Sexual contact or sexual relations between physicians and patients are unethical as this may jeopardize the medical care. Termination of the physician-patient relationship does not eliminate the possibility that sexual contact between a physician and a former patient might be unethical.

Some professional groups and state licensing or disciplinary boards provide designated time limits following the termination of the physician-patient relationship before the treating physician may ethically enter into a sexual relationship with a former patient.

References:
McMurray R, et al. Sexual misconduct in the practice of medicine. Council on Ethical and Judicial Affairs, American Medical Association. *JAMA.* 1991;266(19): 2741-2745. doi:10.1001/jama.1991.03470190089035.
<http://www.aaos.org/CustomTemplates/Content.aspx?id=22300>.

QUESTIONS

1. The science of analyzing human characteristics, capabilities, and limitations to design machines, work flows, and safe environments to improve human safety and efficiency at work is called:
   A. Socioeconomics
   B. Human subjects research
   C. Lean Sigma
   D. Human-factors engineering

2. Human-factors engineering principles include all of the following except:
   A. Strict reliance on scientific methodology and data
   B. Use intuition, logic, and common sense in design
   C. Trial and error methodology typically employed
   D. None of the above

3. Figure 4-1 represents:
   A. Multiple failure mode model
   B. Root cause analysis alignment of errors
   C. Reason's Swiss Cheese model of failure
   D. Precision versus accuracy in detecting holes in a process

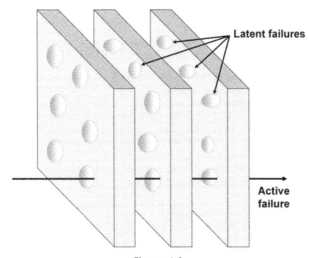

Figure 4-1

4. Instead of injecting contrast dye into a hepatic arteriovenous malformation (AVM), the interventional radiologist trainee injects glue. The human-factors engineering team assesses the problem and recommends:
   A. Assessment of sleep deprivation impact
   B. Only faculty handle the critical component of the study
   C. Creating two different syringes for glue injections and contrast injections
   D. Mandatory training in product recognition by the technologist who handed the syringes to the physician

5. Which of the following would **not** be considered by the human-factors engineering in the case above?
   A. The timing of the solidifying of the glue in the AVM
   B. Lighting in the angiography suite
   C. Ambient noise during procedures
   D. The pressure needed to inject syringes of contrast and glue

6. Professor Nguyen has designed a new injection tubing for angiography. It has a check valve at the injector connector that prevents contrast from entering the tubing if the injection rate exceeds 23 cc/second. This is an example of:
   A. Forcing function
   B. Workarounds
   C. Disruptive technology
   D. Usability testing

7. Professor Nguyen asks the body interventional section at the Mallinkrodt Institute to employ his new setup for their abdominal and thoracic angiograms including pulmonary arteriograms (injected at 15 cc/second) and some aortograms, the latter of which may be done at a flow rate of 25 cc/second. He asks them to test 50 cases of both types. This is an example of:
   A. Forcing function
   B. Workarounds
   C. Disruptive technology
   D. Usability testing

1. **D, Human-factors engineering.** Human-factors engineers employ usability testing, force functions, standardization, and resilience efforts to design products that marry the strengths and limitation of humans with the machines and systems that workers utilize. The goals include the maximization of safety, effectiveness, and ease of use. In short, the idea is to improve system efficiency by minimizing the possibility of human error.

   Human-factors engineering is analogous to ergonomics in that it stresses physical and psychological characteristics of the design of devices and systems for human use. It studies data and principles about human characteristics, habits, capabilities, and limitations in relation to creating more effective, safe, and comfortable machines, jobs, work methods, and environments.

   References:
   <https://psnet.ahrq.gov/primers/primer/20/human-factors-engineering>.
   <http://www.hfes.org/Web/EducationalResources/HFDefinitions.pdf>.

2. **B, Use intuition, logic, and common sense in design.** Human-factors engineering is the science of designing devices and systems for human use, stressing the physical and psychological characteristics that maximize a product's effectiveness. Another term used for this science is ergonomics. The designers emphasize human characteristics, capabilities, and limitations in relation to engineering of machines, jobs, and environments. The science highlights safety, comfort, and efficiency. The designs are, in part, based in intuition, logic, and common sense.

   Reference:
   <https://psnet.ahrq.gov/primers/primer/20/human-factors-engineering>.

3. **C, Reason's Swiss Cheese model of failure.** Reason's Swiss Cheese model of failure points to systemic vulnerabilities that predispose to errors and the ways errors can be prevented with a system of checks and balances. Reason refers to the systemic means of trying to prevent errors as a piece of Swiss cheese with many holes, only these holes are constantly changing and adapting. An example may be the reliance on trainees to prevent a patient fall in musculoskeletal (MSK) radiology when the trainees rotate each month and the diligence of each trainee is variable. If you superimpose the technologist and nurse who also rotate, you have more layers employed that may prevent a slip and fall by a patient with a hip fracture in the MSK area, but inevitably the holes in the slices of Swiss cheese will eventually superimpose such that an error/fall happens. Reason says that to reduce these errors organizations should (1) become preoccupied with the possibility of failures, (2) train employees to recognize failures and study them when they occur, (3) rehearse familiar scenarios of failure, (4) brainstorm to predict new sources of failure, and (5) look for systemic ways to resolve those errors. He recommends that organizations should always be afraid, uneasy, and searching for the next disaster waiting to happen. Investigating and predicting errors make the system more resilient.

   Reference:
   Reason J. Human error: models and management. *BMJ*. 2000;320(7237): 768-770.
   Figure 4-1 Reason's Swiss Cheese model of failure. (From Reason J. Human error: models and management. *BMJ*. 2000 Mar 18; 320(7237): 768-770.)

4. **C, Creating two different syringes for glue injections and contrast injections.** Human-factors engineering tries to take into account human strengths and limitations to design professional systems that ensure safety, effectiveness, and ease of use. This discipline has been utilized to reduce errors and accidents in the aviation and automobile industries and only recently has been introduced into health care. Human-factors engineers take into account concepts such as usability, standardization, and forcing functions (wherein users are forced to enact a defined correct protocol) to prevent the use of workarounds and other error prone methods. Creating a separate syringe that is unique for glue would be what a human-factors engineer would do.

   References:
   Agency for Healthcare Research and Quality. Patient safety primer on human factors engineering. <https://psnet.ahrq.gov/primers/primer/20/human-factors-engineering>. Accessed November 2015.
   The American Board of Radiology. *Noninterpretive Skills Domain Specification and Resource Guide. Part II: Patient Safety, Human Factors.* 2016:15-17. Available at: <http://theabr.org/sites/all/themes/abr-media/pdf/Noninterpretive_Skills_Domain_Specification_and_Resource_Guide.pdf>.

5. **A, The timing of the solidifying of the glue in the AVM.** Human-factors engineers consider real-world, practical factors of the users' environment that may make execution of the procedure more error prone, regardless of the specific details of the procedure, and then try to fix them. Here the engineer would consider the factors that led to the wrong medication being administered, and why the error was not caught before the sentinel event, but would not be concerned with the chemical properties of the glue, which are not under a human's control.

   References:
   Agency for Healthcare Research and Quality. *Patient Safety Primer on Human Factors Engineering.* <https://psnet.ahrq.gov/primers/primer/20/human-factors-engineering>. Accessed November 2015.
   The American Board of Radiology. *Noninterpretive Skills Domain Specification and Resource Guide. Part II: Patient Safety, Human Factors.* 2016:15-17. Available at: <http://theabr.org/sites/all/themes/abr-media/pdf/Noninterpretive_Skills_Domain_Specification_and_Resource_Guide.pdf>.

6. **A, Forcing function.** A forcing function is an aspect of a human-factors engineering system design that prevents an unintended or undesirable action from being performed or allows its performance only if another specific action is performed first. A forcing function makes it impossible to do the wrong thing. For example, the driver cannot start a car that is in gear. Removal of concentrated potassium chloride from patient units is also an example of a (negative) forcing function.

   References:
   PSNet (Patient Safety Network) website. <https://psnet.ahrq.gov/primers/primer/20/human-factors-engineering>.
   Hughes RG, ed. *Patient Safety and Quality: An Evidence-Based Handbook for Nurses.* Rockville, MD: Agency for Healthcare Research and Quality; 2008 Apr. Available at: <http://www.ncbi.nlm.nih.gov/books/NBK2673/>.

7. **D, Usability testing.** In human-factors engineering a testing of new systems and equipment under real-world conditions must be performed as much as possible, in order to identify unintended consequences of new technology. This is usability testing. The overlooked issues in equipment design or system can pose substantial safety risks.

   References:
   PSNet (Patient Safety Network) website. <https://psnet.ahrq.gov/primers/primer/20/human-factors-engineering>.
   PSNet (Patient Safety Network) website. <http://pubs.rsna.org/doi/full/10.1148/rg.2015150107>.

8. After onsite testing, Professor Nguyen develops a checklist to ensure his device is used properly. This is an example of:
   A. Root cause analysis
   B. Workarounds
   C. Standardization
   D. Resiliency efforts

9. Dr. Chung does not like Professor Nguyen's invention. She uses two Y-connectors from the injector back to the catheter to bypass the check valve. This is an example of:
   A. Forcing function
   B. Workarounds
   C. Disruptive technology
   D. Usability testing

10. SBAR (Situation, Background, Assessment, and Recommendation) is The Joint Commission's recommended strategy to standardize:
    A. Performance improvement
    B. An institution's critical findings
    C. Communication
    D. Medication reconciliation

11. Which of the following is an example of the S in SBAR (Situation, Background, Assessment, and Recommendation)?
    A. "Dr. Green, I think we need to call a code for Ms. Greenly's deteriorating respiratory status from a contrast dye reaction".
    B. "Dr. Green, Ms. Greenly is having difficulty breathing after the iodine injection for her CT scan".
    C. "Dr. Green, I think Ms. Greenly is having an allergic reaction to the contrast dye and may be in laryngospasm".
    D. "Dr. Green, Ms. Greenly is a patient with chest pain who was being evaluated for pulmonary embolism. She has lupus and has had no prior iodine injections but is allergic to shellfish. I gave her iohexol 3 minutes ago, and now she's breathing at 30 times a minute".

12. Which of the following is an example of the B in SBAR (Situation, Background, Assessment, and Recommendation)?
    A. "Dr. Green, I think we need to call a code for Ms. Greenly's deteriorating respiratory status from a contrast dye reaction".
    B. "Dr. Green, Ms. Greenly is having difficulty breathing after the iodine injection for her CT scan".
    C. "Dr. Green, I think Ms. Greenly is having an allergic reaction to the contrast dye and may be in laryngospasm".
    D. "Dr. Green, Ms. Greenly is a patient with chest pain who was being evaluated for pulmonary embolism. She has lupus and has had no prior iodine injections but is allergic to shellfish. I gave her iohexol 3 minutes ago, and now she's breathing at 30 times a minute".

13. Which of the following is an example of the A in SBAR (Situation, Background, Assessment, and Recommendation)?
    A. "Dr. Green, I think we need to call a code for Ms. Greenly's deteriorating respiratory status from a contrast dye reaction".
    B. "Dr. Green, Ms. Greenly is having difficulty breathing after the iodine injection for her CT scan".
    C. "Dr. Green, I think Ms. Greenly is having an allergic reaction to the contrast dye and may be in laryngospasm".
    D. "Dr. Green, Ms. Greenly is a patient with chest pain who was being evaluated for pulmonary embolism. She has lupus and has had no prior iodine injections but is allergic to shellfish. I gave her iohexol 3 minutes ago, and now she's breathing at 30 times a minute".

14. Which of the following is an example of the R in SBAR (Situation, Background, Assessment, and Recommendation)?
    A. "Dr. Green, I think we need to call a code for Ms. Greenly's deteriorating respiratory status from a contrast dye reaction and give her epinephrine".
    B. "Dr. Green, Ms. Greenly is having difficulty breathing after the iodine injection for her CT scan".
    C. "Dr. Green, I think Ms. Greenly is having an allergic reaction to the contrast dye and may be in laryngospasm".
    D. "Dr. Green, Ms. Greenly is a patient with chest pain who was being evaluated for pulmonary embolism. She has lupus and has had no prior iodine injections but is allergic to shellfish. I gave her iohexol 3 minutes ago, and now she's breathing at 30 times a minute".

8. **C, Standardization.** The equipment and processes should be standardized to increase reliability, improve information flow, and minimize cross-training needs. The examples of standardization are standardizing equipment across clinical settings as well as standardized processes including the use of checklists. A checklist is an algorithmic listing of actions to be performed in a given clinical setting. By standardizing the list of steps to be followed, and formalizing the expectation that every step will be followed for every patient, checklists have the potential to greatly reduce errors due to slips.

References:
PSNet (Patient Safety Network) website. <https://psnet.ahrq.gov/primers/primer/20/human-factors-engineering>.
PSNet (Patient Safety Network) website. <https://psnet.ahrq.gov/primers/primer/14>.

9. **B, Workarounds.** Workarounds are the shortcuts developed by the frontline personnel for bypassing safety features of medical equipment. Workarounds frequently arise because of flawed or poorly designed systems that increase workers' time input or hamper their ability to complete a task. As a result, frontline personnel work around the system in order to get work done efficiently.

References:
PSNet (Patient Safety Network) website. <https://psnet.ahrq.gov/primers/primer/20/human-factors-engineering>.
<http://pubs.rsna.org/doi/full/10.1148/rg.2015150107>.

10. **C, Communication.** Breakdowns in the verbal and written communication between members of the health care team are not only common occurrences but are also a major source of untoward medical events. Approximately 90% of root cause analyses and 65% of sentinel events at one institution evaluated by the Joint Commission on the Accreditation of Healthcare Organizations included communication as a contributing factor. There are many barriers to effective and safe communication. Differences in communication styles between nurses and physicians, for example, as well as lack of standardization and structure in communicating can all contribute to communication breakdowns. The SBAR technique was devised as a framework of structured communication to help clinicians have a shared mental model for the patient's clinical condition and is especially valuable in regard to critical items that require a clinician's immediate attention.

Reference:
Haig K, Sutton S, Whittington J. SBAR: a shared mental model for improving communication between clinicians. *Jt Comm J Qual Patient Saf.* 2006;32(3):167-715.

11. **B, Dr. Green, Ms. Greenly is having difficulty breathing after the iodine injection for her CT scan.** When calling a physician to discuss critical items using the SBAR technique, one starts by describing the situation (S) by identifying oneself and the patient and briefly stating the problem: what it is and when it happened or started.

Reference:
Guidelines for Communicating with Physicians Using SBAR Process. <http://www.sdfmc.org/ClassLibrary/Page/Information/DataInstances/293/Files/1789/Guidelines_for_Using_SBAR.pdf>.

12. **D, Dr. Green, Ms. Greenly is a patient with chest pain who was being evaluated for pulmonary embolism.** She has lupus and has had no prior iodine injections but is allergic to shellfish. I gave her iohexol 3 minutes ago, and now she's breathing at 30 times a minute. When calling a physician to discuss critical items using the SBAR technique, start by describing the situation (S) by identifying oneself and the patient and briefly stating the problem: what it is and when it happened or started. Then, give the pertinent background (B) information related to the situation, including admitting diagnosis, any recent hospitalizations, pertinent medical history, and a brief synopsis of the treatment given to date.

Reference:
Guidelines for Communicating with Physicians Using SBAR Process. <http://www.sdfmc.org/ClassLibrary/Page/Information/DataInstances/293/Files/1789/Guidelines_for_Using_SBAR.pdf>.

13. **C, Dr. Green, I think Ms. Greenly is having an allergic reaction to the contrast dye and may be in laryngospasm.** When calling a physician to discuss critical items using the SBAR technique, start by describing the situation (S) by identifying oneself and the patient and briefly stating the problem: what it is and when it happened or started. Then, give the pertinent background (B) information related to the situation, including admitting diagnosis, any recent hospitalizations, pertinent medical history, and a brief synopsis of the treatment given to date. Then, give an assessment (A) of the situation (ie, what one thinks is the problem).

Reference:
Guidelines for Communicating with Physicians Using SBAR Process. <http://www.sdfmc.org/ClassLibrary/Page/Information/DataInstances/293/Files/1789/Guidelines_for_Using_SBAR.pdf>.

14. **A, Dr. Green, I think we need to call a code for Ms. Greenly's deteriorating respiratory status from a contrast dye reaction and give her epinephrine.** After describing the situation (S), providing pertinent background (B) and giving an assessment (A) of the situation, one gives a recommendation (R) for what one thinks the next appropriate action should be.

Reference:
Guidelines for Communicating with Physicians Using SBAR Process. <http://www.sdfmc.org/ClassLibrary/Page/Information/DataInstances/293/Files/1789/Guidelines_for_Using_SBAR.pdf>.

15. Mrs. Jones is scheduled for a mammogram and a bone densitometry study for osteoporosis. Her family practice physician Dr. Kim Smith orders the studies electronically as "mammogram and bone scan for screening." Dr. Smith does not see a physician order entry option for bone densitometry so she clicks on "bone scan." Mrs. Jones arrives at the outpatient imaging center and gets a screening mammogram, which shows a 1.5-cm suspicious mass. The radiologist calls Dr. Kim Smith's office in Redwood and leaves a message with the nurse who dutifully takes the information. Unfortunately the office that was called was Dr. Kim Smith in Redwood, but Mrs. Jones' doctor is Dr. Kim Smith in Twin Oaks. The message never gets delivered. At the same imaging center, Mrs. Jones gets a technetium pertechnetate bone scan rather than the bone densitometry. The tech administering the technetium fails to recognize that he has infiltrated the nuclear medicine agent into the subcutaneous tissues. No one asks Mrs. Jones why she is getting the bone scan. If they had, she most likely would have said, "osteoporosis." The error in ordering the mammogram and bone scan by Kim Smith would be termed a(n):
    A. Latent error
    B. Active error
    C. Error of omission
    D. Error of commission

16. The error in injecting the technetium into the subcutaneous tissues is an example of a(n):
    A. Blunt end error
    B. Sharp end error
    C. Error of omission
    D. Error of commission

17. The error in not offering bone densitometry in the physician order entry system would be termed a:
    A. Mistake
    B. Slip
    C. Sharp end error
    D. Blunt end error

18. The error in calling the wrong Dr. Kim Smith because the radiologist did not note that the correct Kim Smith was the one with the office in Twin Oaks is what type of error?
    A. Mistake
    B. Slip
    C. Heuristic error
    D. Identity theft

19. Mrs. Jones calls the correct Dr. Kim Smith for the results of her mammogram at one week. Dr. Smith notes that there is no report back, calls the imaging center, and has the report faxed to her. Upon reading it, she schedules Mrs. Jones for a breast mass biopsy. The whole sequence of events regarding the mammogram reports represents a(n):
    A. Near miss
    B. Slip
    C. Root cause analysis
    D. Sentinel event

20. A patient with a known iodine allergy inadvertently receives iodinated contrast but does not have an allergic reaction that time. This error would be termed:
    A. Adverse event
    B. Potential adverse drug event
    C. Nonpreventable adverse drug event
    D. An ameliorable adverse drug event

15. **B, Active error.** The systems approach to errors has as its premise that most errors reflect predictable human failings in the context of poorly designed systems. Health care systems consist of multiple interacting entities (including providers, patients, support staff, technology, and information) and contain multiple layers (including at the national, state, hospital, and caregiving unit levels). This is in contrast to the traditionally held view in medicine that errors reflect failings on the part of individual providers. Rather than punishing providers for individual errors, the systems approach focuses corrective efforts instead on identifying situations or factors likely to give rise to human error and changing the underlying systems of care to reduce the occurrence of errors or to minimize their impact on patients. One of the insights from the systems approach includes the Swiss Cheese model of errors, which posits that larger more catastrophic safety failures are almost never caused by isolated errors committed by individuals, but rather are the result of many small errors in environments with serious underlying system flaws (overlapping holes within layers of the system).

Active errors in this context consist of errors committed by individuals, typically at the point of contact between a human and some aspect of a larger system (eg, at a human-machine interface). This is the error type that occurred when Kim Smith clicked on bone scan instead of bone densitometry when ordering studies. Latent errors, in contradistinction, refer to system errors and can be thought of as accidents waiting to happen. They relate to active errors in that they represent failures of organization or design.

Reference:
PSNet (Patient Safety Network) website. <https://psnet.ahrq.gov/primers/primer/21/systems-approach>.

16. **B, Sharp end error.** The "sharp end" refers to the location within the system where active errors occur. Therefore, when a physician injects a radiotracer into the subcutaneous tissue instead of the targeted vein, she is committing this active error at the sharp end of the system. The blunt end is where latent errors occur, that is, within the many layers of the health care system not in direct contact with patients, although they influence the personnel and equipment at the sharp end that do come into contact with patients.

Reference:
PSNet (Patient Safety Network) website. <https://psnet.ahrq.gov/primers/primer/21/systems-approach>.

17. **D, Blunt end error.** The blunt end is where latent errors occur—within the many layers of the health care system not in direct contact with patients, although they influence the personnel and equipment at the sharp end that do come into contact with patients. In this case, though it may seem remote, the design of the POE such that bone densitometry was not provided as an option for the ordering physician consists of a blunt end error.

Reference:
PSNet (Patient Safety Network) website. <https://psnet.ahrq.gov/primers/primer/21/systems-approach>.

18. **A, Mistake.** Slips and mistakes are two different kinds of active errors. Slips are more common than mistakes and refer to lapses in concentration during activities we perform reflexively, as if acting on autopilot. These typically occur in the face of competing sensory or emotional distractions, fatigue, or stress. Mistakes, on the other hand, relate to errors during attentional behavior, which is characterized by conscious thought, analysis, or planning. Mistakes in this sense reflect incorrect choices and typically reflect lack of experience, insufficient training, or outright negligence.

To call the error in this question a mistake would be to imply that the radiologist called the wrong Dr. Smith and consciously considered that this location was the correct location from which the order was placed, instead of the more likely scenario, in which the radiologist absentmindedly called the first Dr. Smith she could find and didn't consider the fact that this could be the wrong Dr. Smith due to fatigue, stress, and the growing number of studies on her reading list. A common example of a slip is the surgeon operating on the wrong side of the body, typically due to a lapse in concentration. Timeouts were devised to safeguard against such lapses in the operating room.

Reference:
PSNet (Patient Safety Network) website. <https://psnet.ahrq.gov/primers/primer/21/systems-approach>.

19. **A, Near miss.** Near misses are events that occurred but that either did not reach the patient because they were discovered in time or did not cause harm to the patient. Sentinel event alerts are issued by The Joint Commission in response to unexpected incidents involving death or serious physical or psychological injury. Root cause analysis is a retrospective method of analyzing errors. A slip is a common type of active error caused by a lapse in concentration that typically occurs in the face of competing sensory or emotional distractions, fatigue, or stress.

References:
Kessels-Habraken M, et al. Defining near misses: towards a sharpened definition based on empirical data about error handling processes. *Social Sci & Med.* 2010;79(9):1301-1308.
PSNet (Patient Safety Network) website. <https://psnet.ahrq.gov/resources/resource/1337/sentinel-event>.

20. **B, Potential adverse drug event.** Potential adverse drug events are defined by the Agency for Healthcare Research and Quality as medication errors that reached the patient but by good fortune did not cause any harm. Drug errors that were intercepted before the order was actually carried out are also in this category. For instance, delivery of penicillin to a patient despite a known allergy to penicillin but the patient does not develop any allergic reaction is considered a potential adverse drug event.

References:
PSNet (Patient Safety Network) website. <http://www.psnet.ahrq.gov/glossary.aspx>.
Bates DW, Cullen DJ, Laird N, et al. Incidence of adverse drug events and potential adverse drug events. implications for prevention. ADE prevention study group. *JAMA.* 1995;274(1):29-34.

21. A patient on Coumadin has it held for 5 days before a catheter angiogram. The patient develops a large retroperitoneal hematoma that requires surgical intervention. This error would be termed:
    A. Adverse event
    B. Potential adverse drug event
    C. Nonpreventable adverse drug event
    D. An ameliorable adverse drug event

22. Dr. Smith conducts an analysis of how Mrs. Jones' mammogram report went awry. She wants to know all the potential missteps that occurred or could have occurred from the time the report was generated to the time she read it. She lists all the steps in the process and next to each she writes all the potential ways things could go wrong, their likelihood of happening, consequences, and then solicits ideas on how to prevent those potential errors. This is an example of:
    A. Lean Sigma
    B. Six Sigma
    C. Failure Mode and Effects Analysis (FMEA)
    D. Plan Do Study Act (PDSA) [alternative is PDCA (Plan Do Check Act)]

23. Root cause analysis as a means of preventing errors has been criticized because:
    A. Its effectiveness has infrequently been validated
    B. It does not look at system errors
    C. It emphasizes individual persons' mistakes
    D. It uses shaky statistics if at all

24. The Joint Commission has mandated the use of root cause analysis to analyze:
    A. Potential adverse drug events
    B. Near misses
    C. Latent errors
    D. Sentinel events

25. Sentinel events are defined by The Joint Commission as:
    A. A near miss that could have caused a drug-drug interaction
    B. Any unanticipated event resulting in death or serious physical or psychological injury to a patient or patients, unrelated to the natural course of the patient's disease
    C. Episodes of potential injury that occur before an actual catastrophic event occurs which, if dealt with correctly, prevent the serious injury
    D. Events which are caught in the nick of time by monitoring devices

21. **D, An ameliorable adverse drug event.** An *ameliorable* adverse drug effect (ADE) is defined as the harm from a medication that, while not completely preventable, could have been mitigated. A classic example would be a patient taking a cholesterol-lowering agent (statin) who develops muscle pains and eventually progresses to rhabdomyolysis. Failure to regularly check a blood test that assesses muscle damage or failure to recognize the signs of muscle damage would count as the harm from medical care that could have been prevented with earlier, appropriate management. The initial development of a problem is not preventable, but the eventual harm can be lessened. In patients who are at low risk for thrombotic complications and who need a temporary interruption of anticoagulation for an invasive procedure, a 5-day withdrawal is recommended. In the question scenario, Coumadin was appropriately held for 5 days prior to a low bleeding risk procedure. The targeted INR for such procedures is ideally <1.5. If the INR was checked appropriately prior to the elective catheter angiogram and kept at <1.5 the retroperitoneal hematoma could have been mitigated and perhaps the surgical intervention would have been deferred.

References:
PSNet (Patient Safety Network) website. <http://www.psnet.ahrq.gov/glossary.aspx>.
Douketis JD, Berger PB, Dunn AS, et al. The perioperative management of antithrombotic therapy: American College of Chest Physicians Evidence-Based Clinical Practice Guidelines (8th Edition). *Am Coll Chest Physicians Chest.* 2008;133(6 suppl):299S-339S.

22. **C, Failure mode and effects analysis (FMEA).** Failure analysis is the process of collecting and analyzing data to determine the multidimensional causes of failure to provide a road map for corrective actions or liability. FMEA was one of the first systematic techniques developed by reliability engineers in the late 1950s to study problems that might arise from malfunctions of military systems and adopted by the health care industry. FMEA is a step-by-step assessment that identifies and improves steps in a process, thereby reasonably ensuring a safe and clinically desirable outcome. The analysis not only has the information of what and why the process went wrong but also defines what potentially could have gone wrong and the likelihood of consequences of each failure, aiming to develop ways to prevent those potential errors. The Joint Commission designed a worksheet to include the intended process, the actual process, and discrepancies between which of the results form the components of potential failure modes and potential effects graded with severity, probability, invisibility, and criticality. The final step is to summarize the failure mode with actionable causes and potential solutions/redesigns.

References:
American Society for Quality website. *Failure Mode Effects Analysis (FMEA).* <http://asq.org/learn-about-quality/process-analysis-tools/overview/fmea.html>.
The Joint Commission website. *Failure Mode, Effect, and Criticality Analysis (FMECA) Worksheet.* <http://www.jointcommission.org/assets/1/18/Fmeca.pdf>.

23. **A, Its effectiveness has infrequently been validated.** Root cause analysis (RCA) is a systematic approach to problem solving used for analyzing serious adverse events. It is one of the most widely used retrospective methods for detecting safety hazards. Initially developed to analyze industrial accidents, RCA is now applied as an error analysis tool in health care to identify both active errors (errors occurring at the point of interface between humans and a complex system) and latent errors (the hidden problems within health care systems that contribute to adverse events). RCA identifies the underlying problems that increase the likelihood of errors while avoiding the trap of focusing on mistakes by individuals.

The ultimate goal of RCA is to prevent future harm by eliminating factors—the latent errors in health care that underlie the adverse events. A factor is considered a root cause if removal from the problem-fault-sequence prevents the final undesirable event from recurring, whereas a causal factor is one that affects an event's outcome but is not a root cause. Removing a causal factor but not the root cause can benefit an outcome, but it does not prevent its recurrence with any certainty.

References:
Taiichi O. *Toyota Production System: Beyond Large-Scale Production.* Portland, OR: Productivity Press; 1988:17.
PS Net (Patient Safety Network) website. *Root Cause Analysis.* August 2014. <https://psnet.ahrq.gov/primers/primer/10/root-cause-analysis>.

24. **D, Sentinel events.** The Joint Commission developed a Root Cause Analysis and Action Plan tool in response to a sentinel event. The framework has 24 analysis questions to provide a template and aid in organizing the steps in a root cause analysis. For each finding the reader is recommended to continue to ask "Why?" and drill down further to uncover why parts of the process occurred or didn't occur when they should have. A root cause is typically a finding related to a process or system that has a potential for redesign to reduce risk. If a particular finding relevant to the event is not a root cause, it is addressed later in the analysis with a "Why?" question whether it contributed to the likelihood or the severity of the event. Each finding that is identified as a root cause should be addressed in the action plan and considered for a risk reduction strategy.

Reference:
The Joint Commission website. *Framework for Conducting a Root Cause Analysis and Action Plan.* March 22, 2013. <http://www.jointcommission.org/framework_for_conducting_a_root_cause_analysis_and_action_plan/>.

25. **B, Any unanticipated event resulting in death or serious physical or psychological injury to a patient or patients, unrelated to the natural course of the patient's disease.** A sentinel event is a Patient Safety Event that reaches a patient and results in death, permanent or severe temporary harm, and/or requires an intervention to sustain life. Such events are called "sentinel" because of the need for immediate investigation and response. Each accredited organization is strongly encouraged, but not required, to report sentinel events to The Joint Commission. (TJC). The Joint Commission adopted a formal Sentinel Event Policy in 1996 to help hospitals that experience serious adverse events improve safety and learn from those sentinel events. Careful investigation and root cause analyses of Patient Safety Events (events not primarily related to the natural course of the patient's illness or underlying condition) and evaluation of corrective actions are essential to reduce risk and prevent patient harm. Organizations benefit from self-reporting in the following ways:

1. The Joint Commission can provide support and expertise during the review of a sentinel event.
2. The opportunity to collaborate with a patient safety expert in The Joint Commission's Sentinel Event Unit of the Office of Quality and Patient Safety.
3. Reporting raises the level of transparency in the organization and promotes a culture of safety.

Reference:
The Joint Commission website. *Sentinel Event Policy and Procedures.* April 13, 2016. <http://www.jointcommission.org/sentinel_event_policy_and_procedures/>.

26. The three manageable behaviors of the Just Culture model are:
    A. Human errors, mechanical errors, communication errors
    B. Human errors, at-risk behaviors, reckless behavior
    C. Perceptual, conceptual, effectual
    D. Malicious, neutral, benevolent

27. In the Just Culture model, conscious disregard for substantive risk is:
    A. A human error
    B. Malicious behavior
    C. Reckless behavior
    D. A push defect

28. In the Just Culture model, the appropriate response to a human error such as lack of training is:
    A. Coaching
    B. Consoling
    C. Collaborating
    D. Punishing

29. After a patient is administered 10 times the correct dose of FDG PET because of a mechanical error, the manufacturer is sued, the technologist using the isotope is fired, and the root cause analysis director is commended. In this scenario, the "second victim" is the:
    A. Patient
    B. Manufacturer
    C. Technologist
    D. RCA director

30. "Speak up /speak out" refers to a program whereby:
    A. Educational materials are shared in a group setting by having each participant teach a part of the course
    B. Employees are commended for acknowledging good work
    C. Leadership encourages its employees to report safety concerns
    D. Employees are encouraged to contact CMS when or if they identify Medicare fraud

31. The principal purpose for employing a checklist is to:
    A. Prevent/reduce errors
    B. Improve efficiency
    C. Ensure compatibility
    D. Grade students' papers

32. Which of the following was the most common sentinel event reported between 2004 and 2014?
    A. Delay in treatment
    B. Wrong patient, wrong site, wrong procedure
    C. Fall
    D. Medication error

33. Which of the following was the least common sentinel event reported between 2004 and 2014?
    A. Drug overdose
    B. Fire
    C. Radiation overdose
    D. Medication error

34. Does a sentinel event have to result in death or serious injury to be considered a "sentinel event"?
    A. Yes
    B. No
    C. It depends on the setting
    D. All of the above

35. The consistent bypassing of radiation safety procedures by neurosurgeons who perform interventional procedures is called a(n):
    A. Active error remediation
    B. Latent error remediation
    C. Workaround
    D. Resilience effort

26. **B, Human errors, at-risk behaviors, reckless behavior.** The Just Culture model as introduced by David Marx describes the three behaviors that are key to comprehending the interrelationship between discipline and patient safety: human error, at-risk behavior, and reckless behavior. The concept tries to achieve a balance between the traditional punitive culture and a totally blame-free culture by holding individuals accountable for reckless behavior, coaching them when at-risk behavior is identified, and consoling them when unintentional errors are made as in a case where a lack of training may lead to error. Human error is described as an unintentional slip or momentary lapse that leads to an undesired outcome. At-risk behaviors describe a situation where minimal or no risk is perceived by the individual and workarounds or shortcuts are used that then leave the process and individual vulnerable to error.

References:
Marx D. Patient safety and the "just culture": a primer for health care executives. April 17, 2001. Available at: <http://www.mha-apps.com/media/maps/Marx_Primer.pdf>.
Bruno MA, Nagy P. Fundamentals of quality and safety in diagnostic radiology. *J Am Coll Radiol.* 2014;11(12 Pt A):1115-1120.

27. **C, Reckless behavior.** The Just Culture model as introduced by David Marx describes the three behaviors that are key to comprehending the interrelationship between discipline and patient safety: human error, at-risk behavior, and reckless behavior. Reckless behavior is defined as a conscious disregard of a visible, significant risk.

References:
Marx D. Patient safety and the "just culture": a primer for health care executives. April 17, 2001. Available at <http://www.mha-apps.com/media/maps/Marx_Primer.pdf>.
Bruno MA, Nagy P. Fundamentals of quality and safety in diagnostic radiology. *J Am Coll Radiol.* 2014;11(12 Pt A):1115-1120.

28. **B, Consoling.** The Just Culture model tries to achieve a balance between the traditional punitive culture and a totally blame-free culture by holding individuals accountable for reckless behavior, coaching them when at-risk behavior is identified, and consoling them when unintentional errors are made as in a case where a lack of training led to that error.

References:
Marx D. Patient safety and the "just culture": a primer for health care executives. April 17, 2001. Available at <http://www.mha-apps.com/media/maps/Marx_Primer.pdf>.
Bruno MA, Nagy P. Fundamentals of quality and safety in diagnostic radiology. *J Am Coll Radiol.* 2014;11(12 Pt A):1115-1120.

29. **C, Technologist.** "Second victims" are those health care workers directly involved with the patient when an adverse event occurs who then struggle to cope emotionally. When handling patient adverse events, it is important to understand all those affected, and support strategies should be in place to offer comfort and emotional help to second victims.

Reference:
Edrees HH, Paine LA, Feroli ER, et al. Health care workers as second victims of medical errors. *Pol Arch Med Wewn.* 2011;121(4):101-108.

30. **C, Leadership encourages its employees to report safety concerns.** The Joint Commission launched its "Speak Up" patient safety program, which has many campaigns that are centered on patients being active participants in their health care. In the "Speak up" campaign directed at preventing medical errors, doctors, health care executives, nurses, and health care technicians are advised to speak up if there is a safety concern.

Reference:
The Joint Commission website. *Speak Up: Preventing Medical Errors.* http://www.jointcommission.org/topics/speakup_preventing_medical_errors.aspx.

31. **A, Prevent/reduce errors.** Checklists can accomplish many objectives including, for example, the standardization of a procedure, a basis for memory recall, or a framework for evaluation. Nevertheless, the principal purpose of having a checklist is to reduce errors and ensure best practice adherence, leading to improved performance.

Reference:
Hales BM, Provonost PJ. The checklist—a tool for error management and performance improvement. *J Crit Care.* 2006;21(3):321-325.

32. **B, Wrong patient, wrong site, wrong procedure.** Invasive procedures that were performed on the wrong patient, at the wrong site, or that were unintended (wrong procedure) were the most commonly reported sentinel events to The Joint Commission between 2004 and 2014, totaling 1162 cases (10% of reported events). Note that hospitals are encouraged but not required to report sentinel events to The Joint Commission; therefore, the relative frequency of reported events may not parallel the frequency of actual event occurrences.

Reference:
The Joint Commission. Summary Data of Sentinel Events Reviewed by the Joint Commission. July 9, 2015. <http://www.jointcommission.org/assets/1/18/2004-2015_2Q_SE_Stats-Summary.pdf>. Accessed December 8, 2015.

33. **C, Radiation overdose.** Of the listed events, radiation overdose was the least commonly reported, totaling only 39 cases, or 0.3% of all sentinel events reported to The Joint Commission between 2004 and 2014. Medication error, fire, and drug overdose totaled 452, 130, and 102 cases, respectively.

Reference:
The Joint Commission. Summary Data of Sentinel Events Reviewed by the Joint Commission. July 9, 2015. <http://www.jointcommission.org/assets/1/18/2004-2015_2Q_SE_Stats-Summary.pdf>. Accessed December 8, 2015.

34. **B, No.** In January 2015, The Joint Commission updated its definition of a sentinel event. A sentinel event is now defined as either (1) a patient safety event that results in death or serious harm to a patient; or (2) any event from a list of approximately 20 additional scenarios, including prolonged fluoroscopy delivering >1500 rads to a single site; fire or unanticipated smoke during patient care regardless of whether it causes injury; and wrong patient/wrong site/wrong procedure events regardless of outcome.

Reference:
The Joint Commission. Comprehensive Accreditation Manual for Hospitals Update 2. January 2015. <http://www.jointcommission.org/assets/1/6/CAMH_24_SE_all_CURRENT.pdf>. Accessed December 8, 2015.

35. **C, Workaround.** Workarounds are compensatory steps people take to accomplish a goal in a dysfunctional system of broken work processes. The ingenuity of the employees is demonstrated by all the ways people figure out how to complete the task by bypassing the constraints that would normally rule the process maps. Workarounds make it easier to get something done, but also raise the possibility of error. They also breed a system of breaking rules and a lack of confidence/respect for the work group as rules are disregarded. Another example of a workaround might be the example of someone figuring out that the best way to ensure that he/she will get to order a barium enema using decision support is to add an ICD-10 code for rectal bleeding. It might not be "kosher" but it gets around the hard stop of decision support for a study the referring physician desires.

Reference:
Turnbull JE. Process management and systems thinking for patient safety. In: *The Business of Health Care: A Journal of Innovative Management Collection.* Salem, NH: Goal/QPC; 2002:3-77 <https://www.goalqpc.com/cms/docs/journals/Fall2001.pdf>.

36. When a new catheter comes out in the market that no longer fits the previous sheath system and the hospital committee has to adapt a new process to account for it, it's termed a(n):
    A. Active error remediation
    B. Latent error remediation
    C. Workaround
    D. Resilience effort

37. When an operator tries to insert a catheter into a sheath that does not allow its passage and in so doing dissects the vessel, it's termed a(n):
    A. Active error
    B. Latent error
    C. Workaround
    D. Resilience effort

38. When a new catheter is measured in millimeters instead of "French," leading to the person ordering the catheter to fail to realize it will not fit through a sheath, it's termed a(n):
    A. Active error remediation
    B. Latent error remediation
    C. Workaround
    D. Resilience effort

39. What is it called when you do tests to see whether a catheter will be easily employable through a sheath to perform an angioplasty?
    A. Workaround
    B. Usability testing
    C. Forcing function
    D. Standardization

40. If all sheaths purchased in a department are capable of handling all angioplasty catheters it's called:
    A. Workaround
    B. Usability testing
    C. Forcing function
    D. Standardization

41. What is it called when you require a catheter to be filled with saline before it is to be inserted into the sheath?
    A. Workaround
    B. Usability testing
    C. Forcing function
    D. Standardization

36. **D, Resilience effort.** System resilience can be defined as "the ability of systems to anticipate and adapt to the potential for surprise and failure." In this case, the hospital has to adapt to a new product that is incompatible with a former setup, and they make the reformation to do so. When people refer to "system mindfulness" it's in the realm of being able to predict failures and to have processes in place to prevent failures or to adjust as soon as one untoward error occurs so that it will not be repeated. The idea that >200 patients may have received eight times the expected radiation from a CT perfusion study should be unfathomable in a resilient system. If sensors had been in place and the radiation tube was malfunctioning, it would have been picked up before several patients were burned by the machinery.

References:
Carayon P, Xie A, Kianfar S. Human factors and ergonomics as a patient safety practice. *BMJ Qual Saf.* 2014;23(3):196-205.
<http://www.aboutlawsuits.com/radiation-exposure-lawsuit-filed-over-ct-scans-at-la-hospital-6558/>.

37. **A, Active error.** An "active error" generally refers to a human error where the fault lies with the way the human interacts with the overall system. In this case, the physician has forced the catheter into a tight space that was not the right size and in so doing injured the patient. It took the human to realize what he/she was doing wrong. This is sometimes referred to as the sharp end of the system where it literally is the person holding the offending agent in hand when the error takes place. For remediation of the active error issues, one has to address the human failure.

References:
<https://psnet.ahrq.gov/primers/primer/21/systems-approach>.
Keers RN, Williams SD, Cooke J, et al. Understanding the causes of intravenous medication administration errors in hospitals: a qualitative critical incident study. *BMJ Open.* 2015;5(3):e005948.

38. **B, Latent error remediation.** Latent errors are failures of design that allow active errors to cause harm. This is like the classic case of the space program's disaster where a part on the Hubble telescope was measured in meters instead of feet, leading to its not being in focus. Having a system that prevents such a type of error to occur is essential. Everyone must be on the same page, and all parts must be standardized to the same system. Thus, having the possibility of making this mistake is what is meant by a latent error. If the catalog for ordering catheters ONLY had catheters referred to by French measures, then this error would not occur. When referring to "blunt ends," one is again speaking of latent errors. For remediation of the latent error issues one has to address the system failure.

Reference:
<https://psnet.ahrq.gov/primers/primer/21/systems-approach>.

39. **B, Usability testing.** Usability testing is part of performance improvement based on the assumption that an item that has passed tests for usability by the customer will be more widely accepted and implemented. Having the world's best statistical program that no one can figure out how to use means that program is unlikely to make it to market. This was the genius of Steve Jobs and the Apple team—they made products that were easy to use right out of the box. According to Jaspers, the benefits of usable systems are (1) increased productivity, (2) reduced errors, (3) reduced training, and (4) greater acceptance. They are also likely to lead to greater employee satisfaction and reduced need for "help desk" support.

Reference:
Jaspers MW. A comparison of usability methods for testing interactive health technologies: methodological aspects and empirical evidence. *Int J Med Informatics.* 2009;78(5):340-353.

40. **D, Standardization.** Standardization is highly regarded as a means of reducing errors. Eliminating variability in the performance of a process achieves the goal of Six Sigma. While training can do this, manufacturing design may also allow standardization of techniques. An example may be the automation associated with CT dosage; such standardized protocols for kvP and pitch and mAs for average adults for abdominal imaging can be provided to customers.

The World Health Organization has targeted five high priority arenas where developing standard operating procedures (SOPs) is likely to have high impact. They are effectively taken from The Joint Commission's National Patient Safety Goals. The problem areas the WHO listed are (1) managing concentrated injectable medicines (concentrated injectables), (2) assuring medication accuracy at transitions of care (medication reconciliation), (3) performance of the correct procedure at the correct body sites (correct site surgery), (4) communication during patient care handovers, and (5) improved hand hygiene to prevent health care–associated infections. For each of these important issues, the WHO recommends an SOP that (1) contains a set of instructions for implementing a defined patient care process in a consistent and measurable way, (2) can be revised with user experience after analysis of collected data, (3) summarizes the problems in the SOP, (4) proposes solutions, (5) presents the evidence for the solution, (6) identifies potential barriers to adoption, and (7) delineates potential unintended consequences of the solution. These SOPs employ quality improvement tools to effect processes and systems, address health care professional behaviors, and describe the roles for patients and their families in the patients' health care plans.

Reference:
Wood DL, Brennan MD, Chaudhry R, et al. Standardized care processes to improve quality and safety of patient care in a large academic practice: the Plummer Project of the Department of Medicine, Mayo Clinic. *Health Serv Manage Res.* 2008;21(4):276-280.

41. **C, Forcing function.** Poka-yoke is Japanese for "mistake-proofing." One of the techniques in the Lean Sigma process to prevent (yokeru) mistakes (poka) is by using techniques such as a force function. This is a manufacturing strategy that prevents errors by creating products that are specifically designed so as to not allow mistakes. An example of this might be designing a positive lead on a cable that can only fit on the positive terminal of a car battery, with a different lead for the negative terminal. In this way one can never short out a car battery. Force functions are very effective at preventing errors. They may increase the inconvenience, but they are strong measures that work.

Reference:
Turnbull JE. Process management and systems thinking for patient safety. In: *The Business of Health Care: A Journal of Innovative Management Collection.* Salem, NH: Goal/QPC; 2002:3-77 <https://www.goalqpc.com/cms/docs/journals/Fall2001.pdf>.

42. The process of mapping out a process, identifying how each step of the process could go wrong, and assigning probabilities to each misstep is called:
    A. Root cause analysis
    B. Failure mode and effects analysis
    C. Mistake indexing
    D. Lean Six Sigma

43. The criticality index is a measure of the:
    A. Likelihood of a particular process failure
    B. Chance of detecting a process failure
    C. Impact of the process failure
    D. All of the above

44. One critique of root cause analysis is that:
    A. It has not been validated for its effectiveness
    B. It is more superficial than failure mode and effects analysis
    C. It is too objective
    D. All of the above

42. **B, Failure mode and effects analysis.** FMEA takes a proactive look at procedures in patient care and tries to address potential failures before they happen (as opposed to a root cause analysis, which is usually reactive). To perform an FMEA, one needs (1) a process map that identifies all the steps in a sequence of events, (2) determination of all the ways in which each step can go wrong, (3) the probability that each error will be detected, and (4) the consequences or impact of the error not being detected. Because doing FMEA is time-consuming and expensive from the standpoint of FTE salaries and support in cost and the cost of correcting potential errors, the patient care problem that is addressed must have high impact. Usually both a severity rating scale and a likelihood rating scale are used for each step in a process in FMEA to assess the importance of addressing that single step in the corrective actions. Detectability is also graded and a risk priority score is created from all these factors. The steps that have the highest risk priority scores are given highest priority for reducing the risk.

Reference:
Duwe B1, Fuchs BD, Hansen-Flaschen J. Failure mode and effects analysis application to critical care medicine. *Crit Care Clin*. 2005;21(1):21-30, vii.

43. **D, All of the above.** The criticality index measures the probability that an activity lies on the critical path. It is typically expressed as a ratio between 0 and 1 or as a percentage for how often a particular step in a process is a critical one divided by the total number of trials. The ability to detect a process failure will influence the ratio and its impact is important for calculating the significance of the failure, and are sometimes also in the criticality index. [CAUTION: While nearly all references in the literature include answer A in the definition, some references do not include answers (B) and (C). Overall, we found most include A, B, and C, hence D is the chosen answer.]

In asset management, criticality is the relative risk of an asset from a cost perspective, calculated in order to understand which assets deserve the highest scrutiny to prevent failure. The analysis often includes four factors: (1) failure mode, (2) cost, (3) risk, and (4) relative importance. In addition, when measuring the sensitivity of an activity for its risk, one should consider, besides the criticality index, the (1) significance index, which measures the relative importance of the activity, (2) schedule sensitivity index, which measures the relative importance of an activity taking the criticality index into account, and (3) cruciality index, which measures the correlation between the activity duration and the total project duration.

Reference:
<http://www.assetinsights.net/Glossary/G_Criticality_Index.html (JUST A) versus <https://psnet.ahrq.gov/glossary/fmea>.

44. **A, It has not been validated for its effectiveness.** Some critics of root cause analysis point to the paucity of literature supporting its long- term effectiveness. In part this is because many RCAs are done for very uncommon defects in the system such that measuring them for incidence takes many years to see whether they will recur. Also, because the usual finding is that errors are due to multiple factors or systems or individuals failing at the same time (like the Swiss cheese theory), it is difficult to pinpoint how to address the simultaneous occurrence of multiple errors leading to the bad outcome. In some articles assessing RCA analysis the clinical outcome is the endpoint, whereas in others it is process measures. Most of the criticism of RCA is that, after developing a solution with action plans, there is not usually a controlled trial to show the "solution's" effect and there often are participant biases to ensure the solution's success (so as not to have to go through another RCA!).

Still others note that the RCA process can be performed in a number of ways: (1) retrospective root cause of failure analysis (RCFA), (2) prospective potential failure modes analysis such as opportunity analysis (OA), or (3) failure mode and effects analysis (FMEA).

Reference:
Percarpio KB1, Watts BV, Weeks WB. The effectiveness of root cause analysis: what does the literature tell us? *Jt Comm J Qual Patient Saf*. 2008;34(7): 391-398.

QUESTIONS

1. When a radiologist seeks confirming evidence to support a diagnosis and does not consider evidence to refute it, it's an example of:
   A. Contradiction bias
   B. Availability bias
   C. Confirmation bias
   D. Anchoring bias

2. Having a checklist of anatomic areas to review for pathology for every case may help with:
   A. Sampling bias
   B. Availability bias
   C. Search satisfaction bias
   D. Anchoring bias

3. Reading a case without any history may help with:
   A. Framing bias
   B. Availability bias
   C. Search satisfaction bias
   D. Anchoring bias

4. Doubting an existing diagnosis and not agreeing immediately with an initial impression may help reduce:
   A. Framing bias
   B. Availability bias
   C. Search satisfaction bias
   D. Anchoring bias

5. Generating a differential diagnosis for every case rather than jumping to a final definitive diagnosis would help with:
   A. Contradiction bias
   B. Availability bias
   C. Premature closure bias
   D. Anchoring bias

6. Dr. Moses detects a renal cell carcinoma in a patient being evaluated for hematuria. He describes the relationship of the tumor to the renal vein and the adjacent lymph nodes as well as capsular spread. On the postoperative study, Dr. Henry notes an iliac artery aneurysm that was not reported by Dr. Moses. The likely explanation was an error of:
   A. Lack of knowledge
   B. Poor interpretation of a finding
   C. Satisfaction of search error
   D. Communication error

7. An error where an initial interpretation of renal cell carcinoma, made by Dr. Moses, is carried forward on subsequent studies despite evidence to the contrary is called:
   A. Framing bias
   B. Discriminative bias
   C. Repetition bias
   D. Anchoring bias

8. An error where an initial interpretation of renal cell carcinoma, made by Dr. Moses, is made because the clinical history is "von Hippel-Lindau disease with hematuria" is called:
   A. Framing bias
   B. Discriminative bias
   C. Repetition bias
   D. Anchoring bias

9. An error where an initial interpretation of renal cell carcinoma, made by Dr. Moses, is due to the fact that he had been criticized twice that month at peer review for missing incidental renal cell carcinomas (RCCs) is:
   A. Weber bias
   B. Premonition bias
   C. Availability bias
   D. Anchoring bias

10. An error where the diagnosis of renal cell carcinoma is made after seeing a purely cystic lesion on an unenhanced CT scan of the abdomen after presented with a clinical history of "von Hippel-Lindau disease, pancreatic cysts, hemangioblastomas with hematuria" is:
    A. Premature closure bias
    B. Discriminative bias
    C. Repetition bias
    D. Haberdasher bias

1. **C, Confirmation bias.** Confirmation bias is the process of collecting and interpreting information that confirms rather than refutes a particular hypothesis. For example, a radiologist's initial impression may be to view a vertical line over the chest as a skin fold rather than a pneumothorax, leading to search for additional supporting evidence such as other overlying artifacts or skin folds elsewhere on the image. Subsequently, the possibility of an underlying pneumothorax may be entirely dismissed. Hence, a strategy to avoid this bias is to examine and reexamine the evidence, consider alternative possibilities, and state a conclusion that may sometimes require follow-up studies.

Reference:
Lee CS, Nagy PG, Weaver SJ, et al. Cognitive and system factors contributing to diagnostic errors in radiology. *AJR Am J Roentgenol.* 2013;201(3):611-617.

2. **C, Search satisfaction bias.** Satisfaction of search bias occurs when an important and often interesting finding is made, resulting in prematurely closing the study before it is viewed in its entirety. Proper search pattern or a diagnostic checklist often helps to avoid this problem. Alternatively, a secondary search to review additional findings ensures that no incidental findings are missed.

Reference:
Lee CS, Nagy PG, Weaver SJ, et al. Cognitive and system factors contributing to diagnostic errors in radiology. *AJR Am J Roentgenol.* 2013;201(3):611-617.

3. **A, Framing bias.** Clinical history often biases the radiologist to think of certain diagnoses that fit within a particular "frame" of clinical context. As an example, history of a biopsy-proven prostate nodule will predispose a radiologist to upgrade a bone island to a blastic metastasis. Hence, it is often prudent to preview the images prior to viewing the clinical information.

Reference:
Lee CS, Nagy PG, Weaver SJ, et al. Cognitive and system factors contributing to diagnostic errors in radiology. *AJR Am J Roentgenol.* 2013;201(3):611-617.

4. **D, Anchoring bias.** Viewing the prior reports and correlating the findings to previous studies anchors the radiologist to draw similar conclusions and arrive at a similar diagnosis. Although consistency is important, it is sometimes necessary to raise an alternative diagnosis than what was initially suspected. Hence, an important strategy to avoid anchoring bias is to make individual conclusions before referring to a previous report. It may be necessary at times to challenge the conclusions drawn on the prior studies rather than immediately agreeing with the former impression.

Reference:
Lee CS, Nagy PG, Weaver SJ, et al. Cognitive and system factors contributing to diagnostic errors in radiology. *AJR Am J Roentgenol.* 2013;201(3):611-617.

5. **C, Premature closure bias.** The risk of premature closure is that other diagnoses are not considered. Failing to search the study for clues that might challenge the presumed diagnosis or failing to consider other diagnoses occurs with premature closure. This may occur when one is overly confident in assuming the imaging features are "pathognomonic" for a specific diagnosis. One may fall into the trap of premature closure because of anchoring: focusing on one particular piece of information such as a symptom, sign, or a particular diagnosis early in the diagnostic process, perhaps even because of prior reports suggesting that diagnosis. To reduce premature closure bias one should recognize anchoring, review the EHR to consider other potential diagnoses, consider the impact of imaging findings inconsistent with the preliminary conclusion, ask a friend for a second opinion, or ask oneself, "what else besides the obvious could this be?"

References:
Lee CS, Nagy PG, Weaver SJ, et al. Cognitive and system factors contributing to diagnostic errors in radiology. *AJR Am J Roentgenol.* 2013;201(3):611-617.
<http://www.ganfyd.org/index.php?title=Cognitive_bias#Premature_closure>.

6. **C, Satisfaction of search error.** Satisfaction of search refers to the tendency to terminate the search process after an initial diagnosis has been identified. In this case, Dr. Moses felt cognitively satisfied after making the diagnosis of renal cell carcinoma and did not continue to search for additional abnormalities. A systematic approach to interpreting studies can help reduce diagnostic errors related to satisfaction of search.

References:
Lee CS, Nagy PG, Weaver SJ, et al. Cognitive and system factors contributing to diagnostic errors in radiology. *AJR Am J Roentgenol.* 2013;201(3):611-617.
Bruno MA, Walker EA, Abujudeh HH. Understanding and confronting our mistakes: the epidemiology of error in radiology and strategies for error reduction. *Radiographics.* 2015;35(6):1668-1676.

7. **D, Anchoring bias.** Anchoring bias is the tendency to latch on to an initial impression or diagnosis and to stay grounded to it despite new information that may come to light. In this case, Dr. Moses is cognitively anchored to his initial diagnosis of renal cell carcinoma and fails to revise this interpretation when reviewing subsequent studies with evidence to the contrary.

References:
Lee CS, Nagy PG, Weaver SJ, et al. Cognitive and system factors contributing to diagnostic errors in radiology. *AJR Am J Roentgenol.* 2013;201(3):611-617.
Bruno MA, Walker EA, Abujudeh HH. Understanding and confronting our mistakes: the epidemiology of error in radiology and strategies for error reduction. *Radiographics.* 2015;35(6):1668-1676.

8. **A, Framing bias.** Framing bias refers to the tendency for radiologists to be influenced by how a case is presented or framed. For example, the presence of a leading clinical history such as "von Hippel-Lindau disease with hematuria" increases the likelihood that a renal lesion will be interpreted as renal cell carcinoma.

Reference:
Lee CS, Nagy PG, Weaver SJ, et al. Cognitive and system factors contributing to diagnostic errors in radiology. *AJR Am J Roentgenol.* 2013;201(3):611-617.

9. **C, Availability bias.** Availability bias refers to the tendency to consider a diagnosis more likely if it is more readily "available" in one's mind. For example, a recent encounter with a rare disease may lead a radiologist to propose it as a leading diagnosis for several months afterward. In this case, Dr. Moses was recently criticized for missing two cases of RCC. The next time he encounters a lesion in the kidney, he is more likely to diagnose it as renal cell carcinoma due to his heightened attention to this diagnosis.

References:
Bruno MA, Walker EA, Abujudeh HH. Understanding and confronting our mistakes: the epidemiology of error in radiology and strategies for error reduction. *Radiographics.* 2015;35(6):1668-1676.
Lee CS, Nagy PG, Weaver SJ, et al. Cognitive and system factors contributing to diagnostic errors in radiology. *AJR Am J Roentgenol.* 2013;201(3):611-617.

10. **A, Premature closure bias.** Premature closure refers to settling on a diagnosis prematurely, before its accuracy has been verified. For example, a round lesion detected in a patient with von Hippel-Lindau disease may be quickly diagnosed as renal cell carcinoma, before verifying whether the lesion actually enhances. Framing bias from the highly suggestive clinical history can also contribute to premature closure.

Reference:
Lee CS, Nagy PG, Weaver SJ, et al. Cognitive and system factors contributing to diagnostic errors in radiology. *AJR Am J Roentgenol.* 2013;201(3):611-617.

11. If an investigator in a study reviews medical records to identify a particular disease after having interpreted a diagnostic imaging study for that disease as "probable," it would be considered:
    A. Sampling bias
    B. Interviewer bias
    C. Verification bias
    D. Incorporation bias

12. Dr. Moses spends several hours contemplating why he makes errors. He examines his last 20 errors and separates them into the various error classifications. He then concludes he should check five blind spots in his abdominal search technique. This is an example of:
    A. Peer review
    B. Rogerian analysis
    C. Metacognition
    D. Premature closure bias

13. John sends out an ad in the *Wall Street Journal* to select subjects for a study on their understanding of market forces that influence the Federal Reserve's determination in interest rate setting. He receives 50 volunteers. He has them each read a spreadsheet of values and then separates the subjects by educational levels (college or graduate school educated) and income levels. He does not include less educated subjects. He has them score a likelihood whether the FED will raise or lower rates on a 1-to-10 scale based on made-up scenarios. He then has two different reviewers, one for the collegiate and one for the graduate school graduates, determine whether the subjects accurately predicted FED interest rate changes. He then separates the results based on income levels. He finds that graduate school graduates and wealthy students are able to predict interest rate hikes better than college graduates and lower income students. He concludes that wealthy and highly educated people should be responsible for setting our national interest rates. The way John advertised for subjects in this scenario may lead to:
    A. Selection bias
    B. Sampling bias
    C. Confounding bias
    D. Measurement bias

14. The selection of the variables of education and income level may lead to:
    A. Selection bias
    B. Sampling bias
    C. Confounding bias
    D. Measurement bias

15. The use of a 1-to-10 scale for predicting whether the Fed will raise rates rather than a yes or no determination represents:
    A. Ordinal versus rank decision making
    B. Ordinal versus continuous decision making
    C. Interval ranking versus nominal scaling
    D. Continuous versus ordinal rating

16. The use of a 1-to-10 scale for predicting whether the Fed will raise rates rather than a yes or no determination could lead to:
    A. Shaping bias
    B. Sampling bias
    C. Ordinal bias
    D. Measurement bias

17. Anchoring refers to which example of a cognitive error?
    A. "I just saw a teratoma in the mediastinum so this must be another one."
    B. "Dr. Yousem called this a teratoma on the prior report, so it must be a teratoma."
    C. "There's a teratoma in the mediastinum so the lung mass must be metastatic teratoma."
    D. "I made the amazing diagnosis of a teratoma in the mediastinum. I'm done!"

18. Framing refers to which example of a cognitive error?
    A. "I just saw a teratoma in the mediastinum so this must be another one."
    B. "The history says family history of teratoma with hairy mass in mediastinum."
    C. "There's a teratoma in the mediastinum so the lung mass must be metastatic teratoma."
    D. "I just missed a case of a teratoma. This may be another."

19. Availability bias refers to which example of a cognitive error?
    A. "I made the amazing diagnosis of a teratoma in the mediastinum. I'm done!"
    B. "Dr. Yousem called this a teratoma on the prior report, so it must be a teratoma."
    C. "There's a teratoma in the mediastinum so the lung mass must be metastatic teratoma."
    D. "I just missed a case of a teratoma. This may be another."

11. **B, Interviewer bias.** Interviewer bias occurs when medical records are selectively reviewed by an investigator who has previously reviewed a test for disease. The way that person looks at the medical record, or interviews a patient, will be biased based on the preconceived notion of the interpretation of that prior study. The investigator who reviews the chart should be different from the one interpreting the study.

Verification bias/workup bias refers to applying different methods for how disease is diagnosed in the gold standard. For example, does one use pathology or clinical impression or amyloid imaging as the gold standard for Alzheimer's disease? If the research protocol is variable from study subject to study subject it may lead to verification bias.

Incorporation bias occurs when the results of the study test are used to make the final diagnosis. Thus, if you need an autopsy to make the gold standard diagnosis of Alzheimer's disease but then use a combination of amyloid imaging and clinical findings as the gold standard while the patient is alive in your study, you cannot evaluate the accuracy of amyloid imaging in the study. Because you have introduced verification bias and are looking at the ability of amyloid imaging in the diagnosis, you have effectively incorporated the study in question into the verification of the disease. How can amyloid imaging go wrong then?

Reference:
Sica GT. Bias in research studies. *Radiology.* 2006;238(3):780-789.

12. **C, Metacognition.** Metacognition, or "thinking about thinking," is the process of stepping back and examining one's own cognitive processes. This can aid in identifying sources of error and allow for the development of corrective strategies.

Reference:
Lee CS, Nagy PG, Weaver SJ, et al. Cognitive and system factors contributing to diagnostic errors in radiology. *AJR Am J Roentgenol.* 2013;201(3):611-617.

13. **B, Sampling bias.** Sampling bias refers to the bias that occurs by not sampling a wholly representative portion of the general population. Sampling bias can arise when the intended sample does not adequately reflect the spectrum of characteristics in the target population (in this case education and/or wealth). In this case, the advertisement led to only college or graduate school participants. This bias sample of research subjects does not represent the general population and led to only "highly educated" people being in the study. There were no uneducated participants.

Reference:
Pannucci CJ, Wilkins EG. Identifying and avoiding bias in research. *Plast Reconstr Surg.* 2010;126(2):619-625.

14. **C, Confounding bias.** Confounding bias occurs when association between a factor and an outcome is distorted by the presence of another variable. Thus one might expect that by virtue of higher education one might be expected to have a higher income. Therefore the presence of a relationship between wealth and education in the ability to predict the Fed interest rate, as described in the example, may be due to the confounding effects of the inter-related nature of the two factors.

Reference:
<https://onlinecourses.science.psu.edu/stat507/node/34>.

15. **C, Interval ranking versus nominal scaling.** Nominal scales are used for labeling variables, without any quantitative value. With ordinal scales, it is the order of the values that is important, whereas with interval scales we know not only the order but also the exact differences between the values in a numerical coding. We know the differences between 1, 2, 3, 4, and so on up to 10 in a 1-to-10 scale and that the difference on the scale between 7 and 9 is the same as between 2 and 4 in an interval scale. In a nominal situation we can use a yes or no dichotomy.

Reference:
<http://study.com/academy/lesson/scales-of-measurement-nominal-ordinal-interval-ratio.html>.

16. **D, Measurement bias.** Measurement bias in this case refers to the tendency of graders not to use the extremes of a scale. Therefore the likelihood of individuals choosing the numbers 1 and 10 on a 1-to-10 scale is reduced because of measurement bias.

Reference:
<http://www.ncbi.nlm.nih.gov/pmc/articles/PMC2917255/>.

17. **B, "Dr. Yousem called this a teratoma on the prior report, so it must be a teratoma."** Anchoring bias describes the human tendency to rely on conclusions drawn on prior studies before making individual decisions on a particular case, hence "anchoring" the radiologist to make a similar diagnosis. For example, multifocal brain lesions previously attributed to a demyelinating process may result in an anchoring bias if the radiologist attributes a new focal brain lesion to multiple sclerosis exacerbation rather than lymphoma or other differentials. The ways to avoid this bias are to (1) challenge the findings on the prior report, (2) consider alternative differential diagnoses and avoid premature guesses, and (3) assess interval change and confirm if the finding is concordant with the initial diagnosis.

Reference:
Lee CS1, Nagy PG, Weaver SJ, et al. Cognitive and system factors contributing to diagnostic errors in radiology. *AJR Am J Roentgenol.* 2013;201(3):611-617. doi:10.2214/AJR.12.10375.

18. **B, "The history says family history of teratoma with hairy mass in mediastinum."** Framing bias occurs when the radiologist is strongly influenced by the provided clinical history and subsequently frames the findings to fit a certain diagnosis. For example, if the clinical history is trauma versus known primary malignancy, then the finding of bilateral rib fractures would be attributed to traumatic rib fractures rather than metastatic pathologic fractures. The way to avoid this bias is to (1) preview the images prior to seeking clinical information, (2) obtain more clinical information from electronic medical records or call the referring physicians, and (3) offer multiple appropriate differential considerations when necessary.

Reference:
Lee CS1, Nagy PG, Weaver SJ, et al. Cognitive and system factors contributing to diagnostic errors in radiology. *AJR Am J Roentgenol.* 2013;201(3):611-617. doi:10.2214/AJR.12.10375.

19. **D, "I just missed a case of a teratoma. This may be another."** Availability bias occurs when previous experiences influence diagnostic thinking such that certain thoughts immediately come to mind when viewing a similar study. This is particularly true in situations of recently missed cases or after discussion of an interesting topic. For example, if there was a recent case of intussusception in a patient presenting with abdominal pain, then it is likely for a radiologist to consider intussusception higher on the differential diagnosis in other patients presenting with abdominal pain. The way to avoid this bias is to use objective information before reaching a conclusion and to benchmark diagnostic performance against peers, as is often done in mammography using recall rates.

Reference:
Lee CS, Nagy PG, Weaver SJ, et al. Cognitive and system factors contributing to diagnostic errors in radiology. *AJR Am J Roentgenol.* 2013;201(3):611-617.

20. Satisfaction of search bias refers to which example of a cognitive error?
    A. "I just saw a teratoma in the mediastinum so this must be another one."
    B. "Dr. Yousem called this a teratoma on the prior report, so it must be a teratoma."
    C. "There's a teratoma in the mediastinum so the lung mass must be metastatic teratoma."
    D. "I made the amazing diagnosis of a teratoma in the mediastinum. I'm done!"

21. "I just saw a teratoma in the mediastinum so this must be another one" is an example of:
    A. Sampling bias
    B. Availability bias
    C. Framing bias
    D. Anchoring bias

22. What percentage of lung cancers are seen in retrospect on prior examinations of screening chest radiographs?
    A. 0% to 20%
    B. 21% to 40%
    C. 41% to 60%
    D. >60%

23. In the detection of fractures, most misses occur:
    A. At the beginning of the work day
    B. In the middle of the work day
    C. At the end of the work day
    D. Equally throughout the day

24. The two most common misses that result in radiology lawsuits are:
    A. Aneurysms and fractures
    B. Strokes and cancers
    C. Cancers and fractures
    D. Bleeds and cancers

25. Incorrect interpretation of a malignant lesion as a normal structure after detection is called:
    A. Scanning error
    B. Recognition error
    C. Decision-making error
    D. None of the above

26. Failure of the radiologist to look at all corners of a radiograph is called:
    A. Scanning error
    B. Recognition error
    C. Decision-making error
    D. None of the above

27. Viewing all parts of a radiograph but failing to detect a lesion is called:
    A. Scanning error
    B. Recognition error
    C. Decision-making error
    D. None of the above

20. **D, "I made the amazing diagnosis of a teratoma in the mediastinum.** I'm done!" Particularly well known in the field of radiology, satisfaction of search bias refers to the tendency of a radiologist to prematurely end the study once a particular finding is made and before properly evaluating the remaining structures. This is often the case when a particularly interesting finding is made or if a finding is made that fits the clinical indication. For example, if the indication states that the patient is presenting with facial droop or arm weakness, the radiologist may be eager to diagnose a large middle cerebral artery territory infarction and as a result, overlook the sinuses or inner ear. Hence, to circumvent this problem, it is important to have a search pattern and diagnostic checklist for each study. Sometimes it may be necessary to perform a secondary search for associated findings.

Reference:
Lee CS, Nagy PG, Weaver SJ, et al. Cognitive and system factors contributing to diagnostic errors in radiology. *AJR Am J Roentgenol.* 2013;201(3):611-617.

21. **B, Availability bias.** Availability bias is a tendency to make a diagnosis based on the first thought that comes to mind. These thoughts tend to be about missed cases or interesting cases that were recently viewed. Utilizing objective information or benchmark diagnostic performances such as recall rate are ways to avoid this type of bias. *Availability heuristic* is the term used when recent, more likely, or extraordinary patient diagnoses come to mind and are therefore overcalled when considering a current diagnosis.

Reference:
Lee CS, Nagy PG, Weaver SJ, et al. Cognitive and system factors contributing to diagnostic errors in radiology. *AJR Am J Roentgenol.* 2013;201(3):611-617.

22. **D, >60%.** The retrospectoscope we always say is 20-20. That is why sometimes it is more valuable to have a discrepancy rate, where the answer is not yet known between reviewers, than the bias of hindsight. We know all too well how good lawyers are at reading the films when a lesion has expanded fivefold over a 6-month follow-up period. We also know that, given that very large 5-cm mass now, invariably, we can see it in retrospect. Thus the rate at which lung cancers are seen in retrospect on earlier studies is as high as 71%.

Discrepancy rates are usually much lower. At the Johns Hopkins Hospital we measure these rates frequently. Compared to outside reads, our major finding discrepancy rate was around 8% whereas between members of the neuro-radiology group the rate was about 2%.

Reference:
Brady A, Laoide RÓ, McCarthy P, et al. Discrepancy and error in radiology: concepts, causes and consequences. *Ulster Med J.* 2012;8 1(1):3-9.

23. **C, At the end of the work day.** There is a statistically significant increase in the error rate after a long day of reading cases. Radiologists report eye strain, eye fatigue, and blurred vision after long reading sessions. The maintenance of accommodation and convergence for near vision needed in most viewing settings contributes to the inability to focus as well after a long day of work. The later the day goes in reading cases, the lower the accuracy rate, equally distributed between increased false positives and decreased true positives.

Reference:
Krupinski EA, Berbaum KS, Caldwell RT, et al. Long radiology workdays reduce detection and accommodation accuracy. *J Am Coll Radiol.* 2010;7(9): 698-704.

24. **C, Cancers and fractures.** "Failure to diagnose" is the term used for the majority of lawsuits against radiologists.

This usually means that the radiologist either missed the finding completely or misinterpreted the findings that he/she did see. For the most part, these failures to diagnose predominate in the breast imaging and emergency radiology services. Cancers (breast, lung, colon) and fractures (musculoskeletal wrist and hip and cervical spine) are the most common misses. This is true also in the United Kingdom where their top three misses are breast cancer on mammography, fractures on extremity films, and lung cancers on chest radiographs. The most common lesions missed with breast cancers are nonspecific masses in 19% to 64%, calcifications in 18% to 28%, mass and calcifications in 2%, and architectural distortion in 4% to 12%.

Of interventional cases that come to suits, this usually revolves around biliary, renal, and abscess procedures, although the provision of consent is sometimes at issue.

Reference:
Pinto A, Brunese L. Spectrum of diagnostic errors in radiology. *World J Radiol.* 2010;2(10):377-383.

25. **C, Decision-making error.** Decision-making errors are those in which the radiologist's gaze fixes on the abnormality during the search strategy. It is recognized as not being normal, but the radiologist decides that the abnormality is due to an inconsequential platelike atelectasis rather than a spiculated cancer. The wrong decision has been made. Decision-making errors are the most common of scanning, recognition, and decision-making errors and account for 45% of radiologists' mistakes.

Reference:
Kundel HL, Nodine CF, Carmody D. Visual scanning, pattern recognition and decision-making in pulmonary nodule detection. *Invest Radiol.* 1978;13(3): 175-181.

26. **A, Scanning error.** The scanning of an image by a radiologist may include "blind spots." The chest radiographer who does not look at the costophrenic angles or the middle mediastinal vascular structures begins to notice a preponderance of "misses" in these areas where the eyes have not fixed. This is known as a scanning error, referring not to the modality but to the interpreter of the images who fails to scan the entire field of view with his/her gaze. Because the radiologist never fixates on the abnormality within the visual field, he/she does not report an abnormality. One can think of the terms "glossing over" or "blind spots" for this type of scanning error.

Reference:
Kundel HL, Nodine CF, Carmody D. Visual scanning, pattern recognition and decision-making in pulmonary nodule detection. *Invest Radiol.* 1978;13(3): 175-181.

27. **B, Recognition error.** When one does not have "blind spots" in the search scanning area but, nonetheless, a lesion is not identified (possibly due to overlapping strictures or poor conspicuity or inadequate technique) it is called a recognition error. The radiologist did not recognize the abnormality as such. Recognition errors are the least common of chest radiologists' errors in missing pulmonary nodules. With improved techniques, the recognition of abnormalities has improved, such that a subtle finding on a CT scan for a stroke that is not recognized can be brilliantly and clearly portrayed by an MRI scan using diffusion-weighted imaging that even a first-year trainee can readily notice.

References:
Kundel HL, Nodine CF, Carmody D. Visual scanning, pattern recognition and decision-making in pulmonary nodule detection. *Invest Radiol.* 1978;13(3):175-181.
Krupinski EA. Current perspectives in medical image perception. *Atten Percept Psychophys.* 2010;72(5):1205-1217.

28. Having an infection at the site of a catheter insertion is called:
    A. Scanning error
    B. Recognition error
    C. Decision-making error
    D. None of the above

29. When clinicians and radiologists discuss a case together there is a change in final clinical diagnosis in what percent?
    A. 0% to 20%
    B. 21% to 40%
    C. 41% to 60%
    D. >60%

30. Computer-assisted diagnosis for breast cancer on mammograms:
    A. Performs as well as double reading by humans
    B. Performs better than double reading by humans
    C. Performs less well than double reading by humans
    D. Is not justifiable at this time

28. **D, None of the above.** Scanning errors, recognition errors, and decision-making errors refer to interpretation errors and not procedural errors such as having an infection at a catheter insertion site. Instead this would be classified as a preventable adverse event. A hospital-acquired infection (HAI) is one that occurs more than 48 hours after admission. Catheter insertions are considered predisposing factor to HAIs even as they are used for patient care as supportive measures. An ameliorable adverse event is an event that could have been lessened in severity had preventative or different actions been taken. Contrast that with an unavoidable adverse event, which is one that no one could have predicted would occur.

How common are catheter infections? CMS reported that in 2006 there were 3759 catheter-associated urinary tract infections reported from 433 locations and 2681 vascular catheter-associated infections from 548 locations.

Reference:
Reed D, Kemmerly SA. Infection control and prevention: a review of hospital-acquired infections and the economic implications. *Ochsner J.* 2009;9(1):27-31. PMCID: PMC3096239.

29. **C, 41% to 60%.** In one study of the relationships between clinicians and a 20-member radiology group, the authors found that each radiologist averaged about four contacts with clinicians per day. The time devoted to communication with clinicians for these 20 radiologists per day was one full-time equivalent radiologist. The authors cite the same experience in another department in Oslo, Norway, where the multidisciplinary conferences each day take up one full-time staff equivalent.

The clinicians in the study said that the radiology communications led to a refinement in the diagnostic strategy in 84% of cases and helped derive therapeutic decisions in 67% of cases. This is an acknowledgment of a very important role of the radiologist. The authors found that the diagnosis was changed in 50% of cases and therapy changed in 60% based on the imaging and the communication with the radiologist.

Reference:
Dalla Palma L, Stacul F, Meduri S, et al. Relationships between radiologists and clinicians: results from three surveys. *Clin Radiol.* 2000;55(8):602-605.

30. **C, Performs less well than double reading by humans.** Both double reading and computer-aided detection (CAD) improve the sensitivity of breast cancer detection in screening mammograms. Double reading is more widely practiced in Europe than in the United States. On the other hand, CAD has gained more implementation and utilization in the United States than in Europe.

CAD works by placing marks on potentially suspicious areas on screening mammograms, hence reducing the risk of overlooking a substantial abnormality. However, some studies have shown significant limitations in the performance of CAD compared to double reading. In a prospective study from the United Kingdom in 2004, single reading, single reading with CAD, and double reading were compared in terms of cancer detection rate. Single reading with CAD demonstrated an increased sensitivity over single reading alone by 1.3% while double reading increased sensitivity by 8.2%. Furthermore, a 2010 survey study involving 257 community radiologists participating in the national Breast Cancer Surveillance Consortium, assessed their perceptions related to use of CAD or a second radiologist in their interpretive process. Most of the participating radiologists perceived that double reading improved cancer detection rate compared to CAD. It was also perceived that recall rates increased with CAD compared to double reading. These findings have favored double reading over CAD utilization in the detection of breast cancers on screening mammograms.

References:
Onega T, Aiello Bowles EJ, Miglioretti DL, et al. Radiologists' perceptions of computer aided detection versus double reading for mammography interpretation. *Acad Radiol.* 2010;17(10):1217-1226.

Khoo LA, Taylor P, Given-Wilson RM. Computer-aided detection in the United Kingdom National Breast Screening Programme: prospective study. *Radiology.* 2005;237(2):444-449.

Harvey JA, Nicholson BT, Cohen MA. Finding early invasive breast cancers: a practical approach. *Radiology.* 2008;248(1):61-76.

James JJ, Gilbert FJ, Wallis MG, et al. Mammographic features of breast cancers at single reading with computer-aided detection and at double reading in a large multicenter prospective trial of computer-aided detection: CADET II. *Radiology.* 2010;256(2):379-386.

QUESTIONS

1. The Joint Commission (TJC) National Patient Safety Goals program refers to a "Do Not Use" list. This refers to:
   A. Medications that are off label
   B. Devices that have not been FDA approved
   C. Patient identifiers that may compromise HIPAA rules
   D. Abbreviations

2. Members of the Patient Safety Advisory Group of The Joint Commission (TJC) do NOT include:
   A. Nurses
   B. Engineers
   C. Risk managers
   D. Members of Congress

3. The Joint Commission (TJC) specifies that critical findings must be reported:
   A. Within 30 minutes of study completion
   B. Within 60 minutes of study completion
   C. Within 120 minutes of study completion
   D. According to the institution's policies

4. Dr. Gowdy is performing a lumbar puncture. His technologist supplies a 5 cc syringe for the lidocaine to anesthetize the patient. He then gets a 20 cc syringe and draws up the contrast dye. According to The Joint Commission (TJC) Safety Standards:
   A. The two syringes need not be labeled as to their contents as long as standard procedure is to always have the 5 cc syringe have lidocaine and the 20 cc syringe have contrast dye.
   B. The syringes must be labeled as to their contents.
   C. The syringes need not be labeled as to their contents for this study if they are in the sterile field due to risk of nosocomial infections.
   D. The syringes must be of different colors to comply with The Joint Commission (TJC) guidelines.

5. The Institute of Medicine report "To Err is Human" contested that the number of deaths each year that were attributable to medical error were:
   A. 0–10,000
   B. 10,001–20,000
   C. 20,001–40,000
   D. >40,000

6. Which of the following is not considered a serious reportable event by the National Quality Forum?
   A. Surgery or other invasive procedure performed on the wrong site
   B. Surgery or other invasive procedure performed on the wrong patient
   C. A metal oxygen cylinder entering the MRI magnet bore
   D. Absence of time out performed on a patient

7. The Institute of Medicine has the following opinion about patients' open access to their medical records:
   A. Patients should have unfettered access to their medical record.
   B. Parts of the medical record should be open to the patient.
   C. Patients should not be allowed access to their records because it would prevent open and honest discourse among medical professionals and may harm patients emotionally.
   D. Patients must prove proficiency with English before being allowed access to their record.

8. Dr. Brooks, prior to performing a lumbar nerve root block on Ms. Brown, uses two patient identifiers confirmed by Dr. Brooks and his nurse, marks the left side of the spinal column, reviews the signed consent form, and Ms. Brown confirms with the nurse that it is her understanding that Dr. Brooks will be doing a left L5 nerve root block. Dr. Brooks and his team have thus:
   A. Completed informed consent
   B. Completed The Joint Commission (TJC) Universal Protocol for "Time Out"
   C. Not fulfilled a time out
   D. Established the standard of care

1. **D, Abbreviations.** The Joint Commission's National Patient Safety Goals program was established to help address specific areas of concern for patient safety. The "Do Not Use" list was established in 2004 to reduce misinterpretation of written orders that use abbreviations such as acronyms and symbols that are susceptible to misinterpretation; for instance, "IU" for "international units" may be misinterpreted as "IV" (route of administration) or "10" (dose amount).

Reference:
The Joint Commission website. *Facts about the Official "Do Not Use" List of Abbreviations.* <http://www.jointcommission.org/facts_about_do_not_use_list/>; Accessed November 2015.

2. **D, Members of Congress.** The Patient Safety Advisory Group is composed of widely recognized expert physicians, nurses, pharmacists, engineers, risk managers, and others with real-world patient safety experience. It is unclear what real-world experience members of Congress have.

Reference:
The Joint Commission Patient Safety Advisory Group. *Facts About the Patient Safety Advisory Group.* <http://www.jointcommission.org/facts_about_the_patient_safety_advisory_group/>; Accessed November 2015.

3. **D, According to the institution's policies.** According to The Joint Commission (TJC) Safety Goal NPSG.02.03.01 effective January 1, 2015, "Critical results of tests and diagnostic procedures fall significantly outside the normal range and may indicate a life threatening situation. The objective is to provide the responsible licensed caregiver these results within an established time frame so that the patient can be promptly treated." A specific time window for communication of critical findings is not specified by TJC; this is to be established by the health care institution.

Reference:
ACR Practice Parameter for Communication of Diagnostic Imaging Findings. <http://www.acr.org/~/media/ACR/Documents/PGTS/guidelines/Comm_Diag_Imaging.pdf>; Accessed November 2015.

4. **B, The syringes must be labeled as to their contents.** According to The Joint Commission (TJC) Safety Goal NPSG.03.04.01, in perioperative and other procedural settings, all medications, medication containers, and other solutions on and off the sterile field should be clearly labeled to avoid confusion and misadministration.

Reference:
The Joint Commission. National Patient Safety Goals. <http://www.jointcommission.org/standards_information/npsgs.aspx>; 2015 Accessed November 2015.

5. **D, >40,000.** The 1999 report from the National Academy of Science and Institute of Medicine titled "To Err is Human" suggested that between 44,000 and 98,000 deaths per year could be attributable to medical errors, exceeding the death totals at the time for motor vehicle accidents, breast cancer, or AIDS. These numbers were extrapolated from a study of medical errors in Colorado, Utah, and New York hospitals. These numbers made national headlines and prompted public calls for the health care system to reduce medical errors systematically.

Reference:
The Institute of Medicine Committee on Health Care Quality in America. *To Err is Human.* <https://iom.nationalacademies.org/~/media/Files/Report%20Files/1999/To-Err-is-Human/To%20Err%20is%20Human%201999%20%20report%20brief.pdf>; November 1999.

6. **D, Absence of time out performed on a patient.** A serious reportable event is defined by the National Quality Forum as a "never event" that should not happen in a properly functional health care system. These include: wrong site, wrong patient, or wrong procedure errors; intraoperative or perioperative death in ASA class 1 patients; maternal or neonatal death in low-risk pregnancies; mortality or significant morbidity associated with contaminated drugs/devices, with devices used for or outside their intended purpose, or with device associated air embolism; mortality or significant morbidity associated with medication error, unsafe blood products, or from a fall; and mortality or significant morbidity associated with the delay or failure of communication of laboratory, pathology, or radiology results, or with the introduction of metallic object into the MRI suite.

Reference:
National Quality Forum List of Serious Reportable Events. <https://www.qualityforum.org/Topics/SREs/List_of_SREs.aspx>; Accessed November 3, 2015.

7. **A, Patients should have unfettered access to their medical record.** In 2001, the Institute of Medicine released a report from their Committee on the Quality of Health Care in America that described 6 aims to improve medicine and 10 rules for redesign. The 6 aims centered on making medicine Safe, Effective, Patient-Centered, Timely, Efficient, and Equitable. The 10 rules of redesign were: Care is based on continuous healing relationships; Care is customized according to patient needs and values; The patient is the source of control; Knowledge is shared and information flows freely; Decision making is evidence-based; Safety is a system priority; Transparency is necessary; Needs are anticipated; Waste is continually decreased; and Cooperation among clinicians is a priority. Patients having unfettered open access to their medical data fits with the rules regarding knowledge sharing and that the patient is the source of control. This is also in line with the Department of Health and Human Services' Blue Button Initiative, which seeks to ensure the open access of medical data to patients.

References:
The Institute of Medicine Committee on the Quality of Health Care in America. *Crossing the Quality Chasm: A New Health System for the 21st Century.* <https://www.nationalacademies.org/~/media/Files/Report%20Files/2001/Crossing-the-Quality-Chasm/Quality%20Chasm%202001%20%20report%20brief.pdf>; March 2001 Accessed November 2015.
The Blue Button Initiative. <https://www.healthit.gov/patients-families/blue-button/about-blue-button>; Accessed November 2015.

8. **B, Completed The Joint Commission (TJC) Universal Protocol for "time out."** Many image-guided interventional procedures and invasive diagnostic imaging procedures require adherence to The Joint Commission's Universal Protocol for Preventing Wrong Site, Wrong Procedure, Wrong Person Surgery™. This protocol includes the concept of a "time out," which includes verification of the correct patient identity, the correct site of the procedure, and the procedure to be performed. Conduct a time out immediately before starting the invasive procedure or making the incision. Marking the incision or insertion site on the patient's skin is required "when there is more than one possible location for the procedure and when performing the procedure in a different location would negatively affect quality or safety." When possible, the patient should be involved in the site marking process. The procedure site is marked by a licensed independent practitioner who is ultimately accountable for the procedure and will be present when the procedure is performed.

Reference:
The Joint Commission. *The Universal Protocol for Preventing Wrong Site, Wrong Procedure, and Wrong Person Surgery™ Guidance for health care professionals.* <http://www.jointcommission.org/assets/1/18/UP_Poster.pdf>.

9. Dr. Conn takes over from Dr. Brooks to perform a nerve root ablation, given the positive response to the nerve root block. Ms. Brown has not moved from the fluoroscopy table.
   A. The same time out can be used
   B. The patient must be returned to the waiting area and another time out must be performed
   C. Another time out can be performed in the same location as the first
   D. Only Dr. Brooks can perform the ablation

10. After a second time out is performed, Dr. Conn performs the nerve root ablation. What component of the time out must be documented in the medical record?
    A. That it was completed
    B. The specification of which two patient identifiers were used
    C. The location of the time out and the time of its occurrence
    D. The participants in the time out

11. In the case of an emergency procedure, such as insertion of a chest tube in a patient with a tension pneumothorax, what are the modifications to the time out process?
    A. Site marking and documentation are required
    B. The physician must perform a time out only for the correct patient and correct procedure
    C. The patient still must verify the identifiers
    D. Site marking and documentation are not required, but the physician must document the circumstances around the emergency and verification of the correct patient, correct procedure, and correct site in the progress notes

12. Which of the following should NOT be used as a patient identifier?
    A. Cellphone number
    B. Last 4 digits of the patient's Social Security number
    C. Mother's maiden name
    D. Date of birth

13. Components of informed consent include all of the following EXCEPT:
    A. Benefits
    B. Time out
    C. Alternatives
    D. Risks

14. A patient is given fentanyl and midazolam prior to obtaining consent. The patient seems alert, answers questions appropriately, and signs her name. The consent should be:
    A. Considered invalid
    B. Repeated after the patient is cleared of sedation
    C. Obtained from a legal representative instead
    D. Valid if the patient is competent, able to listen, communicate, and understand her situation, the need for care, the risks, the alternatives, and the benefits

9. **C, Another time out can be performed in the same location as the first.** Even though the patient has not left the table, per The Joint Commission (TJC), another time out needs to be performed. When the patient has two or more procedures AND the person performing the procedure changes, a new time out must be performed before starting each procedure. If Dr. Brooks did both procedures only one time out would be necessary. The patient does not need to be returned to the waiting area (B).

Reference:
The Joint Commission. *The Universal Protocol for Preventing Wrong Site, Wrong Procedure, and Wrong Person Surgery™ Guidance for health care professionals.* <http://www.jointcommission.org/assets/1/18/UP_Poster.pdf>.

10. **A, That it was completed.** The Joint commission (TJC) requires the completion of the time out to be documented. The organization determines the amount and type of documentation. The use of two patient identifiers, the location and time, and the participants is important information to correctly perform the time out. However, documenting this information is not necessary, only that the time out was completed.

Reference:
The Joint Commission. *The Universal Protocol for Preventing Wrong Site, Wrong Procedure, and Wrong Person Surgery™ Guidance for health care professionals.* <http://www.jointcommission.org/assets/1/18/UP_Poster.pdf>.

11. **D, Site marking and documentation are not required, but the physician must document the circumstances around the emergency and verification of the correct patient, correct procedure, and correct site in the progress notes.** In emergency procedures, time is of the essence. It is recommended that the physician performing the procedure document (1) the circumstances that necessitated an emergency procedure, (2) the verification of the correct patient, and (3) correct site in the progress note. This recommendation was proposed in 2012 because performing the standard time out is not always practical in an emergency situation.

Reference:
Pines JM, Kelly JJ, Meisl H, et al. Procedural safety in emergency care: a conceptual model and recommendations. *Jt Comm J Qual Patient Saf.* 2012;38(11):516-526. <http://www.ncbi.nlm.nih.gov/pubmed/23173399>.

12. **C, Mother's maiden name.** Protected health information (PHI) is information in any format that can be reasonably used to identify an individual. The HIPAA privacy rule lists 18 key patient identifiers, including but not limited to the patient's name, location in a region smaller than a state, all elements of dates (except year) directly related to the patient (including date of birth), telephone numbers, email address, Social Security number, photograph, fingerprints, and other unique identifying numbers, characteristics, or codes. Such identifiers must be removed for information to no longer be considered PHI.

Reference:
OSHA website. *HIPAA Definitions and 18 Identifiers.* <http://www.oshpd.ca.gov/Boards/CPHS/HIPAAIdentifiers.pdf>.

13. **B, Time out.** As defined by the American Medical Association (AMA), informed consent should involve discussion of the patient's diagnosis, if known; the nature and purpose of a proposed treatment or procedure; the risks and benefits of a proposed treatment or procedure; alternatives (regardless of their cost or the extent to which the treatment options are covered by health insurance); the risks and benefits of the alternative treatment or procedure; and the risks and benefits of not receiving or undergoing a treatment or procedure. The patient should also have the opportunity to ask questions about any of these elements. A time out is not a component of informed consent.

Reference:
Institute for Health Quality and Ethics website. *What is Informed Consent?* <http://instituteforhealthqualityandethics.com/Informed_Consent.html>.

14. **D, Valid if the patient is competent, able to listen, communicate, and understand his/her situation, the need for care, the risks, the alternatives, and the benefits.** There are common situations when a patient's ability to make decisions about surgery and anesthesia may be questioned, such as a premedicated patient, patient in labor, patient under stress, patient with known mental illness, patient with organic brain disease, immature patient (ie, patient who is minor in age or who has immature mental capacity, such as some forms of mental handicap). It is common to encounter patients who have received sedation and/or pain medication prior to coming to surgery, and it is also common for such medications to be deliberately withheld prior to surgery in anticipation of the necessity to obtain consent. When pain medications are withheld, patients may feel pressured to consent in order to obtain medication to relieve their suffering. In some instances, premedication may actually enhance a patient's ability to make decisions, by providing pain relief or relief from emotional distress, so that they can focus on the choices they are making. Clearly, if premedication has rendered the patient unable to listen, to understand the situation, need for care, risks, and alternatives, or to communicate a decision, then it has negated the informed consent process. But pain medication should never be withheld from a suffering patient under the guise of obtaining informed consent.

A patient who is not sedated can withdraw consent at any time. However, the staff should be aware that consent can be withdrawn after administration of sedation.

Although the consent process would be valid as long as the patient understand the benefits, risks, and alternatives, it may be best to get the informed consent before the administration of midazolam because there are websites to inform patients that midazolam or similar sedative drugs legally invalidate any patient testimony regarding their treatment.

Because the patient must be able to understand the consent process for it to be valid, consent should be obtained before procedure-related sedation is administered. In the situation described in this question, there should be ample documentation that other members of the care team and family agree that the patient was mentally competent at the time of the consent process.

References:
Ethics in medicine, University of Washington School of Medicine website. *Informed Consent in the Operating Room.* <https://depts.washington.edu/bioethx/topics/infc.html#ques1>.

American Society for Gastrointestinal Endoscopy (ASGE) website. Standards of Practice Committee. *Informed consent for GI endoscopy.* <http://www.asge.org/assets/0/71542/71544/279c89a3-4acf-46e1-aaed-24c2b37e70df.pdf>.

Medical Patient Modesty website. *Sedation, Versed and Your Procedure.* When talking to your doctor about your procedure, <http://patientmodesty.org/versed.aspx>.

15. Six people arrive for an MRI at the same time. Patient A is in perfect health. Patient B has a sniffle. Patient C has sickle cell disease and had a crisis last week and has had multiple bone infarcts casing considerable pain. Patient D arrived comatose as a do not resuscitate for ischemic dilated cardiomyopathy. Patient E has cancer and known bone metastases. Patient F has a malignant heart rhythm problem and is being evaluated prior to RF ablation of the aberrant cardiac sinoatrial node obliteration. As far as the American Society of Anesthesiologists Physical Status Classification one would characterize Patient A as:
    A. Class I
    B. Class II
    C. Class III
    D. Class IV

16. Patient B is:
    A. Class I
    B. Class II
    C. Class III
    D. Class IV

17. Patient C is:
    A. Class II
    B. Class III
    C. Class IV
    D. Class V

18. Patient D is:
    A. Class II
    B. Class III
    C. Class IV
    D. Class V

19. Patient E is:
    A. Class II
    B. Class III
    C. Class IV
    D. Class V

20. Patient F is:
    A. Class II
    B. Class III
    C. Class IV
    D. Class V

21. A patient who is brain dead and being evaluated as a kidney donor would be categorized as:
    A. Class III
    B. Class IV
    C. Class V
    D. Class VI

22. After how many hours does the Society of Anesthesiology task force recommend the patient may be discharged upon return to normal level of consciousness after sedation?
    A. 1
    B. 2
    C. 3
    D. 4

23. Which of the following pairs of terms is NOT part of the Institute of Medicine's six improvement aims for the health care system?
    A. Safety and effectiveness
    B. Patient-centeredness and timeliness
    C. Efficiency and equity
    D. None of the above

15. **A, Class I.** According to the American Society of Anesthesiologists (ASA) Physical Status Classification System, Patient A in this example would be classified as ASA I, a normal healthy patient.

    The ASA recommends the physical status classification (Table 6.1) for anesthetic risk assessment

Reference:
American Society of Anesthesiologists. *ASA Physical Status Classification System*. Available at: <https://www.asahq.org/resources/clinical-information/asa-physical-status-classification-system>.

16. **A, Class I.** A sniffle would not qualify as a systemic disease. Examples of mild systemic disease would include pregnancy, obesity, and well-controlled diabetes mellitus or hypertension. Patient B would still be considered an otherwise normal healthy patient. Thus, the appropriate category would be ASA I.

    The ASA recommends the physical status classification (Table 6.1) for anesthetic risk assessment.

Reference:
American Society of Anesthesiologists. *ASA Physical Status Classification System*. Available at: <https://www.asahq.org/resources/clinical-information/asa-physical-status-classification-system>.

17. **B, Class III.** Patient C has a severe systemic disease. Although there are substantive functional limitations related to this condition, they are not considered to be immediately life-threatening. The patient would therefore be classified as ASA III.

    The ASA recommends the physical status classification (Table 6.1) for anesthetic risk assessment.

Reference:
American Society of Anesthesiologists. *ASA Physical Status Classification System*. Available at: <https://www.asahq.org/resources/clinical-information/asa-physical-status-classification-system>.

18. **D, Class V.** The definition of ASA V encompasses a terminal patient who is not expected to survive without the operation. Patient D would fit under this category.

    The ASA recommends the physical status classification (Table 6.1) for anesthetic risk assessment.

Reference:
American Society of Anesthesiologists. *ASA Physical Status Classification System*. Available at: <https://www.asahq.org/resources/clinical-information/asa-physical-status-classification-system>.

19. **B, Class III.** The most appropriate classification of Patient E would be ASA III. The patient has a severe systemic disease, but his life is not in immediate jeopardy.

    The ASA recommends the physical status classification (Table 6.1) for anesthetic risk assessment.

Reference:
American Society of Anesthesiologists. *ASA Physical Status Classification System*. Available at: <https://www.asahq.org/resources/clinical-information/asa-physical-status-classification-system>.

Table 6.1 PHYSICAL STATUS CLASSIFICATION

Class I	Completely healthy and fit patient
Class II	Patient with mild systemic disease
Class III	Patient with severe systemic disease that is not incapacitating
Class IV	Patient with severe systemic disease that is a constant threat to life
Class V	A moribund patient who is not expected to survive without the operation
Class VI	A declared brain death patient whose organs are being removed for donor purposes

20. **C, Class IV.** Preexisting medical conditions and physical status can affect the outcomes of severely injured patients. The American Society of Anesthesiologists (ASA) classification of physical status is a widely used system for preoperative health scaling of surgical patients. In 1941, the ASA asked a committee of three physicians to develop a system that allows anesthesiologists to assess and record the overall health status of patients prior to surgery in order to predict patient operative risk for facilitating collection and tabulation of statistical data in anesthesia.

    The ASA recommends the physical status classification (Table 6.1) for anesthetic risk assessment.

References:
Ringdal KG, et al. Classification of comorbidity in trauma: the reliability of pre-injury ASA physical status classification. *Injury*. 2013;44(1):29-35.
Skaga NO, et al. Pre-injury ASA physical status classification is an independent predictor of mortality after trauma. *J Trauma*. 2007;63(5):972-978.
Sankar A, et al. Reliability of the American Society of Anesthesiologists physical status scale in clinical practice. *Br J Anaesth*. 2014;113(3):424-432.

21. **D, Class VI.** The American Society of Anesthesiologists (ASA) classification of physical status is a system developed to have a subjective scoring system for preoperative comorbidities and general health assessment to predict anesthesia and surgical outcomes. Class VI is the category that includes declared brain death patients whose organs are being removed for donor purposes.

    The ASA recommends the physical status classification (Table 6.1) for anesthetic risk assessment.

Reference:
American Society of Anesthesiologists. *ASA Physical Status Classification System*. Available at: <https://www.asahq.org/resources/clinical-information/asa-physical-status-classification-system>.

22. **B, 2.** The American Society of Anesthesiologists (ASA) Task force 2002 guidelines for sedation and analgesia by nonanesthesiologists recommend that patients undergoing moderate or deep sedation should be monitored until appropriate discharge criteria are satisfied. Level of consciousness, vital signs, and oxygenation should be monitored and recorded regularly. One of the guidelines they proposed for discharging patients was that sufficient time (up to 2 hours) should pass since the last administration of reversal agents (naloxone, flumazenil) to ensure that the patient will not become re-sedated after the effect of reversal agents wears off.

Reference:
American Society of Anesthesiologists Task Force on Sedation and Analgesia by Non-Anesthesiologists. Practice guidelines for sedation and analgesia by non-anesthesiologists. *Anesthesiology*. 2002;96(4):1004-1017.

23. **D, None of the above.** The Institute of Medicine's six improvement aims for the health care system are safety, effectiveness, patient-centeredness, timeliness, efficiency, and equity.

Reference:
http://www.ihi.org/resources/pages/improvementstories/acrossthechasmsixaimsforchangingthehealthcaresystem.aspx

24. Which is not appropriate for skin marking?
    A. Use of a permanent indelible magic marker
    B. Adhesive markers employing superglue
    C. Marks made by physician assistants in the OR
    D. Marks approved before the procedure is performed

25. Which of the following is prohibited by both the CDC and WHO for health care professionals taking care of "high risk" patients?
    A. Chewing gum
    B. Tattoos
    C. Gauges in the ears
    D. Artificial nails

26. TJC says what about alcohol-based hand cleansers?
    A. They are preferred over soap and water
    B. They are not preferred over soap and water
    C. They must be made available for health care workers in accredited facilities
    D. They are not to be used in operating room areas

27. CDC guidelines say that individuals handing food trays to patients:
    A. Must wash their hands after each tray is delivered
    B. Must wash their hands only if the patient is in a high risk area (eg, ICU, OR, ED)
    C. Must wash their hands if they touch a utensil delivered to the patient
    D. Must wash hands if they have direct contact with the patient

28. According to the WHO, how long should hand washing take?
    A. <15 seconds
    B. 15 to 30 seconds
    C. 31 to 60 seconds
    D. >60 seconds

29. According to the WHO, how should faucets be turned off?
    A. Automatically
    B. Without directly touching the handle
    C. By manually turning off the faucet assuming 40 to 60 seconds have been employed to clean the hands
    D. Using the elbow

30. According to the WHO, how long should hand washing using alcohol dispensers take?
    A. <15 seconds
    B. 15 to 30 seconds
    C. 31 to 60 seconds
    D. >60 seconds

31. Hand washing should occur:
    A. Before patient contact
    B. After removing gloves
    C. Before putting on gloves
    D. All of the above

32. Dr. Rogan enters Ms. Tyler's room in the ICU. Dr. Rogan puts on sterile gloves to examine the patient's infected decubitus ulcer. She then adjusts Ms. Tyler's ventilator settings after finding the tidal volume is too low. She then explores the depth of the patient's decubitus ulcer with a sterile metal probe. Having done so, she removes the gloves. She then readjusts the ventilator. As she is leaving, the patient motions that she is sore in her left wrist near an intravenous catheter. Dr. Rogan does a Tinel sign check on the patient and finds it negative. She leaves Ms. Tyler's room. Regarding appropriate hand hygiene:
    A. Dr. Rogan should wash her hands on entering the room
    B. Dr. Rogan should put on gloves upon entering the room
    C. Dr. Rogan need not wash her hands on leaving the room
    D. All of the above

24. **B, Adhesive markers employing superglue.** Operative sites have to be marked at a minimum when there is more than one possible location for the procedure. Site marking should occur before the procedure is performed and if possible with the patient awake and involved. The site has to be marked by a licensed practitioner (physician, PA, or advanced practice RN) who is ultimately accountable for the procedure and who will be present when the procedure is performed. The method of marking the site and the type of mark are unambiguous and are used consistently throughout the hospital. A permanent medical indelible magic marker is the most common and accepted skin marking modality. The mark has to be sufficiently permanent to be visible after the skin is prepped and draped. Adhesive markers are acceptable, but those employing superglue are not because they alter the surgical site and might damage the tissues.

Reference:
The Joint Commission. National Patient Safety Goals Effective January 1, 2016. Retrieved at: <http://www.jointcommission.org/assets/1/6/2016_NPSG_HAP.pdf>.

25. **D, Artificial nails.** Both the CDC and the WHO recommend health care professionals do not wear artificial fingernails or extenders when having direct contact with patients, and natural nails should be kept short (0.5 cm long or approximately $\frac{1}{4}$ inch long). Numerous studies have documented that subungual areas of the hand harbor high concentrations of bacteria, most frequently coagulase-negative staphylococci, gram-negative rods (including *Pseudomonas* spp.), *Corynebacteria*, and yeasts. Case control studies have demonstrated that health care workers who wear artificial nails are more likely to harbor gram-negative pathogens and yeast on their fingertips than are those who have natural nails, both before and after handwashing.

References:
Guidelines for Hand Hygiene in Healthcare Settings. Published October 25, 2002; 51(RR-16). Retrieved at: <http://www.cdc.gov/mmwr/PDF/rr/rr5116.pdf>.
WHO Guidelines on Hand Hygiene in Healthcare. Retrieved at: <http://apps.who.int/iris/bitstream/10665/44102/1/9789241597906_eng.pdf>; 2009.

26. **C, They must be made available for health care workers in accredited facilities.** According to TJC hand hygiene guidelines, when hands have no visible soil, they may be disinfected with either an alcohol-based hand rub (ABHR) or soap and water; however, when visible soiling is evident, soap and water must be used. Staff is encouraged to use ABHR when no soiling is present and hand hygiene guidelines recommend that all health care organizations make ABHR available for staff.

Reference:
The Joint Commission. *Acceptable Practices of Using Alcohol-Based Hand Rub*. Retrieved at: <http://www.jointcommission.org/assets/1/18/Acceptable%20Practices%20of%20Using%20Alcohol2.PDF>.

27. **D, Must wash hands if they have direct contact with the patient.** Inadequate hand hygiene has been linked to outbreaks of food poisoning. CDC guidelines state that individuals handing food trays to patients must wash their hands in case of direct contact with a patient before handing food to the next patient. A 30-second wash is necessary to remove organisms completely from the hands.

Reference:
WHO Guidelines on Hand Hygiene in Healthcare. Retrieved at: <http://apps.who.int/iris/bitstream/10665/44102/1/9789241597906_eng.pdf>; 2009.

28. **C, 31–60 seconds.** According to the WHO, the duration of hand washing with soap and water should be between 40 and 60 seconds. Hand rub has to include palm-to-palm, palm over dorsum with interlaced fingers, and rotational rubbing of thumbs in the opposite palm. Hands should be rinsed thoroughly with water and with a single use towel.

Reference:
WHO Guidelines on Hand Hygiene in Healthcare. Retrieved at: <http://apps.who.int/iris/bitstream/10665/44102/1/9789241597906_eng.pdf>; 2009.

29. **B, Without directly touching the handle.** *Pseudomonas* species, and specifically *P. aeruginosa*, are frequently isolated from taps/faucets in hospitals. The WHO recommends that after hand antisepsis faucets be turned off not by directly touching the handle but instead by using a single use towel. Automated sensor-operated faucets, or faucets that can be activated with a pedal or with the knee are therefore recommended.

Reference:
WHO Guidelines on Hand Hygiene in Healthcare. Retrieved at: <http://apps.who.int/iris/bitstream/10665/44102/1/9789241597906_eng.pdf>; 2009.

30. **B, 15–30 seconds.** According to the WHO, the duration of hand washing with a palmful of an alcohol-based formulation should be between 20 and 30 seconds. Hand rub has to include palm-to-palm, palm over dorsum with interlaced fingers, and rotational rubbing of thumbs in the opposite palm. Hands should be left to dry naturally and not dried with towels.

Reference:
WHO Guidelines on Hand Hygiene in Healthcare. Retrieved at: <http://apps.who.int/iris/bitstream/10665/44102/1/9789241597906_eng.pdf>. 2009.

31. **D, All of the above.** The U.S. Centers for Disease Control and Prevention (CDC) has cited hand washing as the single most effective way to prevent disease transmission. Hand washing should be performed prior to patient contact as well as before and after use of personal protective equipment.

Reference:
Siegel JD, Rhinehart E, Jackson M, et al. Health Care Infection Control Practices Advisory Committee. 2007 guideline for isolation precautions: preventing transmission of infectious agents in health care settings. *Am J Infect Control*. 2007;35(10 suppl 2):S65-S164.

32. **A, Dr. Rogan should wash her hands on entering the room.** Per WHO's 2009 guideline, the five moments for hand hygiene are:
   1. Before touching the patient
   2. Before a clean/aseptic procedure
   3. After body fluid exposure risk
   4. After touching a patient
   5. After touching patient surroundings

   In addition, while not expressly listed in the "five moments for hand hygiene," the WHO 2009 guideline also lists other indications for hand hygiene including before handling an invasive device, before moving from a contaminated body site to another body site, and after removing gloves.

References:
Pittet D, Allegranzi B, Boyce J, World Health Organization World Alliance for Patient Safety First Global Patient Safety Challenge Core Group of Experts. The World Health Organization guidelines on hand hygiene in health care and their consensus recommendations. *Infect Control Hosp Epidemiol*. 2009;30(7):611-622.
Ellingson K, Haas JP, Aiello AE, et al. Strategies to prevent healthcare-associated infections through hand hygiene. *Infect Control Hosp Epidemiol*. 2014;35(8):937-960. doi:10.1086/651677.
<http://www.jointcommission.org/assets/1/18/hh_monograph.pdf>.

33. As far as hand hygiene:
    A. Dr. Rogan should wash her hands after touching the ventilator
    B. Dr. Rogan should wash her hands after taking off her sterile gloves
    C. Dr. Rogan should wash her hands before doing the Tinel sign
    D. All of the above

34. As far as hand hygiene:
    A. Dr. Rogan should wash her hands before touching the ventilator the second time
    B. Dr. Rogan need not wash her hands after taking off her sterile gloves
    C. Dr. Rogan does not need to wash her hands after performing the Tinel sign check
    D. All of the above

35. As far as hand hygiene:
    A. Dr Rogan should wash her hands and put on new gloves after adjusting the ventilator and before probing the decubitus ulcer
    B. Because she put on gloves Dr. Rogan does not have to wash her hands before probing the decubitus ulcer
    C. Because she put on gloves Dr. Rogan does not have to wash her hands after probing the decubitus ulcer
    D. All of the above

36. As far as hand hygiene:
    A. Dr. Rogan should remove her gloves and wash her hands after touching the ventilator
    B. Dr. Rogan should remove her gloves and wash her hands after touching the ventilator and then put on a new set of gloves before probing the decubitus ulcer
    C. Before and after doing the Tinel sign check Dr. Rogan should wash her hands
    D. All of the above

37. As far as hand hygiene:
    A. Dr. Rogan should wash her hands after seeing one patient but need not wash her hands before seeing a new patient
    B. Dr. Rogan should wash her hands before seeing one patient but need not wash her hands after seeing the patient
    C. Dr. Rogan should wash her hands after seeing one patient and before seeing a new patient
    D. All of the above

38. After which pathogen is alcohol-based hand rub ineffective?
    A. *Clostridium difficile*
    B. *Staphylococcus*
    C. *Tuberculosis*
    D. *Streptococcus*

39. Which of the following is not a risk factor for poor hand hygiene?
    A. Male sex
    B. Weekend shift
    C. Physician as opposed to a nurse
    D. Multiple hand hygiene opportunities per hour

33. **D, All of the above.** Per the WHO's 2009 guideline, the five moments for hand hygiene are:
    1. Before touching the patient.
    2. Before a clean/aseptic procedure.
    3. After body fluid exposure risk.
    4. After touching a patient
    5. After touching patient surroundings.

    In addition, while not expressly listed in the "five moments for hand hygiene," the WHO 2009 guideline also lists other indications for hand hygiene including before handling an invasive device, before moving from a contaminated body site to another body site, and after removing gloves.

References:
Pittet D, Allegranzi B, Boyce J, World Health Organization World Alliance for Patient Safety First Global Patient Safety Challenge Core Group of Experts. The World Health Organization guidelines on hand hygiene in health care and their consensus recommendations. *Infect Control Hosp Epidemiol.* 2009;30(7): 611-622.
Ellingson K, Haas JP, Aiello AE, et al. Strategies to prevent healthcare-associated infections through hand hygiene. *Infect Control Hosp Epidemiol.* 2014;35(8):937-960. doi:10.1086/651677.
<https://www.jointcommission.org/assets/1/18/hh_monograph.pdf>.

34. **A, Dr. Rogan should wash her hands before touching the ventilator the second time.** Per the WHO's 2009 guideline and The Joint Commission (TJC) hand hygiene monograph, Dr. Rogan should wash her hands after touching a patient; thus answers B and C are false. The WHO says one must clean hands after touching the patient's ulcer (She then explores the depth of the patient's decubitus ulcer with a sterile metal probe. Having done so, she removes the gloves. She then readjusts the ventilator) and the patient's surroundings.

    The Tinel test or sign is positive if tapping at the site of a division of a peripheral nerve elicits paresthesia in the distal limb, such as median neuropathy from carpal tunnel.

References:
Pittet D, Allegranzi B, Boyce J, World Health Organization World Alliance for Patient Safety First Global Patient Safety Challenge Core Group of Experts. The World Health Organization guidelines on hand hygiene in health care and their consensus recommendations. *Infect Control Hosp Epidemiol.* 2009;30(7): 611-622.
<https://www.jointcommission.org/assets/1/18/hh_monograph.pdf>.

35. **A, Dr Rogan should wash her hands and put on new gloves after adjusting the ventilator and before probing the decubitus ulcer.** Per the WHO's 2009 guideline and The Joint Commission (TJC) hand hygiene monograph, everyone in an acute care setting should always wash their hands before and after touching a patient, every time. The use of gloves does not abrogate the need to wash hands.

References:
Pittet D, Allegranzi B, Boyce J, World Health Organization World Alliance for Patient Safety First Global Patient Safety Challenge Core Group of Experts. The World Health Organization guidelines on hand hygiene in health care and their consensus recommendations. *Infect Control Hosp Epidemiol.* 2009;30(7): 611-622.
<https://www.jointcommission.org/assets/1/18/hh_monograph.pdf>.

36. **D, All of the above.** As previously cited, answer choices A and C are clearly correct. Before moving from a contaminated site to a different site a physician should wash his or her hands. The physician does not want to introduce respiratory and ventilator associated pathogens into the decubitus ulcer.

Reference:
<https://www.jointcommission.org/assets/1/18/hh_monograph.pdf>.

37. **C, Dr. Rogan should wash her hands after seeing one patient and before seeing a new patient.** Per the WHO's 2009 guideline and The Joint Commission (TJC) hand hygiene monograph, everyone in an acute care setting should always wash their hands before and after touching a patient, every time. The use of gloves does not abrogate the need to wash hands.

References:
Pittet D, Allegranzi B, Boyce J, World Health Organization World Alliance for Patient Safety First Global Patient Safety Challenge Core Group of Experts. The World Health Organization guidelines on hand hygiene in health care and their consensus recommendations. *Infect Control Hosp Epidemiol.* 2009;30(7): 611-622.
<https://www.jointcommission.org/assets/1/18/hh_monograph.pdf>.

38. **A, *Clostridium difficile*.** *C. difficile* spores are not killed or removed from a caregiver's hands as effectively by an alcohol-based hand sanitizer as with soap and water (provided good hand washing technique). In addition to situations where *C. difficile* is suspected or proven, hand washing with soap and water instead of alcohol-based hand rubs is preferred when the hands are visibly dirty, visibly soiled with blood or other body fluids, or after using the toilet. In other situations, an alcohol-based hand cleanser is preferred over hand washing with soap and water.

Reference:
Pittet D, Allegranzi B, Boyce J, World Health Organization World Alliance for Patient Safety First Global Patient Safety Challenge Core Group of Experts. The World Health Organization guidelines on hand hygiene in health care and their consensus recommendations. *Infect Control Hosp Epidemiol.* 2009;30(7): 611-622.

39. **B, Weekend shift.** Observational studies on hand hygiene have documented a number of risk factors for poor adherence to hand hygiene practices. These have included physician status, nursing assistant status, male gender, working during the week, wearing gowns/gloves, and having a high number of opportunities for hand hygiene per hour of patient care. Studies have shown the higher the demand for hand hygiene, the lower the adherence.

Reference:
Centers for Disease Control and Prevention. Guideline for hand hygiene in healthcare settings: recommendations of the Healthcare Infection Control Practices Advisory Committee and the HICPAC/SHEA/APIC/IDSA Hand Hygiene Task Force. *MMWR Recomm Rep.* 2002;51(RR-16):1-48.

QUESTIONS

1. The Medicare incentive program for reporting quality clinical data on prescribed treatments for smoking cessation is called:
   A. Meaningful use
   B. Decision support
   C. Physician Quality Reporting System (PQRS)
   D. Quality Data Analysis Program (QDAP)

2. Use of the electronic health record to understand health disparities in large populations and improve outcomes is encompassed in:
   A. Meaningful use
   B. Health Disparities Outcomes Program (HDOP)
   C. National Practitioner's Data Base (NPDB)
   D. Quality Data Analysis Program (QDAP)

3. The AMA eliminated the CPT code 72069: Radiologic examination, spine, thoracolumbar, standing (scoliosis). This is an example of:
   A. Bundling
   B. Component coding
   C. Deletion
   D. Editorial change

4. The AMA combined the KUB charge of an abdominal radiograph with the intravenous urogram study that follows it. This is an example of:
   A. Bundling
   B. Component coding
   C. Deletion
   D. Editorial change

5. The AMA changed the terminology of several CPT codes replacing the term "film(s)" with the term "image(s)." This is an example of:
   A. Bundling
   B. Component coding
   C. Deletion
   D. Editorial change

6. CMS separated the supervision and interpretation code for nephrostomy tube placement into separate codes. This is an example of:
   A. Bundling
   B. Component coding
   C. Deletion
   D. Editorial change

7. Regarding the charging of multiple CPT codes, which modifier should be used to designate a service that is distinct because it occurred during a separate session?
   A. XE
   B. XP
   C. XU
   D. XS

1. **C, Physician Quality Reporting System (PQRS).** According to CMS, the Physician Quality Reporting System (PQRS) is "a quality reporting program that encourages individual eligible professionals and group practices to report information on the quality of care to Medicare." Such items as smoking and drinking habits and weight reduction counseling are the types of things that further patients' health and may be part of the PQRS.

   Meaningful use refers specifically to using an Electronic Health Record (EHR) to improve quality, safety, and efficiency.

   Decision support is a feature of EHR systems, part of Patient Protection and Affordable Care Act (PPACA) Meaningful Use, Phase 2 requirements, which uses "person-specific information, intelligently filtered and organized … to enhance health." This can include disease-specific order sets and automatic templates, triggered by data within the medical record. "Quality Data Analysis Program" is not a term in use within Medicare.

   References:
   <www.cms.gov/PQRI/>.
   <www.cms.gov/Regulations-and-Guidance/Legislation/EHRIncentivePrograms/downloads/MU_Stage1_ReqOverview.pdf>.
   Patient Protection and Affordable Care Act (PPACA), Federal Register 75 FR 44350 and 77 FR 53997.

2. **A, Meaningful use.** Meaningful use refers specifically to using an electronic health record (EHR) to improve quality, safety, and efficiency. It also specifies the goal to reduce health disparities and improve population and public health.

   "Health Disparities Outcomes Program" is not a phrase in common use. Although the Centers for Disease Control and Prevention publish the annual CDC Health Disparities & Inequalities Report (CHDIR), this report is unrelated to EHR.

   The NPDB is a confidential information clearinghouse created by Congress to improve health care quality, protect the public, and reduce health care fraud. It contains records of medicolegal actions against physicians.

   "Quality Data Analysis Program" is also not a phrase in common use by CMS.

   References:
   <www.cms.gov/Regulations-and-Guidance/Legislation/EHRIncentivePrograms/downloads/MU_Stage1_ReqOverview.pdf>.
   <www.cdc.gov/minorityhealth/CHDIReport.html>.
   .

3. **C, Deletion.** A deletion of a CPT code is when CMS will no longer pay for a particular CPT code. This may be because another one supersedes it or because it is no longer deemed an appropriate test. Sometimes CMS will delete a temporary CPT code when they decide to make it a permanent code that they have decided to reimburse.

   Reference:
   Healthcare Common Procedure Coding System (HCPCS) Level II Coding Procedures. <https://www.cms.gov/medicare/coding/medhcpcsgeninfo/downloads/hcpcsleveliicodingprocedures7-2011.pdf>.

4. **A, Bundling.** When two codes are linked by virtue of their frequent performance together and CMS decides to fold one of the studies into the other, it is called bundling. It used to be that, for CTA, one could use the CPT code for the CTA and then add a 3D reconstruction code to that charge. Then CMS decided that the 3D analysis is part and parcel of the CTA study and no longer paid for it separately—instead it got bundled into the CTA total payment.

   In a similar fashion they have recently decided that doing a non-contrast CT scan before the CTA should not be charged separately but should be combined as part of the overall CTA study. Hence it too is now bundled into the CTA CPT code and its reimbursement.

   References:
   <http://www.acr.org/Advocacy/Economics-Health-Policy/Billing-Coding/Coding-Source-List/2015/Mar-Apr-2015/CPT-2016-Anticipated-Code-Changes>.
   <http://www.acr.org/Advocacy/Economics-Health-Policy/Billing-Coding/Coding-Source-List/2015/Mar-Apr-2015/CPT-2016-Anticipated-Code-Changes>.

5. **D, Editorial change.** An editorial change by CMS does not change the CPT code or the reimbursement for the study. It simply is a means for updating the descriptors of studies. As an example, in 2009 there was an editorial change for CPT code 74270, the "barium enema":

   "An editorial change has been made to the narrative description of code 74270, Radiologic examination, colon; contrast (e.g., barium enema) enema, with or without KUB, to clarify that it should be used to report any type of contrast enema procedure, such as barium, water-soluble contrast, or other contrast media."

   Reference:
   <http://library.ahima.org/xpedio/groups/public/documents/ahima/bok1_042414.hcsp?dDocName=bok1_042414>.

6. **B, Component coding.** When two procedures are unbundled and are charged as separate events, it is called component coding. For example, in 2009 there was a change in interventional radiology. Surgical interventional radiology services that may be performed in the operating room must separate the surgical procedure from the radiological component. An example may be the performance by a neuroradiologist of an intraoperative arteriogram for confirmation of the appropriate location of an aneurysm clip during transcranial surgery. Separating the radiology study from the surgical procedure is component coding even though they may be concurrent events.

   Reference:
   <https://www.oxhp.com/secure/policy/reimbursement_for_comprehensive_and_component_cpt_codes.pdf>.

7. **A, XE.** Modifier 59 is useful because it designates that a procedure or service was distinct or independent from other services performed on the same day. Modifier 59 is used to identify procedures/services that are not normally reported together but are appropriate under the circumstances. This might be the situation with a poly-trauma case in which a wrist fracture occurs at the same time as a subdural hematoma and a bowel perforation. Documentation must support a different session, different procedure or surgery, different site or organ system, separate incision/excision, separate lesion, or separate injury (or area of injury in extensive injuries) not ordinarily encountered or performed on the same day by the same individual. This may be accompanied (or replaced) by an XE code that states that there was a separate encounter with the patient. Therefore seeing the orthopod is distinct from seeing a neurosurgeon for subdural evaluation. This might be the same in radiology with a breast examination by the mammographer, separate from the MRI of the cervical spine for neck pain.

   References:
   American Medical Association. Appendix A–Modifiers. *Current Procedural Terminology (CPT) 2016 Professional Edition.* Chicago: AMA Press.
   <https://www.modahealth.com/pdfs/reimburse/RPM027.pdf>.

8. Regarding the charging of multiple CPT codes, which modifier should be used to designate an infrequent non-overlapping service (one that is distinct because it does not overlap the usual components of the main service)?
   A. XE
   B. XP
   C. XU
   D. XS

9. Regarding the charging of multiple CPT codes, which modifier should be used for a service that is distinct because it was performed by a different health care provider?
   A. XE
   B. XP
   C. XU
   D. XS

10. Regarding the charging of multiple CPT codes, which modifier should be used to designate a service that is distinct because it was performed on a separate body part?
    A. XE
    B. XP
    C. XU
    D. XS

11. The image in Figure 7-1 represents:
    A. Meaningful use
    B. Value modifier
    C. ACR Select
    D. MACRA

12. MACRA refers to:
    A. Medicare Authorization and CPT Reimbursement Assessment
    B. Medicaid Accountability and Component Reimbursement Act
    C. Medicare Access and CHIP Reauthorization Act
    D. Medicare Accountability and Cost Reimbursement Act

13. The Medicare Sustainable Growth Rate (SGR) formula was repealed in April 2015 by the Medicare Access and Children's Health Insurance Program Reauthorization Act (MACRA), resulting in:
    A. No further cuts to physician fees on the basis of the overall growth of the Medicare budget since 1997
    B. Annual increase for fee-for-service physician reimbursements of 0.5% annually until 2020
    C. The merit-based incentive payment system (MIPS), phasing in physician reimbursement bonuses and penalties on the basis of various quality measures
    D. All of the above

14. One of the most important components of MACRA is that:
    A. It fixed the sustainable growth rate "fix"
    B. It required meaningful use
    C. It added value modifiers
    D. It initiated the PQRS system

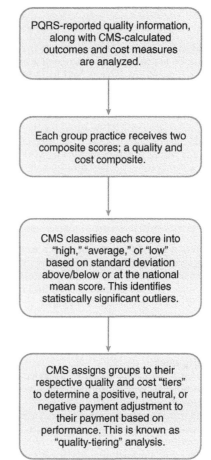

Figure 7-1 Value modifier.

8. **C, XU.** XU designates an unusual nonoverlapping service, such as if an ultrasound of the abdomen is performed on a child and in so doing an intussusception is discovered. The radiologist decides to attempt a reduction of the intussusception via a contrast enema study. Even if this occurs in the same procedure room during the same session it may be performed and reimbursed under the XU designation.

References:
American Medical Association. Appendix A–Modifiers. *Current Procedural Terminology (CPT) 2016 Professional Edition.* Chicago: AMA Press.
<https://www.modahealth.com/pdfs/reimburse/RPM027.pdf>.

9. **B, XP.** In the preceding example where the ultrasound of the abdomen led to the performance of a bowel-reducing contrast enema study, what would happen if the ultrasonographer was not the same person as the pediatric GI radiologist? One might have two procedures in the same room in the same session performed by two different people. In that case the XP designation may be employed.

A CMS description of XP is: "The patient is seen in the office by a family practice physician, who in the course of the visit encounters a problem outside their scope of ability so calls in a specialist physician at the same time to perform the needed service."

Reference:
American Medical Association. Appendix A-Modifiers. *Current Procedural Terminology* (CPT) *2016 Professional Edition.* Chicago: AMA Press.

10. **D, XS.** When two different procedures are performed on different anatomic parts at the same time, one can use the XS designation. Thus when the MSK radiologist performs a left shoulder MR arthrogram and a right knee MR arthrogram, it is considered as an XS modifier.

To summarize:

Modifier XE: separate encounter, a service that is distinct because it occurred during a separate encounter

Modifier XS: separate structure, a service that is distinct because it was performed on a separate organ/structure

Modifier XP: separate practitioner, a service that is distinct because it was performed by a different practitioner

Modifier XU: unusual nonoverlapping service, the use of a service that is distinct because it does not overlap usual components of the main service

Reference:
American Medical Association. Appendix A-Modifiers. *Current Procedural Terminology (CPT) 2016 Professional Edition.* Chicago: AMA Press.

11. **B, Value modifier.** According to CMS: "The Value Modifier provides for differential payment to a physician or group of physicians under the Medicare Physician Fee Schedule based upon the quality of care furnished compared to the cost of care during a performance period. In the future, the Value Modifier will be used to adjust Medicare PFS payments to non-physician eligible professionals, in addition to physicians. The Value Modifier is an adjustment made on a per claim basis to Medicare payments for items and services under the Medicare PFS."

CMS calculates the 2016 value modifier using a quality-tiering approach based on their 2014 performance. Under quality-tiering, physicians can earn an upward payment adjustment for demonstrating higher quality and/or lower cost. The use of value modifier must be budget-neutral, so for every upward adjustment there must be reduction to other physicians' payments based on "lower value" care.

Reference:
<https://www.cms.gov/Medicare/Medicare-Fee-for-Service-Payment/Physician-FeedbackProgram/Downloads/2016-VM-Fact-Sheet.pdf>.

12. **C, Medicare Access and CHIP Reauthorization Act.** The Medicare Access and CHIP Reauthorization Act of 2015 introduces a new pay-for-performance program: the Merit-Based Incentive Payment System (MIPS). The MIPS program adjusts payment to coincide with performance on clinical quality, resource use, meaningful use electronic health record information technology, and clinical practice improvement activities. In addition, it encourages health systems to share risk and reward for quality and quantity of health services provided.

Reference:
<https://www.cms.gov/Newsroom/MediaReleaseDatabase/Fact-sheets/2015-Fact-sheets-items/2015-10-30-2.html>.

13. **D, All of the above.** In April 2015 the Medicare Access and CHIP Reauthorization Act of 2015 (MACRA) was signed into law. Prior to this legislation, the sustainable growth rate (SGR) formula had been slated to enact large cuts to reimbursement (about 21% in 2015). However, there had historically been legislation passed by Congress each fiscal year to offset or defer these cuts. In addition to repealing the SGR, MACRA set fee-for-service reimbursement increases of 0.5% annually for 2015-2019.

Finally, there is a new Merit-Based Incentive Payment System (MIPS), which phases in bonuses and penalties for physician reimbursement rates. In 2019, MIPS can adjust reimbursements from −4% up to +12%, and by 2022, the range goes from −9% to +27%. MIPS will include quality measures from the Physician Quality Reporting System (PQRS), EHR incentives from Meaningful Use measures, and the Physician Value-Based Modifier.

References:
<www.congress.gov/bill/114th-congress/house-bill/2/>.
Hirsch JA, Boswell MV, Staats PS, et al. Analysis of the carrot and stick policy of repeal of the sustainable growth rate formula: the good, the bad, and the ugly, health policy review. *P Phys J.* 2015;18(3):E273-E292.
<www.cms.gov/Medicare/Quality-Initiatives-Patient-Assessment-Instruments/Value-Based-Programs/MACRA-MIPS-and-APMs/MACRA-MIPS-and-APMs.html>.

14. **A, It fixed the sustainable growth rate "fix."** MACRA is also commonly referred to as the Permanent Doc Fix because it repeals the Medicare Part B Sustainable Growth Rate (SGR) reimbursement formula that had plagued Congress since 1997 when the federal budget law tied doctors' Medicare fees to overall economic growth. Because medical costs have far exceeded inflation year after year, Congress was forced to block reimbursement cuts 17 times since 2002. MACRA eliminated that flawed process of adjusting physician CMS fees. Instead, it proposed a new means of reimbursing physicians that emphasized value over volume.

References:
<https://www.rt.com/usa/244461-house-medicare-reform-bill/>.
<https://www.cms.gov/Medicare/Quality-Initiatives-Patient-Assessment-Instruments/Value-Based-Programs/MACRA-MIPS-and-APMs/MACRA-MIPS-and-APMs.html>.

15. MACRA created the merit-based incentive payment system, which consolidated parts of the:
    A. Physician Quality Reporting System
    B. Value-based Payment Modifier
    C. Medicare Electronic Health Record incentive program
    D. All of the above

16. MACRA's goal is to pay for:
    A. Value
    B. Results
    C. Reductions
    D. All of the above

17. Which is not considered an alternate payment model by CMS?
    A. Bundled payments
    B. Capitated payments
    C. Fee-for-service payments
    D. All of the above

18. The merit-based incentive payment system (MIPS) assesses physicians based on:
    A. Quality
    B. Resource use
    C. PQI initiatives
    D. All of the above

19. MIPS does not allow adjustments to payments:
    A. Upward
    B. Downward
    C. Based on outcomes
    D. Based on electronic health record utilization

20. The CHIP program:
    A. Allocates money to pay for Medicaid beneficiaries less than 18 years old
    B. Help states insure low-income children who are ineligible for Medicaid but cannot afford private insurance
    C. Allows low-income children to apply for Medicare benefits
    D. None of the above

15. **D, All of the above.** The physician's quality reporting system applies to individuals and group practices. They must select at least nine individual measures across three National Quality Strategy domains or one measures group to report on measures to CMS and one cross-cutting measure (measures that are broadly applicable across multiple clinical settings within a variety of specialties, eg, time outs, medication reconciliation, health directives) if they have at least one Medicare patient with a face-to-face encounter.

The value modifier pays physicians at different reimbursement levels based on the quality of care furnished to CMS patients compared to the cost of care during a performance period.

The Medicare Electronic Health Record incentive program provides payments to physicians and hospitals for the "meaningful use" of certified electronic health care record technology.

Reference:
<https://www.cms.gov/Medicare/Quality-Initiatives-Patient-Assessment-Instruments/Value-Based-Programs/MACRA-MIPS-and-APMs/MACRA-MIPS-and-APMs.html>.

16. **A, Value.** MACRA sets the priority for payment based on value and not volume. Therefore reimbursement will be based on an increased percentage of alternate payment models besides fee for service, leading to more shared risk and reward by health care systems. These will likely include more capitated models of fixed payments for patients seen or bundled payments for services provided. These models will focus also on quality of care, resource utilization, quality improvement activities, and optimized use of EHR technology.

Clinicians will receive a grade, a Composite Performance Score, that evaluates them on the parameters listed above. Based on this grade, payments may be adjusted higher, lower, or unchanged. The object is to incentivize, via these adjustments, health care that creates a better, smarter, and healthier system than the current CMS system of fee for service.

Reference:
<http://healthaffairs.org/blog/2015/09/28/macra-new-opportunities-for-medicare-providers-through-innovative-payment-systems-3/>.

17. **C, Fee-for-service payments.** Examples of alternate payment models include risk-based or budget-based payment models. These include capitation, bundled payments, and shared savings arrangements. Currently the state of Maryland is using the "waiver" global budget revenue system in which all inpatient technical fees for in-state patients are paid as a lump sum at the beginning of the year. The hospitals are told to manage that money for the technical fees. Professional fees, for now, are still as a fee-for-service solution. The onus is on the hospital to be able to manage expected utilization and related practice expenses for treatment and to avoid add-on costs such as rehospitalizations and iatrogenic infections. If the hospitals do not exceed the budgeted amount, they get to keep the savings. Depending upon shifts in volumes and exigency of care, the State of Maryland may flex more or fewer dollars to a hospital within a 3% to 4% range. When a practice shares in a percentage of any savings, it's called "upside risk," but if they exceed the budgeted amount and lose money it's called "downside risk."

Risk-based contracts entail insurance risk: the financial costs of diseases, accidents, or injury spread out over a covered population (ie, insured members). Performance or utilization risk involves managing the rates of utilization of medical services by a defined population. This may incentivize radiology groups to reduce redundant imaging and to focus on more cost-effective imaging.

Reference:
<https://www.cms.gov/Medicare/Quality-Initiatives-Patient-Assessment-Instruments/Value-Based-Programs/MACRA-MIPS-and-APMs/MACRA-MIPS-and-APMs.html>.

18. **D, All of the above.** MIPS is part of the CMS Physician Quality Reporting Programs Strategic Vision in which (1) quality reporting programs are guided by input from patients, caregivers, and health care professionals, (2) feedback and data drive rapid cycle quality improvement, (3) public reporting of results provides meaningful, transparent, and actionable information that patients can use in choosing caregivers, (4) quality reporting programs rely on an aligned measure portfolio, and (5) quality reporting and value-based purchasing program policies are aligned (ie, payments are aligned with value added).

The components of MIPS for which physicians will be judged (and in part reimbursed for) are quality of care based on adherence/performance on CMS derived good care measures, resource utilization (influenced by CDS software that can "grade" a physician for appropriateness), and Practice Quality Improvement (PQI) initiatives (generally mandated by subspecialty societies for certification.

Reference:
<https://www.cms.gov/Newsroom/MediaReleaseDatabase/Fact-sheets/2015-Fact-sheets-items/2015-10-30.html>.

19. **C, Based on outcomes.** MIPS may adjust reimbursement up or down and in fact is designed to be revenue neutral. Under the Value Modifier program, also revenue neutral, increased payments to physicians who provide high quality, efficient care and decreased payment will be made to those for low-performing physicians with poor quality and overutilization. The MIPS program begins in calendar year 2019. It will base payments on quality reporting, use of the HER in meaningful use and other factors but not outcomes of the patient.

Reference:
<https://www.cms.gov/Newsroom/MediaReleaseDatabase/Fact-sheets/2015-Fact-sheets-items/2015-10-30.html>.

20. **B, Help states insure low-income children who are ineligible for Medicaid but cannot afford private insurance.** The Children's Health Insurance Program (CHIP) serves uninsured children up to age 19 in families with incomes too high to qualify them for Medicaid. The income eligibility standard varies from state to state, but 46 states and the District of Columbia cover children up to or above 200% of the Federal Poverty Level (FPL) ($44,700 for a family of four in 2011). Partial coverage in 24 states is provided if income is at 250% of the FPL or higher.

Reference:
<http://www.ncsl.org/research/health/childrens-health-insurance-program-overview.aspx>.

21. With regard to the Affordable Care Act and CHIP, the ACA:
    A. Raised the eligible income level for CHIP
    B. Reduced the eligible income level for CHIP
    C. Maintained the eligible income level for CHIP
    D. All of the above

22. The legislation that generally prohibits a physician from making referrals for Medicare-covered designated health services to an entity with which the physician or an immediate family member has a "financial relationship" is called:
    A. Tort reform
    B. Omnibus Reconciliation 1987
    C. Stark Law
    D. Qui Tam provision

23. The Stark Law exceptions apply to:
    A. Prepaid plans
    B. Intra-family rural referrals
    C. Academic medical centers
    D. All of the above

24. A 2010 revision to the Stark Law required that a physician within a group practice referring his/her patient for MRI, CT, or PET provided by the same group practice must:
    A. Provide the patient, at the time of the referral, written notice that the physician owns the imaging equipment
    B. Provide the patient with a list of alternative suppliers in the area where the patient resides
    C. Bill the study at Medicare fee schedule even if not a CMS patient
    D. All of the above

25. Stark I, as opposed to Stark II:
    A. Applied to CMS patients
    B. Applied to Medicare patients
    C. Applied to Medicaid and Medicare patients
    D. Applied to all patients

26. If a diagnostic equipment leasing company "Dr Y Rents" owned by Dr. Yousem leases equipment to General Hospital on a per-click basis and Dr. Yousem then refers patients to that General Hospital site:
    A. It would violate Stark I
    B. It would be permissible under the Freedom of Commerce Act
    C. It would violate the Stark Law Final Rule
    D. It would only be permissible if Dr. Yousem was a radiologist

27. When urologists perform IVPs in their office, this is an example of:
    A. Violation of the Stark Laws
    B. In-office exemption
    C. Qui tam violation
    D. Medicare fraud

21. **C, Maintained the eligible income level for CHIP.** The ACA and its recent updated laws require states to maintain the existing income eligibility levels for CHIP through September 30, 2019. States are prohibited from implementing eligibility standards, methodologies, or procedures that are more restrictive than those in place as of March 23, 2010, when the ACA was initially implemented. Those income requirements include, for a family of three, monthly income of $3451 or less or a yearly income of $41,406 or less. The child must be a legal U.S. resident to get the benefits. Benefits vary state by state, but generally include routine check-ups, immunizations, doctor visits, prescriptions, dental and vision care, hospital care, emergency services, and lab and X-ray services.

Reference:
<https://chipmedicaid.org/en/Benefits>.

22. **C, Stark Law.** The Stark Law, named after Pete Stark, democratic congressman from California, aims to limit self-referral leading to overutilization. This is a part of the CMS code that has the greatest pertinence to nonradiologists performing imaging procedures. The most egregious offenders include cardiologists performing nuclear medicine tests, neurologists who own their own MRI machines, urologists doing IVPs, and orthopedic surgeons with their own extremity MRI magnets. The Stark Law prohibits physician referrals of designated health services (DHS) for Medicare and Medicaid patients if the physician (or an immediate family member) has a financial relationship with that entity. In other words, it tries to curtail self-referral that leads to a conflict of interest in deciding whether or not to order a DHS because of one's financial self-interest.

References:
Social Security website. *Compilation of the Social Security Laws.* <https://www.ssa.gov/OP_Home/comp2/F101-239.html>. Omnibus Budget Reconciliation Act Of 1989.
<https://aishealth.com/sites/all/files/comp_lsta_ch400.pdf>.

23. **D, All of the above.** There are certain situations where it is appropriate for the Stark Law to NOT APPLY. Academic medical centers (AMC) often have clinical practice associations that encompass huge numbers of physicians. To prohibit the University of Florida nephrologist from referring to the University of Florida's radiology department where the University of Florida's radiology group does or does not have an ownership interest in the imaging equipment on campus may not make sense. This is particularly true in those settings where AMC employees are salaried and therefore not incentivized to increase utilization. Similarly, in those situations of prepaid plans or capitation, because CMS pays the physicians up front without regard to volume (ie, NOT on a fee-for-service basis) then the utilization of more services by the physician group is NOT tied to remuneration. In that case, self-referral does not result in added cost to the Medicare program and does not result in added compensation to the physicians. This then would not result, one would hope, in overutilization. The paucity of physicians in the rural setting is the impetus for the intra-family rural referrals exception. One would not want the patient to have to drive 60 miles to the next imaging center and incur that burden. The fear is that, if very inconvenient, the patient will not get the proper care/test. Hence the rural exception.

Reference:
<https://www.law.cornell.edu/cfr/text/42/411.355>.

24. **B, Provide the patient with a list of such alternative suppliers in the area where the patient resides.** Slow and steady erosion of some of the exceptions provided under the initial Stark Law has occurred to reduce the chance that financial self-interest influences the referral of CMS patients for designated health services. It is recognized that imaging studies are a potential financial boon for the owners and a contributing factor in the rise of health care costs for CMS. A 2010 In-Office Ancillary Services Exception was made applicable only to MRI, CT, and PET studies. It states that if a physician within a group practice refers his/her patient for MRI, CT, or PET to be performed by members of that same group practice, that physician must provide the patient, at the time of referral with (1) written notice that the patient may obtain these imaging services from imaging centers other than the one owned by the group practice and (2) a list of alternative imaging sites in the area where the patient resides.

Reference:
<http://starklaw.org/>.

25. **B, Applied to Medicare patients.** The Omnibus Budget Reconciliation Act of 1989 (OBRA 1989) prohibited self-referrals for clinical laboratory services for Medicare patients effective January 1, 1992. This provision, named for U.S. Congressman Pete Stark who sponsored the bill, is known as Stark I. The law, however, contained many exceptions to this rule, supported by pro-business Republicans, who wanted to enable legitimate business arrangements. OBRA 1993 expanded the rules to include Medicaid patients under Stark II. Both of these provisions support the notion that physicians are barred from referring a Medicare patient for designated health care services (including radiology examinations) to an entity with which the physician (or his/her immediate family member) has a financial relationship through ownership or compensation.

Reference:
<http://starklaw.org/stark_law.htm>.

26. **C, It would violate the Stark Law Final Rule.** As of October 1, 2009, CMS, via the Stark Law's Final Rule, prohibits the use of unit-of-service (per-click) fee payments for the use of space/equipment where the physician directly or indirectly leases space/equipment to another entity that the physician refers to. So if a neurologist leases a CT scanner to an outpatient imaging center on a per-click basis and then the neurologist refers patients to that outpatient imaging center, it is prohibited. However, per-click compensation arrangements involving non-physician-owned lessors are allowed (as they do not self-refer), as are per-click payments to physician lessors for services rendered to patients who were not referred to the lessee by the physician lessors.

Reference:
<http://www.thehealthlawpartners.com/diagnostic-imaging-arrangements.html>.

27. **B, In-office exemption.** Stark Laws refer to legislation that sought to limit self-referral of Medicare and Medicaid patients. These laws have several exceptions. The in-office ancillary services exception is perhaps the most important of these exceptions for physicians, across multiple specialties (internists, cardiologists, urologists, etc.), who provide imaging services within their practices to their patients. Without this exception, a number of in-office imaging services (such as a urologist performing an IVP in office) would not be possible.

References:
<www.thehealthlawpartners.com/diagnostic-imaging-arrangements.html>.
<www.radiologytoday.net/archive/rt0811p20.shtml>.
Yousem D. *Radiology Business Practice: How to Succeed.* Philadelphia: Elsevier Health Sciences; 2007.

28. When radiologists perform an unenhanced scan on an 80-year-old for Alzheimer's disease but charge CMS for an enhanced scan, this is an example of:
    A. Violation of the Stark Laws
    B. In-office exemption
    C. Qui tam violation
    D. Medicare fraud

29. There are separate codes for CT scans of the brain, CTAs of the intracranial circulation, and 3D reformatting on an independent workstation. What is the term used for rolling all of these procedures into a single code?
    A. Bundling
    B. Multiple procedure payment reduction (MPPR)
    C. Multiple procedure reduction
    D. Multiple procedure parcellation

30. The goals of the "meaningful use" initiative in the electronic health record (EHR) are to:
    A. Improve quality, safety, efficiency, and reduce health disparities
    B. Reduce cost
    C. Standardize terminology
    D. All of the above

31. Which of the following patient characteristics is included in meaningful use objectives for patient charting?
    A. Smoking history for children less than 13 years of age
    B. Body mass index
    C. Eye color
    D. All of the above

32. Meaningful use specifications require implementation of at least how many clinical decision support rules for high priority hospital conditions?
    A. One
    B. Three
    C. Five
    D. No CDS systems are required to meet meaningful use specifications

28. **D, Medicare fraud.** It is fraudulent for a radiologist or other health care professional to bill Medicare for services that he or she did not provide. The most common areas of fraud include billing for services not rendered, billing for services not medically necessary, double billing, upcoding, or unbundling (using multiple codes instead of a single code to obtain greater reimbursement). In this example, the radiologist is charging for a scan with contrast (a more expensive test) when a non-contrast scan was actually performed. There are multiple examples available of physicians committing Medicare fraud that can be found on a generic online search.

References:
Eisenberg Ronald L. *Radiology and the Law: Malpractice and Other Issues.* New York: Springer; 2004.
<http://www.wsaz.com/news/headlines/BREAKING_NEWS_Coal_Grove_Office_Being_Raided_in_Multi-Million_Dollar_Billing_Fraud_Investigation_124353274.html>.
Yousem D. *Radiology Business Practice: How to Succeed.* Philadelphia: Elsevier Health Sciences; 2007.

29. **A, Bundling.** Bundling is reimbursing for multiple individual services with a single unit of payment. According to the Congressional Budget Office, "bundled payments offer providers an incentive to reduce the costs of the services within each component of the bundle and to increase the efficiency with which they provide medical care." This accounts for the single payment for a CTA of the brain that also includes a preliminary non-contrast CT (NCCT) of the brain as part of the study. One cannot charge for each separately. They are "bundled."

Multiple procedure payment reduction (MPPR) is the process by which the Center for Medicare (and Medicaid) Services (CMS) identified potentially "misvalued codes by examining multiple codes that are frequently billed in conjunction with furnishing a single service," according to Medicare Learning Network publication MM7050 12/21/2010. Meanwhile, multiple procedure reduction has the inevitable result of reducing payment. It accounts for a reduction in payment for CT scanning of adjacent body parts such as a CT of the head and CT of the neck. "Multiple procedure parcellation" is not a term in common use within CMS billing.

Reference:
<www.cbo.gov/sites/default/files/110th-congress-2007-2008/reports/12-18-healthoptions.pdf>.

30. **A, Improve quality, safety, efficiency, and reduce health disparities.** The "meaningful use" initiative in the electronic health record (EHR) was put forth by the governmental Office of the National Coordinator for Health Information Technology (ONC), part of the Department of Health and Human Services, in association with the Centers for Medicare and Medicaid Services (CMS). Meaningful use employs the EHR to achieve the following functions:
1. Improve quality, safety, efficiency, and reduce health disparities
2. Engage patients and family
3. Improve care coordination and population and public health
4. Maintain privacy and security of patient health information

Reducing health care costs and standardizing medical terminology are not stated goals of meaningful use, although these may be fringe benefits of compliance.

References:
<https://www.healthit.gov/providers-professionals/meaningful-use-definition-objectives>.
Blumenthal D, Tavenner M. The "meaningful use" regulation for electronic health records. *N Engl J Med.* 2010;363(6):501-504.
Slight SP, Berner ES, Galanter W, et al. Meaningful use of electronic health records: experiences from the field and future opportunities. *JMIR Med Inform.* 2015;3(3):e30.

31. **B, Body mass index.** The EHR incentive program provides a list of objectives for eligible professionals who take part in patient charting. Such objectives include drug interaction checks, verifying patient allergies, performing a medication reconciliation, recording demographic characteristics, and recording changes in specified vital signs. Body mass index is specified to be recorded at every visit. Smoking status is recorded for patients aged 13 years or older but not less than 13 years of age. Eye color is not a demographic recommended to be recorded.

Reference:
<https://www.cms.gov/Regulations-and-Guidance/Legislation/EHRIncentivePrograms/downloads/EP-MU-TOC.pdf>.

32. **A, One.** Computerized clinical decision support can prevent medical errors, decrease inappropriate treatment variability, and allow for patient-specific care. The EHR incentive program requires clinicians to implement at least one clinical decision support rule for high priority hospital conditions and track compliance with that rule over time. Providers who adhere to such meaningful use guidelines will ultimately be eligible for reimbursement. Those who do not may be subject to financial penalties.

References:
<https://www.cms.gov/Regulations-and-Guidance/Legislation/EHRIncentivePrograms/downloads/Hosp_CAH_MU-TOC.pdf>.
Roshanov PS, Fernandes N, Wilczynski JM, et al. Features of effective computerised clinical decision support systems: meta-regression of 162 randomised trials. *BMJ.* 2013;346:f657.

QUESTIONS

1. The typical resuscitative dose of epinephrine in an allergic reaction is:
   A. Epinephrine SC or IM (1:1000) at 0.1-0.3 cc or 1:10,000 IV 1-3 cc
   B. Epinephrine SC or IM (1:10,000) at 1-3 cc or 1:1000 IV 1-3 cc
   C. Epinephrine SC or IM (1:10,000) at 1-3 cc or 1:1000 IV 0.1-0.3 cc
   D. Epinephrine SC or IM (1:1000) at 1-3 cc or 1:10,000 IV 0.1-0.3 cc

2. The typical resuscitative starting dose of atropine in a vasovagal reaction is:
   A. 0.6-1 mg IV
   B. 1-2 mg IV
   C. 2-3 mg IV
   D. 3-5 mg IV

3. The typical antiseizure starting dose of lorazepam after a contrast dye reaction is:
   A. 1 mg IV
   B. 2-4 mg IV
   C. 5-10 mg IV
   D. >10 mg IV

4. The best pretreatment to avoid contrast-induced nephropathy is:
   A. Without concurrent intravenous hydration
   B. Hydration
   C. Mucormyst
   D. Sodium bicarbonate

5. Patients on chronic hemodialysis who receive iodinated contrast should:
   A. Follow their regular schedule of dialysis
   B. Be dialyzed within 24 hours after the iodinated contrast injection
   C. Be dialyzed within 48 hours after the iodinated contrast injection
   D. Should not be dialyzed until they are evaluated by their referring physicians

6. Deposition of gadolinium in the basal ganglia and dentate nuclei is more common in gadolinium based contrast media (GBCM) that are:
   A. Linear and nonionic
   B. Linear and ionic
   C. Macrocyclic
   D. They are actually all the same in risk

7. Regarding the risk of gadolinium injection in patients with sickle cell disease:
   A. It should be avoided at all costs due to potential of precipitating a sickle crisis
   B. It should only be administered for emergency indications due to potential of precipitating a sickle crisis
   C. It is acceptable but only if the patient has a hematocrit above 20
   D. It is safe to administer

8. Gadolinium agents should be:
   A. Administered at room temperature
   B. Warmed to 20 degrees Celsius
   C. Warmed to 30 degrees Celsius
   D. Warmed to 40 degrees Celsius

9. Dr. Ames is starting to provide conscious sedation to a patient. The patient arrived having already taken diazepam to relieve his anxiety. The patient is subsequently sedated with pentobarbital and unable to communicate or respond to verbal commands without arrousal, but he does not need airway protection and can be aroused by shaking. However, after an extra bolus of midazolam, Dr. Ames notes the respiratory rate drops from a baseline of 12 breaths per minute to 4 breaths per minute. The patient no longer responds to a sternal rub and is unconscious. After about 5 minutes of providing bag ventilation to the patient, the patient is awake, alert, and responding to verbal commands. The patient arrived to the procedure (prior to pentobarbital):
   A. Unsedated
   B. Under minimal sedation
   C. Under moderate sedation
   D. Under deep sedation

1. **A, Epinephrine SC or IM (1:1000) at 0.1-0.3 cc or 1:10,000 IV 1-3 cc.** Patients who have a history of previous allergy-like reaction to contrast media are associated with up to 5 times increased likelihood of experiencing a subsequent reaction. A history of atopy increases risk up to two to three times baseline. Patients experiencing severe allergic reaction to contrast media should receive epinephrine via IV or IM routes.

Reference:
ACR Committee on Drugs and Contrast Media. *ACR manual on contrast media*, version 10.1. Reston, VA: American College of Radiology; 2015.

2. **A, 0.6-1 mg IV.** Vasovagal reactions are common, presenting with bradycardia and hypotension. While the majority of reactions are mild and self-limited, close clinical observation is suggested until resolution of symptoms with no medication administered. In severe cases (ie, persistent symptoms) atropine may be required.

Reference:
ACR Committee on Drugs and Contrast Media. *ACR manual on contrast media*, version 10.1. Reston, VA: American College of Radiology; 2015.

3. **B, 2-4 mg IV.** Seizures rarely occur secondary to iodinated contrast media, although they may be related to contrast media–related hyperosmolality and/or calcium binding leading to hypocalcemia. In some cases, patients who have had intrathecal iodinated contrast agents instilled may seize. This risk may be lessened by withholding psychotropic medications that reduce the threshold for seizures. Past editions of the ACR contrast manual suggest treating seizures with 5 mg IV diazepam, but current recommendations suggest 2-4 mg IV lorazepam in the setting of unremitting seizures.

Reference:
ACR Committee on Drugs and Contrast Media. *ACR manual on contrast media*, version 10.1. Reston, VA: American College of Radiology; 2015.

4. **B, Hydration.** The literature surrounding contrast induced nephropathy continues to evolve. Many of the prior studies did not include a control group of patients not receiving contrast, limiting assessment for physiologic variation in creatinine measurement. More recent large studies have shown contrast induced nephropathy is less common than originally thought. Regardless, volume expansion prior to contrast medium administration remains the main preventative action to mitigate risk of contrast induced nephropathy. Studies on other methods, including mucormyst and sodium bicarbonate, have been inconclusive.

Reference:
ACR Committee on Drugs and Contrast Media. *ACR manual on contrast media*, version 10.1. Reston, VA: American College of Radiology; 2015.

5. **A, Follow their regular schedule of dialysis.** While a theoretical risk of converting oliguric dialysis patients to anuria has been posited, no conclusive outcomes data have been published to substantiate this theory. Additional theoretical risks include increased osmotic load due to difficulty clearing excess intravascular volume, potentially leading to pulmonary edema and anasarca; in such patients low osmolality or iso-osmolality contrast media should be used in as low a dose as possible to achieve a diagnostic result. Unless an unusually large volume of contrast is provided, or there is substantial cardiac dysfunction, urgent dialysis is not required.

Reference:
ACR Committee on Drugs and Contrast Media. *ACR manual on contrast media*, version 10.1. Reston, VA: American College of Radiology; 2015.

6. **A, Linear and nonionic.** Gadolinium based contrast agents are widely used in MR examinations because of the paramagnetic properties of gadolinium. However, the toxicity of gadolinium requires chelation to nontoxic ions for safe excretion. These chelates range in stability from macrocyclic (most stable) to linear nonionic (least stable). Recent studies have suggested that increased signal seen in the dentate nuclei and basal ganglia in patients who have prior history of contrast enhanced MR examinations can be due to gadolinium based contrast agent deposition. One study comparing the deposition of macrocyclic chelates and linear nonionic chelates showed macrocyclic agents did not deposit in the basal ganglia and dentate nuclei, suggesting increased signal in these regions may in fact be due to free gadolinium ions. If so, the least stable gadolinium chelates (linear nonionic) would be most likely to result in gadolinium deposition in the basal ganglia and dentate nuclei.

Reference:
Kanda T, Osawa M, Oba H, et al. High signal intensity in dentate nucleus on unenhanced T1-weighted MR images: association with linear versus macrocyclic gadolinium chelate administration. *Radiology*. 2015;275(3):803-809.

7. **D, It is safe to administer.** The administration of gadolinium based contrast media (GBCM) to patients with sickle cell disease is considered safe. Initial data suggested that the alignment of deoxygenated sickle erythrocytes could be induced in a magnetic field. There is no current evidence to indicate that GBCM is associated with an increased risk of vaso-occlusive or hemolytic adverse events in sickle cell patients.

Reference:
Brody AS, et al. AUR Memorial Award. Induced alignment of flowing sickle erythrocytes in a magnetic field. A preliminary report. *Invest Radiol*. 1985;20(6):560-566.

8. **A, Administered at room temperature.** Gadolinium based contrast media are administered at room temperature. Gadolinium is a chemical element with strong paramagnetic properties. It is one of only four elements that can be magnetized at room temperature (the other three being cobalt, iron, and nickel). Gadolinium becomes ferromagnetic below temperatures of 20 degrees Celsius.

Reference:
Nigh HE, Legvold S, Spedding FH. Magnetism and electrical resistivity of gadolinium single crystals. *Phys Rev*. 1963;132(3):1092-1097.

9. **B, Under minimal sedation.** Conscious sedation/analgesia is defined as combinations of pharmacological agents administered by one or more routes to produce a minimally depressed level of consciousness and satisfactory analgesia while retaining the ability to independently and continuously maintain an airway and respond to physical stimulation and verbal commands.

Under minimal sedation, the patient responds to verbal commands. Cognitive function and coordination may be impaired, but respiration and cardiovascular functions are unaffected.

Combining drugs, such as benzodiazepines and opioids, may potentiate adverse effects, such as sedation and respiratory depression. When a benzodiazepine and an opioid are combined and excessive sedation occurs during a procedure, it is recommended that the dose of the benzodiazepine be decreased before decreasing the dose of the opioid. Because benzodiazepines have no analgesic properties, decreasing the dose will not affect pain control.

Reference:
McCaffery M, Pasero C. *Policy and procedure on conscious sedation/analgesia for adults*. <http://prc.coh.org/html/Paserosedation.htm>.

10. Once the patient was unable to respond to verbal commands the patient was under:
    A. General anesthesia
    B. Minimal sedation
    C. Moderate sedation
    D. Deep sedation

11. When the patient lost airway protection and was unconscious the patient was under:
    A. General anesthesia
    B. Minimal sedation
    C. Moderate sedation
    D. Deep sedation

12. The difference between deep sedation and general anesthesia is that:
    A. Ventilatory function is impaired with general anesthesia, not deep sedation
    B. The deep sedation patient responds purposefully with stimulation
    C. Cardiovascular function is not usually maintained in general anesthesia
    D. The sedated patient can speak purposefully

13. The use of diphenhydramine in anaphylaxis prophylaxis is mostly based on its:
    A. Sedative effect
    B. Antihistamine effect
    C. Antibasophile effect
    D. Antieosinophil effect

14. Intravenous steroids have been shown to have limited effectiveness for preventing anaphylaxis:
    A. Only before 2 hours after administration
    B. Before 4 hours after administration
    C. Without diphenhydramine co-administered
    D. In patients with diabetes

15. The American College of Radiology recommends that, for anaphylaxis prophylaxis, oral steroids be started:
    A. 24 hours prior to iodinated contrast administration
    B. 6-8 hours prior to iodinated contrast administration
    C. 12-13 hours prior to iodinated contrast administration
    D. At the same time as diphenhydramine administration

16. For anaphylaxis prophylaxis, diphenhydramine is best administered:
    A. 30 minutes prior to iodinated contrast administration
    B. 60 minutes prior to iodinated contrast administration
    C. 30 minutes prior to iodinated contrast administration if given intravenously but 60 minutes if given orally
    D. 30 minutes prior to iodinated contrast administration if given orally but 60 minutes if given intravenously

17. For treatment of one or two hives that appear after a gadolinium injection the best treatment would be:
    A. Observation
    B. Cold compress
    C. Diphenhydramine
    D. Atropine

10. **D, Deep sedation.** During moderate sedation, there is depression of consciousness, but patients respond purposefully to verbal commands, either alone or accompanied by light tactile stimulation. The patient maintains protective reflexes and a patent airway. Spontaneous ventilation and cardiovascular function are unaffected. When a patient is unable to respond to verbal commands but respond purposefully following repeated or painful stimulation, he/she is under deep sedation.

Independent ventilator function may be impaired and patients may need assistance in maintaining a patent airway. Cardiovascular function is usually maintained.

During general anesthesia, there is complete loss of protective reflexes, and impaired ability to maintain a patent airway independently and respond appropriately to painful situation.

References:
An Updated Report by the American Society of Anesthesiologists Task Force on Sedation and Analgesia by Non-Anesthesiologists. Practice guidelines for sedation and analgesia by non-anesthesiologists. *Anesthesiology.* 2002;96(4):1004-1017.
<http://www.asahq.org/~/media/Sites/ASAHQ/Files/Public/Resources/standards-guidelines/continuum-of-depth-of-sedation-definition-of-general-anesthesia-and-levels-of-sedation-analgesia.pdf>.

11. **A, General anesthesia.** During general anesthesia there is a state of unconsciousness and complete loss of protective reflexes. The patient is unarousable, even with painful stimulus. Spontaneous ventilation is frequently inadequate, requiring assistance to maintain a patent airway. Cardiovascular function may be impaired.

Reference:
An Updated Report by the American Society of Anesthesiologists Task Force on Sedation and Analgesia by Non-Anesthesiologists. Practice guidelines for sedation and analgesia by non-anesthesiologists. *Anesthesiology.* 2002;96(4):1004-1017.

12. **B, The patient in deep sedation responds purposefully with stimulation.** During deep sedation, the patient gives purposeful response after repeated or painful stimulation. However, during general anesthesia the patient is unarousable, even with painful stimulus. Spontaneous ventilation is often inadequate, and interventions to protect the airway are required for both deep sedation and general anesthesia. Cardiovascular function should be maintained in both.

Reference:
An Updated Report by the American Society of Anesthesiologists Task Force on Sedation and Analgesia by Non-Anesthesiologists. Practice guidelines for sedation and analgesia by non-anesthesiologists. *Anesthesiology.* 2002;96(4):1004-1017.

13. **B, Antihistamine effect.** The majority of allergic-type reactions to intravenous contrast (including urticaria, angioedema, and some respiratory symptoms) are thought to be mediated by direct release of histamine and other minor factors from mast cells and basophils. Diphenhydramine is a competitive inhibitor of the H-1 receptor, thus decreasing the physiologic response to the circulating histamines. Corticosteroids function via independent mechanisms to decrease the total number of circulating basophils and eosinophils.

References:
Dunsky EH, Zweiman B, Fischler E, et al. Early effects of corticosteroids on basophils, leukocyte histamine, and tissue histamine. *J Allergy Clin Immunol.* 1979;63(6):426-432.
ACR Committee on Drugs and Contrast Media. *ACR manual on contrast media,* version 10.1. Reston, VA: American College of Radiology; 2015.

14. **B, Before 4 hours after administration.** Corticosteroids decrease the total number of circulating basophils and eosinophils and function independently from the antihistamine effects of H-1 receptor blockers such as diphenhydramine. Though the effects of corticosteroids on decreasing circulating basophils are noticeable after 1-2 hours, the maximal effect is not seen until 4 hours after administration. Diabetes does not decrease the effects of corticosteroids on circulating basophils and eosinophils, but corticosteroids may have adverse effects on blood sugar levels in diabetic patients.

References:
Dunsky EH, Zweiman B, Fischler E, et al. Early effects of corticosteroids on basophils, leukocyte histamine, and tissue histamine. *J Allergy Clin Immunol.* 1979;63(6):426-432.
Lasser EC. Pretreatment with corticosteroids to prevent reactions to i.v. contrast material: overview and implications. *AJR Am J Roentgenol.* 1988;150(2):257-259.
Lasser EC, Berry CC, Mishkin MM, et al. Pretreatment with corticosteroids to prevent adverse reactions to nonionic contrast media. *AJR Am J Roentgenol.* 1994;162(3):523-526.

15. **C, 12-13 hours prior to iodinated contrast administration.** The ACR recommends premedication with oral prednisone or methylprednisolone 12-13 hours prior to the examination. The PO route is preferred over IV due to increased incidence of adverse reactions to corticosteroids administered intravenously. Alternative premedication strategies with IV corticosteroids may be warranted in emergency situations or in patients unable to take PO medications.

References:
ACR Committee on Drugs and Contrast Media. *ACR manual on contrast media,* version 10.1. Reston, VA: American College of Radiology; 2015.
Lasser EC. Pretreatment with corticosteroids to prevent reactions to i.v. contrast material: overview and implications. *AJR Am J Roentgenol.* 1988;150(2):257-259.

16. **B, 60 minutes prior to iodinated contrast administration.** The ACR recommends administration of either PO or IV diphenhydramine 1 hour prior to the contrast-enhanced examination. The peak plasma concentrations of the medication are achieved after 2-3 hours and effects last 4-5 hours. There is no significant difference in the safety or pharmacokinetics of intravenously or orally administered diphenhydramine.

References:
ACR Committee on Drugs and Contrast Media. *ACR manual on contrast media,* version 10.1. Reston, VA: American College of Radiology; 2015.
Hardman JG, Limbird LE, eds. *Goodman & Gilman's The Pharmacological Basis of Therapeutics.* New York, NY: McGraw-Hill; 1996.

17. **A, Observation.** Mild allergic-type reactions to both iodinated and gadolinium based intravenous contrast agents include hives, mild angioedema, and paroxysmal sneezing, which are usually self-limited and do not require medical treatment. Rarely, these symptoms may progress to moderate or severe allergic reactions. Thus, the ACR recommends monitoring vital signs and observing patients for 20 to 30 minutes or until the symptoms resolve.

Reference:
ACR Committee on Drugs and Contrast Media. *ACR manual on contrast media,* version 10.1. Reston, VA: American College of Radiology; 2015.

18. For treatment of diffuse hives that appear and enlarge after an iodinated contrast agent injection the best treatment would be:
    A. Observation
    B. Cold compress
    C. Diphenhydramine
    D. Atropine

19. For treatment of diffuse hives (Figure 8-1) that appear and enlarge after a gadolinium injection, the best treatment would be:
    A. Observation
    B. Cold compress
    C. Diphenhydramine
    D. Atropine

20. For treatment of the awake and alert patent who is wheezing and drooling after a gadolinium injection (Figure 8-2) the best treatment would be:
    A. Observation
    B. Oxygen, bronchodilators, and epinephrine
    C. Oxygen, diphenhydramine, steroids, epinephrine
    D. Oxygen, atropine, steroids

21. For treatment of an awake and alert patient with hypotension, tachycardia, and anaphylaxis after a gadolinium injection (Figure 8-3) the initial treatment would be:
    A. Oxygen, Trendelenburg, fluids, epinephrine
    B. Oxygen, Trendelenburg, fluids
    C. Oxygen, diphenhydramine, steroids, epinephrine
    D. Oxygen, Trendelenburg, fluids, atropine, steroids

22. For treatment of an awake and alert patient with hypotension and bradycardia after a gadolinium injection the best treatment would be:
    A. Oxygen, Trendelenburg, fluids, epinephrine
    B. Oxygen, Trendelenburg, fluids, steroids
    C. Oxygen, diphenhydramine, steroids, epinephrine
    D. Oxygen, Trendelenburg, fluids, atropine

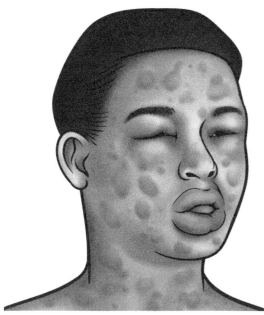

Figure 8-1 Diffuse urticaria

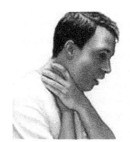

Figure 8-2 Airway distress (without choking)

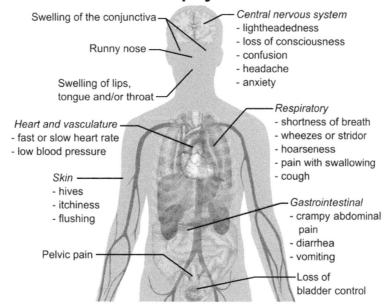

Signs and symptoms of
Anaphylaxis

Swelling of the conjunctiva

Runny nose

Swelling of lips, tongue and/or throat

Heart and vasculature
- fast or slow heart rate
- low blood pressure

Skin
- hives
- itchiness
- flushing

Pelvic pain

Central nervous system
- lightheadedness
- loss of consciousness
- confusion
- headache
- anxiety

Respiratory
- shortness of breath
- wheezes or stridor
- hoarseness
- pain with swallowing
- cough

Gastrointestinal
- crampy abdominal pain
- diarrhea
- vomiting

Loss of bladder control

Figure 8-3 Anaphylaxis systemic effects

18. **C, Diphenhydramine.** Moderate allergic-type reactions including diffuse hives should receive prompt treatment with antihistamine agents such as diphenhydramine, which may decrease adverse symptoms and decrease the risk of progression into more life-threatening allergic reactions. Close clinical monitoring of these patients is especially important. Cold or warm compresses may be considered for symptomatic relief in patients with uncomplicated injection site contrast extravasation. Atropine may be considered for vasovagal reactions presenting with hypotension and bradycardia.

Reference:
ACR Committee on Drugs and Contrast Media. *ACR manual on contrast media,* version 10.1. Reston, VA: American College of Radiology; 2015.

19. **C, Diphenhydramine.** Allergic-type reactions to both iodinated and gadolinium based contrast agents are mediated by the same mechanisms. Gadolinium-mediated moderate allergic-type reactions are therefore most appropriately treated with the same H-1 receptor blockers (diphenhydramine) used to treat the reactions to iodinated contrast material. A targeted physical assessment must be performed on all patients suspected of a contrast reaction. Reactions can be minor, including urticaria, or severe such as seizures and pulmonary edema. A most appropriate treatment option must be determined at the time of assessment. Urticarial reactions are allergic-like and most often mild and self-limited. There is a risk of progression in severity or number of hives as well as progression to more serious symptoms such as angioedema. Typically medical treatment is not necessary although observation for 30 to 60 minutes may be prudent. Oral antihistamines such as diphenhydramine are often the first-line treatment, although if refractory and progressive, second-line treatment such as intravenous antihistamines, beta agonist inhalers, epinephrine, atropine, and oxygen may be required.

Reference:
ACR Committee on Drugs and Contrast Media. *ACR manual on contrast media,* version 10.1. Reston, VA: American College of Radiology; 2015.

20. **B, Oxygen, bronchodilators, and epinephrine.** The patient description here displays signs of laryngeal edema and bronchospasm. These patients will often wheeze and are unable to swallow oral secretions. Oxygen via a face mask at 6 to 10 L/min, cardiopulmonary monitoring to include EKG, pulse oximetry, and blood pressure, administration of a beta-agonist such as albuterol, and epinephrine (SC or IM (1:1000) 0.1-0.3 mL (= 0.1-0.3 mg) or, if hypotensive, epinephrine (1:10,000) slowly IV 1 mL (= 0.1 mg) repeat up to 1 mg) is the most appropriate treatment protocol.

Reference:
<http://www.acr.org/~/media/ACR/Documents/PDF/QualitySafety/Resources/Contrast%20Manual/2015_Contrast_Media.pdf>.

21. **A, Oxygen, Trendelenburg, fluids, epinephrine.** The basic treatment for all patients with hypotension following the administration of gadolinium based contrast agents includes maintenance of IV access, vital sign monitoring, administration of O_2 by mask 6 to 10 L/min, elevation of their legs at least 60 degrees, and administration of IV fluids (0.9% normal saline 1000 mL rapidly or lactated Ringer's 1000 mL rapidly). Additionally, in this patient with tachycardia who is suffering an anaphylactoid reaction, epinephrine IV or IM should be administered.

References:
<http://emedicine.medscape.com/article/135065-treatment#d9>.
<http://www.acr.org/~/media/ACR/Documents/PDF/QualitySafety/Resources/Contrast%20Manual/2015_Contrast_Media.pdf>.

22. **D, Oxygen, Trendelenburg, fluids, atropine.** The basic treatment for all patients with hypotension following the administration of gadolinium based contrast agents includes maintenance of IV access, vital sign monitoring, administration of O_2 by mask 6 to 10 L/min, elevation of their legs at least 60 degrees, and administration of IV fluids (0.9% normal saline 1000 mL rapidly or lactated Ringer's 1000 mL rapidly). Additionally, in this patient with bradycardia, if unresponsive to the aforementioned treatment, atropine (IV) 0.6 to 1.0 mg should be administered into a running IV infusion of fluids and repeated as necessary up to 3 mg. This is the best treatment for a patient as described with a vasovagal reaction.

Reference:
<http://www.acr.org/~/media/ACR/Documents/PDF/QualitySafety/Resources/Contrast%20Manual/2015_Contrast_Media.pdf>.

23. Contrast-induced nephropathy:
    A. Currently is widely accepted as the cause of creatinine elevation within 24 hours after iodinated contrast injection
    B. Currently is widely accepted as the cause of creatinine elevation within 4 days after iodinated contrast injection
    C. Currently is widely accepted as the cause of creatinine elevation within 1 week after iodinated contrast injection
    D. Currently is being scrutinized as to whether it exists at all

24. Risk factors for contrast-induced nephropathy include:
    A. Preexisting kidney disease
    B. Iodine allergy
    C. Gadolinium allergy
    D. Metformin use

25. If you have had a previous hypersensitivity reaction to iodinated contrast, what is your repeat risk rate (assuming no premedication):
    A. 0-20%
    B. 21-40%
    C. 41-60%
    D. >60%

26. The rate of anaphylactic reactions to gadolinium based contrast agents compared to iodinated contrast agents is approximately:
    A. 1 : 1
    B. 1 : 10
    C. 1 : 100
    D. 1 : 1000

27. Gadolinium contrast administrated is contraindicated in:
    A. Early trimester pregnant patients
    B. Patients with moderate kidney failure
    C. Patients with iodine contrast dye allergies
    D. Patients on dialysis

28. Risk factors for nephrogenic systemic fibrosis do NOT include:
    A. Severe chronic kidney failure
    B. Acute hepatorenal failure
    C. Multiple high doses of gadolinium
    D. Use of macrocyclic gadolinium agents

29. Nephrogenic systemic fibrosis has been eliminated by withholding gadolinium agents in patients with an estimated glomerular filtration rate of:
    A. <60 cc/min
    B. <30 cc/min
    C. 30-60 mL/min/1.73 m^2
    D. <30 mL/min/1.73 m^2

23. **D, Currently is being scrutinized as to whether it exists at all.** There is recent evidence that nephrotoxicity following the administration of iodinated contrast is unusual for both inpatients and outpatients. Nephrotoxicity following contrast administration for CT occurs less frequently than after cardiac catheterization procedures, and comorbid conditions may be the strongest factor of renal dysfunction. Contrast-related nephrotoxicity is not likely to be an important clinical event, is unlikely to occur among healthy patients, and is usually limited to a transient elevation of serum creatinine.

Reference:
<http://www.appliedradiology.com/articles/the-myth-and-reality-of-contrast-induced-nephropathy>.

24. **A, Preexisting kidney disease.** Severe preexisting kidney disease is probably the strongest risk factor for nephrotoxicity following the administration of iodinated contrast. Allergies to iodinated contrast or gadolinium based contrast, although potentially serious, do not affect renal function primarily. Metformin is not a risk factor. In fact, does contrast induced nephrotoxicity even exist? Some say no.

References:
<http://www.appliedradiology.com/articles/the-myth-and-reality-of-contrast-induced-nephropathy>.
<http://www.acr.org/~/media/ACR/Documents/PDF/QualitySafety/Resources/Contrast%20Manual/2015_Contrast_Media.pdf>.

25. **B, 21–40%.** The risk of repeat immediate hypersensitivity reaction to a contrast agent is 30% in patients who experienced prior allergic reaction. Immediate hypersensitivity reaction ("allergic reaction") occurs less frequently with low-osmolar nonionic iodinated contrast media used for computed tomography, ranging from 0.17% to 2.4% with a mean incidence of 0.079%. The incidence rate per person is approximately 0.12%. Most of these reactions result in mild urticarial rash. Patients with history of allergy or asthma are at 2.3 to 3.7 times increased risk of developing immediate hypersensitivity reactions. Therefore, ACR guidelines on contrast media recommend premedication with corticosteroids in patients with history of prior hypersensitivity reaction to contrast agent.

References:
Jung JW, Kang HR, Kim MH, et al. Immediate hypersensitivity reaction to gadolinium-based MR contrast media. *Radiology.* 2012;264(2):414-422.
American College of Radiology. *ACR manual on contrast media*, version 10.1, 2015. <http://www.acr.org/~/media/ACR/Documents/PDF/QualitySafety/Resources/Contrast%20Manual/2015_Contrast_Media.pdf>. Published 2015. Accessed 01.11.15.

26. **C, 1:100.** Risk of anaphylaxis following MR contrast media administration averages 0.008%, but ranges in various epidemiological studies from 0.004% to 0.01%. Mortality rate from such reactions is approximately 0.0019%, with approximately 40 reported deaths per 51 million administered doses. Signs and symptoms include hypotension, angioedema, urticaria, dyspnea, bronchospasm, hypoxia, decreased consciousness, headache, nausea, and vomiting. Treatment includes supportive care including hydration, antihistamines, vasopressors, beta-2 agonists, and glucocorticoids.

References:
Jung JW, Kang HR, Kim MH, et al. Immediate hypersensitivity reaction to gadolinium-based MR contrast media. *Radiology.* 2012;264(2):414-422.
Prince MR, Zhang H, Zou Z, et al. Incidence of immediate gadolinium contrast media reactions. *AJR Am J Roentgenol.* 2011;196(2):W138-W143.
American College of Radiology. *ACR manual on contrast media*, version 10.1, 2015. <http://www.acr.org/~/media/ACR/Documents/PDF/QualitySafety/Resources/Contrast%20Manual/2015_Contrast_Media.pdf>. Published 2015. Accessed 01.11.15.

27. **A, Early trimester pregnant patients.** Because there no randomized controlled human subject studies to date using gadolinium based contrast agents, the exact effect of gadolinium-based contrast agent (GBCA) on fetuses is unknown. Primate studies have demonstrated GBCA to cross the placenta and thus are assumed to cross the human placenta. GBCA are excreted via the urinary tract into the amniotic fluid and are not "effectively" removed because they remain within the amniotic fluid. As such, GBCA are contraindicated in early pregnancy, unless there is a medical emergency necessitating utilization of GBCA.

References:
American College of Radiology. *ACR manual on contrast media*, version 10.1, 2015. <http://www.acr.org/~/media/ACR/Documents/PDF/QualitySafety/Resources/Contrast%20Manual/2015_Contrast_Media.pdf>. Published 2015. Accessed 01.11.15.
Beckett KR, Moriarity AK, Langer JM. Safe use of contrast media: What the radiologist needs to know. *Radiographics.* 2015;35(6):1738-1750.

28. **D, Use of macrocyclic gadolinium agents.** Risk factors for nephrogenic systemic fibrosis (NSF) include chronic kidney disease with glomerular filtration rate less than 30 mL/min and are highest in patients with end-stage renal disease on hemodialysis. NSF does not appear to be related to duration or etiology of renal failure. High risk agents associated with NSF include gadodiamide (Omniscan), gadoversetamids (OptiMARK), gadopentetate dimeglumine (Magnevist). Intermediate risk agents include gadofosveset (Ablavar), gadoxetate disodium (Eovist), and gadoenate dimeglumine (MultiHance). Low risk agents include gadoteridol (ProHance), gadoterate meglumine (Dotarem), and gadobutrol (Gadavist). The potential dissociation of gadolinium from the parent compound, which is seen most commonly with linear nonionic agents, has led to their characterization as agents with the highest potential risk for NSF. Dialysis does not appear to prevent NSF. Hepatic failure is not considered a risk factor for NSF. In patients at risk for NSF, GBCA should be avoided.

References:
American College of Radiology. *ACR manual on contrast media*, version 10.1, 2015. <http://www.acr.org/~/media/ACR/Documents/PDF/QualitySafety/Resources/Contrast%20Manual/2015_Contrast_Media.pdf>. Published 2015. Accessed 01.11.15.
Beckett KR, Moriarity AK, Langer JM. Safe use of contrast media: What the radiologist needs to know. *Radiographics.* 2015;35(6):1738-1750.

29. **D, <30 mL/min/1.73 m².** Estimated rate of NSF in end-stage renal disease (ESRD; stage V chronic kidney disease, GFR <15 mL/min/1.73 m²) and with stage IV renal disease (GFR less than 30 mL/min/1.73 m²) is 1% to 7%. NSF is most commonly reported in patients on dialysis. Patients with stage IV CKD comprise 3% of all reported cases of NSF. To date, only one case of NSF has been in a patient with GFR greater than 30 mL/min/1.73 m². Because renal failure is the main determinant factor for development of NSF, withholding gadolinium in patients with stage IV renal disease (GFR less than 30 mL/min/1.73 m²) is the single most effective way of preventing NSF.

References:
American College of Radiology. *ACR manual on contrast media*, version 10.1, 2015. <http://www.acr.org/~/media/ACR/Documents/PDF/QualitySafety/Resources/Contrast%20Manual/2015_Contrast_Media.pdf>. Published 2015. Accessed 01.11.15.
Beckett KR, Moriarity AK, Langer JM. Safe use of contrast media: What the radiologist needs to know. *Radiographics.* 2015;35(6):1738-1750.

30. The two biggest issues associated with extravasated contrast agents are:
    A. Cellulitis and necrosis
    B. Cellulitis and nephrogenic systemic fibrosis
    C. Compartment syndrome and necrosis
    D. Compartment syndrome and cellulitis

31. Recommended treatments for extravasation do not include:
    A. Elevation
    B. Cold compresses
    C. Warm compresses
    D. Aspiration of contrast from site

32. Which of the following is an example of "off-label" use?
    A. Magnevist for children under 2 years of age
    B. Iohexol for children under 2 years of age
    C. Penicillin for tonsillitis
    D. Technetium pertechnetate for bone scanning

33. Off-label use is:
    A. Extremely risky
    B. Frequently utilized
    C. Regulated by IRBs
    D. Not utilized

34. Using off-label drugs in a research protocol requires:
    A. Nondisclosure agreements
    B. An investigational device exemption
    C. Double blind randomized trials
    D. Acknowledgments

35. You are employing off-label use of methacrylate for fibroid obliterations.
    A. You can advertise for this online
    B. You can advertise for this within your medical magazine
    C. You cannot advertise for this
    D. You cannot use that agent for that indication

36. The American College of Radiology the National Radiology Data Registry (NRDR) Intravenous Contrast Extravasation (ICE) Registry provides:
    A. Biannual reports on interventional radiology procedures' radiation dosage ranges
    B. Annual reports on interventional radiology complication rates
    C. Biannual reports on intravenous contrast dye extravasation
    D. None of the above

37. The goal(s) of ICE is/are to:
    A. Reduce contrast extravasation rates
    B. Reduce the radiation exposure during IR procedures
    C. Identify intravenous contrast agents that do not cause kidney damage
    D. All of the above

30. **C, Compartment syndrome and necrosis.** The rate of intravenous contrast extravasation (ICE) ranges from 0.1% to 0.9% and extravasation can occur with a power injection or hand injection. Patients may be asymptomatic or experience pain (burning or stinging), swelling, and/or tightness after ICME. Local inflammatory response to ICME peaks between 24 and 48 hours. Most patients recover without complications following ICME. However, rarely compartment syndrome, skin ulceration, and tissue necrosis can complicate ICME. These complications are more likely to occur following large volumes of contrast media extravasation, and these can be seen as early as 6 hours following ICME.

References:
American College of Radiology. *ACR manual on contrast media*, version 10.1, 2015. <http://www.acr.org/~/media/ACR/Documents/PDF/QualitySafety/Resources/Contrast%20Manual/2015_Contrast_Media.pdf>. Published 2015. Accessed 01.11.15.
Beckett KR, Moriarity AK, Langer JM. Safe use of contrast media: What the radiologist needs to know. *Radiographics*. 2015;35(6):1738-1750.

31. **D, Aspiration of contrast from site.** Prompt recognition of ICME is especially important in cases with large volume ICME because these patients are more at risk of developing complications including skin ulceration, compartment syndrome, or tissues necrosis. Close clinical follow-up is recommended in patients following ICME. Recommended treatments for ICME include elevation of the affected extremity above the level of the heart to promote resorption of contrast media. Warm or cold compresses can be used. Warm compresses reportedly aid in resorption of extravasated contrast while the cold compresses reportedly aid in alleviation of pain. Because there is paucity of data supporting benefit of aspiration of contrast media, it is not recommended by the ACR.

Reference:
American College of Radiology. *ACR manual on contrast media*, version 10.1, 2015. <http://www.acr.org/~/media/ACR/Documents/PDF/QualitySafety/Resources/Contrast%20Manual/2015_Contrast_Media.pdf>. Published 2015. Accessed 01.11.15.

32. **A, Magnevist for children under 2 years of age.** Magnevist usage with magnetic resonance imaging is indicated for detection of lesions with abnormal vascularity in the central nervous tissue and extracranial/extraspinal tissues and the body in adults and pediatric patients who are 2 years of age and older. Therefore, usage of Magnevist for children under 2 years of age is considered "off-label." Although in a study in children between 2 months and 2 years of age, the pharmacokinetics of Magnevist were similar to adults, safety and efficacy in this population have not been established.

Reference:
Magnevist—gadopentetate dimeglumine injection [FDA Label]. Bayer HealthCare Pharmaceuticals Inc. Whippany, NJ 07981: 2014 June. <http://www.accessdata.fda.gov/spl/data/640b8995-8945-4f87-b40d-733786fdc88e/640b8995-8945-4f87-b40d-733786fdc88e.xml>.

33. **B, Frequently utilized.** Off-label drug use is very common. In a study by Radley et al in 2006, 21% of prescriptions for commonly used medications were for off-label use. In another study by Shah et al, it was reported that 78.9% of children who were discharged from an emergency department in 2004 were taking at least one medication for off-label use. Off-label drugs can actually become common treatments for certain conditions, an example being tricyclic antidepressants for the treatment of neuropathic pain.

References:
Radley DC, et al. Off-label prescribing among office-based physicians. *Arch Intern Med.* 2006;166(9):1021-1026.

Shah SS, et al. Off-label drug use in hospitalized children. *Arch Pediatr Adolesc Med.* 2007;161(3):282-290.
Wittich CM, et al. Ten common questions (and their answers) about off-label drug use. *Mayo Clin Proc.* 2012;87(10):982-990. doi:10.1016/j.mayocp.2012.04.017; [Epub 2012 Aug 6].

34. **B, An investigational device exemption.** Off-label use of drugs by a physician for the "practice of medicine" does not require an Investigational New Drug Application, Investigational Device Exemption, or review by institutional review board. However, in the setting of a research protocol in which there will be off-label use of the drug, an Investigational Device Exemption or Investigational New Drug Application is required.

Reference:
"Off-Label" and Investigational Use of Marketed Drugs, biologics, and medical devices - Information Sheet. US Food and Drug Administration. 2014. <http://www.fda.gov/RegulatoryInformation/Guidances/ucm126486.htm>.

35. **C, You cannot advertise for this.** Off-label use of medications by physicians is permitted for the "practice of medicine" on the basis of sound medical evidence and scientific rationale. In addition, physicians should keep records of these medications' use and side effects. However, advertising for off-label indications is prohibited under the "false claims act." Under this act, marketing for off-label indications is subject to civil liability and criminal penalties. According to 21 CFR 312.2(b)(1), an Investigational New Drug Application (IND) may be needed for promotion of off-label indications.

References:
Ventola CL. Off-label drug information. *Pharm Therapeutics.* 2009;34(8):428-440.
"Off-Label" and Investigational Use of Marketed Drugs, biologics, and medical devices—Information Sheet. US Food and Drug Administration. 2014. <http://www.fda.gov/RegulatoryInformation/Guidances/ucm126486.htm>.

36. **C, Biannual reports on intravenous contrast dye extravasation.** The ACR intravenous contrast extravasation initiative is limited to the issues surrounding inadvertent extravasation of contrast agents outside the vascular system. Participation in the ICE initiative can fulfill a practice quality improvement program but requires that participants provide 6 months of data on practice extravasation events. The ICE team provides feedback comparing the participants' extravasation rates with national benchmarks.

Reference:
The American College of Radiology. *IV contrast extravasation registry user guide.* 2014. <http://www.acr.org/~/media/ACR/Documents/PDF/QualitySafety/NRDR/ICE/UserGuideICE.pdf>.

37. **A, Reduce contrast extravasation rates.** The ACR intravenous contrast extravasation initiative encourages creation of remediation efforts to reduce the rate of extravasation. Before and after data sets are provided leading to assessment of the effectiveness of the intervention. The model is the Plan Do Study Act cycle that allows revisiting an issue after an "act" to see its impact on the issue studied. The participant can repeat the cycle as many times as desired, but PQI credit for American Board of Radiology Maintenance of Certification can be earned as a PQI project only once.

Reference:
The American College of Radiology. *IV contrast extravasation registry user guide.* 2014. <http://www.acr.org/~/media/ACR/Documents/PDF/QualitySafety/NRDR/ICE/UserGuideICE.pdf>.

38. What is the earliest time period in which patients with thyroid cancer can receive I-131 treatment after iodinated contrast has been given?
    A. The next week
    B. >2 weeks
    C. >4 weeks
    D. >6 weeks

39. The reason for this delay is:
    A. Iodinated contrast prevents I-131 scanning
    B. Non-contrast scans are sufficient for imaging thyroid cancers
    C. It blocks I-131 therapeutic uptake
    D. It blocks Tc pertechnetate surveillance

40. As far as gadolinium in lactating mothers, the most recent literature suggests:
    A. Pumping for 24 hours and then resume breast feeding
    B. Pumping for 48 hours and then resume breast feeding
    C. Pumping for 24 hours and then resume breast feeding
    D. No need to pump. Continue breast feeding

38. **D, >6 weeks.** Prior to I-131 therapy a state of iodine deficiency should be induced in patients to increase I-131 uptake. Current recommendations suggest I-131 treatment should be delayed at least 6 to 8 weeks after the most recent water-soluble iodinated contrast administration.

Reference:

Silberstein EB, Alavi A, Balon HR, et al. The SNM practice guideline for therapy of thyroid disease with I-131 3.0. *J Nucl Med.* 2012;53(10):1633-1651.

39. **C, It blocks I-131 therapeutic uptake.** High levels of exogenous iodine can block uptake of radioactive iodine used for treatment of the cancer. Patients with carcinoma of the thyroid considered for I-131 treatment should therefore not receive IV or oral administration of iodinated contrast media (ionic or nonionic) for 6 to 8 weeks before the I-131 treatment.

References:

Robbins RJ, Schlumberger MJ. The evolving role of I-131 for the treatment of differentiated thyroid carcinoma. *J Nucl Med.* 2005;46:28S-37S.

Pluijemn MJ, Eustatia-Rutten C, Goslings BM, et al. Effects of low-iodide diet on postsurgical radioiodide ablation therapy in patients with differentiated thyroid carcinoma. *Clin Endocrinol.* 2003;58(4):428-435.

40. **D, No need to pump.** Continue breast feeding. Only a small percentage of GBCA is excreted in breast milk and absorbed by the infant. There are no reported adverse effects of GBCA in pregnant or lactating females or infants, including hypersensitivity reactions or direct toxicity of GBCA. As such, as per ACR guidelines, lactating females need not stop breast feeding. However, if the mother is concerned about any potential presently unknown adverse effect of GBCA on infants, she may withhold breast feeding for 12 to 24 hours and express and discard breast milk during this time interval.

References:

American College of Radiology. *ACR manual on contrast media*, version 10.1, 2015. <http://www.acr.org/~/media/ACR/Documents/PDF/QualitySafety/Resources/Contrast%20Manual/2015_Contrast_Media.pdf>. Published 2015. Accessed 01.11.15.

Beckett KR, Moriarity AK, Langer JM. Safe use of contrast media: What the radiologist needs to know. *Radiographics.* 2015;35(6):1738-1750.

QUESTIONS

1. What components of a medicolegal suit must be established for a successful litigation against a physician?
   A. Informed consent, breach of standard of care, negligence, harm
   B. A doctor-patient relationship, deviation from the standard of care, a cause and effect relationship between the deviation and harm to the patient, damages
   C. A doctor-patient relationship, a negligent act, harm (economic and/or emotional) to the patient, and expert witness confirmation that negligence existed in that locale
   D. Jurisdiction, statute of limitations, effective representation, Miranda rights

2. Dr. Dodd performs a fluoroscopically guided lumbar puncture successfully on a patient. The patient does well immediately thereafter and has no long-term consequences from the study. Dr. Dodd realizes that evening he forgot to get consent on the patient. Which is true?
   A. He cannot be held liable based on the gross negligence in failure to obtain consent
   B. He could be held liable in this case despite no apparent damages
   C. Failure to obtain consent is NOT considered battery in the United States
   D. He should get the consent form filled out after the procedure

3. With regard to expert witness testimony, the ACR's policy suggests:
   A. One should testify as an expert witness
   B. One should only testify for physicians' defense
   C. One should testify equally for plaintiffs and defendants
   D. One should not testify as an expert witness

4. Which of these is unethical?
   A. Testifying against members of your own profession
   B. Testifying only in cases where you can defend physicians
   C. Testifying such that you receive a portion of the damages awarded
   D. Testifying for $1500 per hour

5. Dr. Sewell agrees to testify and says that he only expects to get paid if the verdict comes out in favor of his "side." This is:
   A. Generous
   B. Impartial
   C. Commendable
   D. Unethical

6. Dr. Trudeau has been sued successfully six times for negligence.
   A. She should be disqualified as an expert witness
   B. She is eligible as an expert witness
   C. She should be banned from practice
   D. Her experience in the courtroom should make her a better witness

7. Experts should let the jury know, with respect to the physician sued:
   A. What a reasonably prudent individual in a similar situation might have been expected to do
   B. What they (the expert) would have done in a similar situation
   C. What the patient had reason to expect to have done in that situation
   D. All of the above

1. **B, A doctor-patient relationship, deviation from the standard of care, a cause and effect relationship between the deviation and harm to the patient, damages.** Successful litigation against a physician requires four components: (1) There must be an established doctor patient relationship (duty), (2) there must be a deviation from the standard of care (negligence), (3) this deviation from the standard must be the cause of harm to the patient (causation), and (4) the patient has to suffer damages, which includes actual economic loss (lost income, the cost of future medical care) and noneconomic losses (pain and suffering). Therefore the correct answer is B.

Reference:
Bal BS. Legal elements of medical malpractice. In: An Introduction to Medical Malpractice in the United States. *Clin Orthop Relat Res.* 2009;467(2):339-347. <http://www.ncbi.nlm.nih.gov/pmc/articles/PMC2628513/>.

2. **B, He could be held liable in this case despite no apparent damages.** Even though there were no long-term consequences to the patient, Dr. Dodd did deviate from the standard of care (forgetting to obtain consent prior to the procedure). It may be possible to prove harm at a later point, and thus Dr. Dodd can still be held liable (correct answer B). The statute of limitation varies by state as do the implications of not obtaining consent (A, gross negligence, B, battery). Documenting consent after the procedure (D) could help Dr. Dodd show he is attempting to adhere to the standard of care, but won't exonerate him.

Reference:
Bal BS. Legal elements of medical malpractice. In: An Introduction to Medical Malpractice in the United States. *Clin Orthop Relat Res.* 2009;467(2):339-347. <http://www.ncbi.nlm.nih.gov/pmc/articles/PMC2628513/>.

3. **A, One should testify as an expert witness.** The ACR Practice Parameter on the Physician Expert Witness in Radiology and Radiation Oncology serves as a tool to assist practitioners rather than an inflexible rule or requirement of practice. It states that medical expert witness testimony is indicated in any legal proceeding in which the court needs an objective physician who is not a party to the case, has no personal interest in the outcome of the case, and has expertise in the matter at hand to explain the issues.

References:
The ACR practice parameter on the physician expert witness in radiology and radiation oncology. <http://www.acr.org/~/media/ACR/Documents/PGTS/guidelines/Expert_Witness.pdf>.
Berlin L. Can a radiologist be compelled to testify as an expert witness? *AJR Am J Roentgenol.* 2005;185(1):36-42.

4. **C, Testifying such that you receive a portion of the damages awarded.** The ACR Code of Ethics states "the diagnostic radiologist, radiation oncologist, interventional radiologist, nuclear medicine physician, or medical physicist shall not accept compensation that is contingent upon the outcome of litigation." Compensation of the expert witness should not be linked to the amount of the award that is provided to the plaintiff. Regarding compensation of the expert witness, the ACR Practice Parameter on the Physician Expert Witness in Radiology and Radiation Oncology recommends that it should reflect the time and effort involved.

References:
2015-2016 ACR Code of Ethics. <http://www.acr.org/~/media/ACR/Documents/PDF/Membership/Governance/2015_2016 Code of Ethics.pdf>.
The ACR practice parameter on the physician expert witness in radiology and radiation oncology. <http://www.acr.org/~/media/ACR/Documents/PGTS/guidelines/Expert_Witness.pdf>.

5. **D, Unethical.** The ACR Code of Ethics states "the diagnostic radiologist, radiation oncologist, interventional radiologist, nuclear medicine physician, or medical physicist shall not accept compensation that is contingent upon the outcome of litigation." Regarding compensation of the expert witness, the ACR Practice Parameter on the Physician Expert Witness in Radiology and Radiation Oncology recommends that it should reflect the time and effort involved.

References:
2015-2016 ACR Code of Ethics. <http://www.acr.org/~/media/ACR/Documents/PDF/Membership/Governance/2015_2016 Code of Ethics.pdf>.
The ACR practice parameter on the physician expert witness in radiology and radiation oncology. <http://www.acr.org/~/media/ACR/Documents/PGTS/guidelines/Expert_Witness.pdf>.

6. **B, She is eligible as an expert witness.** The ACR Practice Parameter on the Physician Expert Witness in Radiology and Radiation Oncology states that the expert witness should be a physician with the following qualifications:
   - Licensure and active engagement at the time of the incident and for a reasonable period of time in the practice of the radiologic specialty relating to the testimony
   - Certification by the appropriate board
   - Education, training, and practical experience, as well as current knowledge and skill, concerning the subject matter of the case, including in a medical liability case, the relevant standard of care

   In this question, the fact that the doctor has been successfully sued six times for negligence would not affect her eligibility to act as an expert witness.

References:
2015-2016 ACR Code of Ethics. http://www.acr.org/~/media/ACR/Documents/PDF/Membership/Governance/2015_2016 Code of Ethics.pdf.
The ACR practice parameter on the physician expert witness in radiology and radiation oncology. <http://www.acr.org/~/media/ACR/Documents/PGTS/guidelines/Expert_Witness.pdf>.

7. **A, What a reasonably prudent individual in a similar situation might have been expected to do.** The role of the expert witness is to help the fact finder analyze the issues in dispute necessary to decide the case. He/She is expected to give an opinion regarding the reasonableness of the conduct of the parties at hand. The standard of care centers on whether the physician exercised a reasonable and ordinary degree of care and skill. It is not recommended that the expert witness speculate on what he/she would have done or what the patient had reason to expect in that situation. It is about what a reasonably prudent individual in a similar situation might have been expected to do.

References:
The ACR practice parameter on the physician expert witness in radiology and radiation oncology. <http://www.acr.org/~/media/ACR/Documents/PGTS/guidelines/Expert_Witness.pdf>.
Berlin L. Standard of care. *AJR Am J Roentgenol.* 1998;170(2):275-278.

8. With respect to expert witness testimony:
   A. It cannot be questioned after the fact
   B. It can lead to sanctions by the expert's medical society
   C. It cannot lead to review by a medical board
   D. It is protected

9. Two experts are opining about a case of a woman who had a possible 2-mm right MCA aneurysm identified on a CTA performed for a family history of aneurysms. During the subsequent digital subtraction angiogram, the right vertebral artery was injected as part of a four-vessel study. The vertebral artery was dissected during the angiogram. The patient suffered a devastating brainstem stroke. The plaintiff expert said that, given a normal CTA of the vertebrobasilar circulation, the neurointerventionalist should not have been catheterizing that vessel. The defense expert disagreed. This is an example of disagreement on:
   A. Duty
   B. Standard of care
   C. Causation
   D. Principles

10. The plaintiff expert argued that the clinician who ordered the conventional angiogram had no business requiring that study because CTAs are as good as DSA for aneuryms. The defense expert said DSA is the gold standard. This is an example of a disagreement on:
    A. Duty
    B. Standard of care
    C. Causation
    D. Evidence-based medicine

11. The defense attorney argued that the brainstem stroke was due to a reaction to the propofol given and not to the dissected vertebral artery. The plaintiff attorney said this was "hogwash." This is an example of a disagreement on:
    A. Duty
    B. Standard of care
    C. Causation
    D. Probability

12. The defense attorney argued that the attending neurointerventionalist, because he was outside the room directing the fellow in the room but not performing the procedure, should not be considered responsible for the vertebral artery dissection because he did not perform the actual study. The plaintiff lawyer said this was absurd. This is an example of a disagreement on:
    A. Duty
    B. Standard of care
    C. Causation
    D. Probability

13. The plaintiff attorney argued that the neurologist who ordered the study was responsible for the unfortunate outcome of the study because the risks and benefits had to be considered before ordering the study. The defense attorney answered, "Balderdash." This is an example of a disagreement on:
    A. Duty
    B. Standard of care
    C. Informed consent
    D. Intended agent

14. The plaintiff attorney argued that despite the complete recovery from the brainstem stroke by his client, the patient should receive money for the days of work missed. The defense attorney noted that the patient received disability insurance remuneration after the patient exhausted 30 days of paid sick leave. This is an example of a disagreement on:
    A. Causation
    B. Damages
    C. Punitive remuneration
    D. None of the above

8. **B, It can lead to sanctions by the expert's medical society.** The ACR Practice Parameter on the Physician Expert Witness in Radiology and Radiation Oncology states that the expert witness can be held accountable for statements made during a legal proceeding. They should be prepared to explain the basis of their opinion and should take care that their proffered testimony will be scientifically valid, can be or has been tested, and has withstood or could reasonably withstand a peer review.

The ACR Committee on Ethics reviews expert witness complaints, decides whether to investigate complaint, and in some cases imposes disciplinary sanctions against a member.

References:
The ACR practice parameter on the physician expert witness in radiology and radiation oncology. <http://www.acr.org/~/media/ACR/Documents/PGTS/guidelines/Expert_Witness.pdf>.
Berlin L, Hoffman TR, Shields WF, et al. American College of Radiology. When does expert witness testimony constitute a violation of the ACR Code of Ethics? The role of the ACR Committee on Ethics. *J Am Coll Radiol.* 2006;3(4):252-258. Review.
Berlin L. Bearing false witness. *AJR Am J Roentgenol.* 2003;180(6):1515-1521.

9. **B, Standard of care.** Standard of care is what a reasonable and prudent physician would exercise under similar circumstances. In this question there is disagreement as to what was the appropriate course of action during the care of a patient. Duty refers to a contractual agreement between patient and physician regarding the provision of health care; the lawyers are not arguing whether the physician was contractually obligated to care for the patient. Causation refers to damages being directly attributable to the action (or inaction) of the physician providing care; the lawyers are not arguing whether the catheterization caused the stroke but that injection should not have been performed. The last answer, principles, is a moral and not a legal term.

References:
Skeffington v. Bradley, 366 Mich. 552, 115 N.W.2d 303 (1962).
Brenner RJ. Breast cancer evaluation: medical legal issues. *Breast J.* 2004;10(1):6-9.

10. **B, Standard of care. Standard of care is what a reasonable and prudent physician would exercise under similar circumstances.** In this question there is disagreement as to what was the most appropriate study for the patient. Duty refers to a contractual agreement between patient and physician regarding the provision of health care; the lawyers are not arguing whether the physician was contractually obligated to care for the patient. Causation refers to damages being directly attributable to the action (or inaction) of the physician providing care; the lawyers are not arguing whether the catheterization caused the stroke but that the study should not have been ordered in the first place. "Evidence based medicine" is not a term used routinely in negligence litigation.

References:
Skeffington v. Bradley, 366 Mich. 552, 115 N.W.2d 303 (1962).
Brenner RJ. Breast cancer evaluation: medical legal issues. *Breast J.* 2004;10(1):6-9.

11. **C, Causation.** Causation is the direct correlation between damages and their cause. The lawyers are debating whether the fundamental insult leading to the patient's stroke was due to medication rather than catheterization/injection. Standard of care is what a reasonable and prudent physician would exercise under similar circumstances. Whether catheterization/injection is appropriate is no longer being discussed, nor is the appropriateness of propofol argued. Duty refers to a contractual agreement between patient and physician regarding the provision of health care; the lawyers are not arguing whether the physician was contractually obligated to care for the patient. "Probability" is a mathematical term and not a term routinely used in negligence law.

References:
Skeffington v. Bradley, 366 Mich. 552, 115 N.W.2d 303 (1962).
Brenner RJ. Breast cancer evaluation: medical legal issues. *Breast J.* 2004;10(1):6-9.

12. **A, Duty.** The lawyers are debating about the presence of duty of the attending physician to the patient. Duty refers to the contractual obligation of the physician to care for the patient. The defendant's attorney is trying to dissociate the neurointerventionalist from the agreement to provide care, or duty, because he did not personally perform the procedure. Standard of care is what a reasonable and prudent physician would exercise under similar circumstances; whether the procedure was appropriate is not being discussed. Causation is the direct correlation between damages and their cause; the lawyers are no longer debating whether the procedure caused the stroke. "Probability" is a mathematical term and not a term routinely used in negligence law.

References:
Skeffington v. Bradley, 366 Mich. 552, 115 N.W.2d 303 (1962).
Brenner RJ. Breast cancer evaluation: medical legal issues. *Breast J.* 2004;10(1):6-9.

13. **A, Duty.** The main disagreement is with regard to duty of care. Under this concept, the first thing that has to be established is the existence of a doctor-patient relationship. This usually begins once the physician pursues diagnostic or therapeutic options for the patient. Upon establishment of this relationship, the physician is expected to provide care that is consistent with his/her level of training. The relationship exists until either the physician or the patient terminates it. Given that there is an established doctor-patient relationship in this example, the plaintiff attorney is suggesting that it was the family practitioner's duty to look into the risks and benefits of the study.

Reference:
Rozovsky F. *Duty of care.* Legal Medicine—Virginia Commonwealth University School of Medicine. <http://www.medschool.vcu.edu/legalmedicine/duty_of_care/index.html>; 2015 June.

14. **B, Damages.** Damages can be described as either economic or noneconomic. Economic damages include medical expenses and loss of earnings or earning capacity. Noneconomic damages include mental distress, loss of ability to enjoy life's pleasures, and loss of function. In this case, the patient's inability to go to work falls under economic damages due to loss of earnings. Causation is the concept that the doctor's actions directly caused the patient's damage. Punitive remuneration is intended in cases where the defendant's behavior was considered "grossly negligent or intentional." Neither causation nor punitive remuneration applies to the disagreement in this question.

References:
Coppolo G. *Damages—medical malpractice.* Connecticut General Assembly. <https://www.cga.ct.gov/2004/rpt/2004-R-0002.htm>; January 2, 2004.
Bal BS. An introduction to medical malpractice in the United States. *Clin Ortho Related Res.* 2009;467(2):339-347.
Cohen Thomas H, Harbacek K. *Punitive damage awards in state courts, 2005.* U.S. Department of Justice, Bureau of Justice Statistics. <http://www.bjs.gov/content/pub/pdf/pdasc05.pdf>; 2011 March.

15. The defense lawyer argued that the patient had a 33% chance of the aneurysm rupturing during the angiogram because of its shape. That might have led to a brainstem stroke because of vasospasm, and therefore the outcome might have been the same no matter what. The plaintiff lawyer said, "That's bonkers!" This is an example of a disagreement based on:
    A. Duty
    B. Standard of care
    C. Consent
    D. None of the above

16. The plaintiff lawyer argued that the risks of a brainstem stroke were not adequately explained to his client or she would not have undergone the angiogram. Brainstem stroke is never specifically listed on the consent form although "stroke" is. He demands to see the consent forms used by all the defense experts' institutions. The defense lawyer said, "That's just wrong!" This is an example of a disagreement based on:
    A. Duty
    B. Standard of care
    C. Causation
    D. None of the above

17. In his final statements, the plaintiff lawyer argued that the performance of the angiogram by the neuroradiology fellow without the presence of an attending directly in the room is such an egregious deviation that the jury should "send a message to the plaintiff." The defense lawyer looked astounded and said, "I don't even know what to say about that." This would represent a disagreement on:
    A. Duty
    B. Standard of care
    C. Causation
    D. Damages

18. The main role of an institutional review board (IRB) is to:
    A. Ensure good science
    B. Protect the rights and welfare of human research subjects
    C. Assist investigators
    D. Ensure adequate informed consent is obtained

19. Outside IRBs (not within one's own institution):
    A. Are forbidden
    B. Are encouraged widely
    C. Are mandated by the CDC
    D. May approve studies at another institution

20. Qui tam refers to:
    A. The concept of "who knows": a wide swath of accusations
    B. Whistle blowing
    C. Medicare fraud
    D. Retaliation

21. "The failure to (a) establish an accurate and timely explanation of the patient's health problem(s) or (b) communicate that explanation to the patient" is the definition of what according to the Institute of Medicine?
    A. Malpractice
    B. Deviation from the standard of care
    C. Diagnostic error
    D. Deliberative failure

22. How do errors made in medicine harm patients?
    A. By preventing or delaying appropriate treatment
    B. By providing unnecessary or harmful treatment
    C. By resulting in psychological or financial repercussions
    D. All of the above

15. **D, None of the above. Duty of care refers to a physician's established relationship with a patient and the physician's obligation to provide care to the patient until either party terminates the relationship.** Standard of care refers to the principle that the physician is expected to provide care that would have been provided by another similarly situated physician with similar training. Causation is the concept that the doctor's actions directly caused the patient's damage. The lawyer may be arguing on the basis of causation that the damages were not caused by his client or he may be arguing about the damages: Would the damages have occurred no matter what?

References:
Rozovsky F. Duty of care. Legal Medicine—Virginia Commonwealth University School of Medicine. <http://www.medschool.vcu.edu/legalmedicine/duty_of_care/index.html>; 2015 June.
Bal BS. An introduction to medical malpractice in the United States. *Clin Ortho Related Res.* 2009;467(2):339-347.

16. **B, Standard of care.** Standard of care refers to the principle that a physician is expected to provide care that would have been provided by another similarly situated physician with similar training. In this case, the plaintiff lawyer is likely demanding to see all the consent forms used by the defense institutions to establish what the standard of care is regarding consent forms for angiograms at that institution compared to national norms. Causation is the concept that the physician's actions directly caused the patient's damage. Duty of care refers to a physician's established relationship with a patient and the physician's obligation to provide care to the patient until either party terminates the relationship.

References:
Bal BS. An introduction to medical malpractice in the United States. *Clin Ortho Related Res.* 2009;467(2):339-347.
Rozovsky F. Duty of care. Legal Medicine—Virginia Commonwealth University School of Medicine. <http://www.medschool.vcu.edu/legalmedicine/duty_of_care/index.html>; 2015 June.

17. **D, Damages. Damages can be compensatory or punitive.** Compensatory damages can further be broken down into economic and noneconomic damages. Economic damages include medical expenses and loss of earnings or earning capacity. Noneconomic damages include mental distress, loss of ability to enjoy life's pleasures, and loss of function. Punitive damages are intended in cases where the defendant's behavior was considered "grossly negligent or intentional." The purpose of punitive damages is to punish the defendant for his/her behavior and reform or deter the defendant from similar behavior in the future. In this case, the plaintiff lawyer wanting to "send a message to the plaintiff" for his egregious deviation is an example of truing to argue for punitive damages.

Reference:
Coppolo G. *Damages—medical malpractice.* Connecticut General Assembly. <https://www.cga.ct.gov/2004/rpt/2004-R-0002.htm>; Jan 2, 2004.

18. **B, Protect the rights and welfare of human research subjects.** As per the IRB Guidebook, the IRB is "established to protect the rights and welfare of human research subjects recruited to participate in research activities." While getting informed consents is part of the IRB review process, it is one of the many roles of an IRB and comes under "protecting the rights and welfare" of research subjects. Ensuring good science and assisting investigators are not the main roles of the IRB.

Reference:
Institutional Administration. *Institutional Review Board Guidebook*, Chapter 1. <http://www.hhs.gov/ohrp/archive/irb/irb_chapter1.htm>; Feb 5, 1993.

19. **D, May approve studies at another institution.** Although institutions that have their own IRBs will generally have jurisdiction over all studies performed solely within that institution, there are two cases in which outside IRBs typically are permitted. One is if the scope of the project is greater than that single institution, and the other is if the expertise to examine the study is not available from the local IRB. Outside IRBs may even be from another country. But there are caveats: In addition to expertise on conditions in which the proposed research is conducted and the risks to participants [Rules from FDA bulletin 21 CFR 56.111] an outside IRB must have an understanding of the "local community attitudes" in the locations in which proposed research would take place.

Therefore, while outside IRBs are not forbidden, encouraged, or required, they are permitted in certain circumstances.

Reference:
FDA Regulatory Information, Non-local IRB Review Information Sheet, published 2014-06-25. <www.fda.gov/regulatoryinformation/guidances/ucm126423.htm>. Accessed November 16, 2015.

20. **B, Whistle blowing.** The False Claims Act is a federal law conferring liability to those who would commit fraud against the government. When someone reports such fraud within his own organization it is referred to as "whistleblowing." Such whistleblowing often results in legal action against the organization, the individual, or both. Qui tam is an abbreviation for a Latin phrase translating to "he who prosecutes for himself as well as for the King." In the United States, qui tam provisions allow the whistleblower to receive a percentage of the funds the government recovers from the prosecution of a fraud case.

Reference:
Doyle C. *Qui tam: The False Claims Act and related federal statutes.* Congressional Research Service, 7-5700. R40784. <https://www.fas.org/sgp/crs/misc/R40785.pdf>; August 6, 2009.

21. **C, Diagnostic error.** The institute of medicine defines diagnostic errors as "The failure to (a) establish an accurate and timely explanation of the patient's health problem(s) or (b) communicate that explanation to the patient." The multifaceted definition serves to explain that a diagnosis consists of more than simply labeling a patient as having a particular disease. It also serves to note that the process of arriving at a diagnosis is a complex one. The term, as defined, has an emphasis on the patient and the error's impact on the patient, in order to keep in mind that the ultimate consequence of diagnostic errors can be patient harm.

Reference:
Institute of Medicine. Improving Diagnosis in Health Care, Quality Chasm Series. *Report in Brief.* <http://iom.nationalacademies.org/~/media/Files/Report%20Files/2015/Improving-Diagnosis/DiagnosticError_ReportBrief.pdf>; September 2015.

22. **D, All of the above. Diagnostic errors are a common occurrence.** In fact, most patients will experience one at some point in their lifetime, and 5% of outpatients per year will be exposed to one. The results of such errors can be significant and include the prevention or delay of appropriate treatment. Alternatively, an inaccurate diagnosis can result in the patient receiving unnecessary treatment with potentially harmful results. Any of these negative results can have potentially adverse psychological and financial repercussions.

Reference:
Institute of Medicine. Improving Diagnosis in Health Care, Quality Chasm Series. *Report in Brief.* <http://iom.nationalacademies.org/~/media/Files/Report%20Files/2015/Improving-Diagnosis/DiagnosticError_ReportBrief.pdf>; September 2015.

23. Postmortem studies show that diagnostic errors contribute to patients deaths in what percent of cases?
   A. 0% to 3%
   B. 3% to 6%
   C. 6% to 9%
   D. >9%

24. Which of the following is not an accurate statement?
   A. Approximately 35% to 50% of all radiologists practicing today have been sued
   B. Approximately 50% of neuroradiologists who have been sued have been sued more than once
   C. Between 1% and 5% of all radiology reports have errors in them
   D. 40% of lung nodules that are missed are seen in retrospect

25. Among radiologists, which of the following is more common?
   A. Failure to interpret correctly
   B. Failure to detect an abnormality
   C. Failure to provide an adequate differential diagnosis
   D. Failure to suggest the next step in the workup

26. Which of the following is true?
   A. Failure to interpret correctly is three times more common than failure to detect
   B. Failure to interpret correctly is two to four times less common than failure to detect
   C. Failure to interpret correctly is equally as common as failure to detect
   D. Failure to interpret correctly is less than two times less common than failure to detect

23. **D, >9%.** Medical errors can account for between 6% and 17% of adverse events in hospitals. Postmortem examinations have shown that errors contribute to approximately 10% of patient deaths. Perhaps not unexpectedly, diagnostic errors are thus the #1 type of paid medical malpractice claims. The Institute of Medicine notes that more attention needs to be paid to studying and understanding medical errors, how they occur, and how they can be prevented. Their recommendations include facilitating more effective teamwork among health care professionals and patients/families. They also recommend improved IT systems, and developing reporting systems without the threat of liability, in order to analyze and learn from errors and near misses.

Reference:

Institute of Medicine. Improving Diagnosis in Health Care, Quality Chasm Series. *Report in Brief.* <http://iom.nationalacademies.org/~/media/Files/Report%20 Files/2015/Improving-Diagnosis/DiagnosticError_ReportBrief.pdf>; September 2015.

24. **D, 40% of lung nodules that are missed are seen in retrospect.** The missed lung nodule rate was reported to be as low as 19% in a cohort of observed non-small cell lung cancer in the Netherlands form 1992 to 1995. The pulmonary system is the third most common organ system involving radiologists surveyed in an article from 2014. In that article, nondetection of a lesion was the leading cause of the plaintiff complaint.

References:

Quekel LG, et al. Miss rate of lung cancer on the chest radiograph in clinical practice. *Chest.* 1999;115(3):720-724.

Pereira NP, Lewin JS, Yousem KP, et al. *Medical malpractice: An American Society of Neuroradiology survey.* <http://www.ajnr.org/content/35/4/638. full.pdf>; July 22, 2013. Accessed December 13, 2013.

25. **B, Failure to detect an abnormality.** Diagnostic error is by far the most common cause for malpractice litigation against radiologists. In comparison, failure of communication (such as failure to provide an adequate differential diagnosis, as in answer choice C) and failure to recommend more testing (answer choice D) are much rarer reasons for malpractice suits.

Diagnostic errors in radiology can be classified as either perceptual errors, where the radiologist fails to detect an abnormal finding (answer choice B), or cognitive errors, where a detected abnormality is interpreted incorrectly (answer choice A). Of these, perceptual errors are much more common, accounting for 60% to 80% of diagnostic errors. Therefore, answer B is correct.

References:

Whang JS, Baker SR, Patel R, et al. The causes of medical malpractice suits against radiologists in the United States. *Radiology.* 2013;266(2):548-554.

Bruno MA, Walker EA, Abujudeh HH. Understanding and confronting our mistakes: the epidemiology of error in radiology and strategies for error reduction. *Radiographics.* 2015;35(6):1668-1676.

26. **B, Failure to interpret correctly is two to four times less common than failure to detect.** Diagnostic errors in radiology can be classified as either perceptual errors, where the radiologist fails to detect an abnormal finding, or cognitive errors, where a detected abnormality is interpreted incorrectly. Perceptual errors are much more common, accounting for 60% to 80% of diagnostic errors, while cognitive errors account for only 20% to 40% of diagnostic errors. Therefore, cognitive errors are two to four times less common than perceptual errors (answer choice B).

Reference:

Bruno MA, Walker EA, Abujudeh HH. Understanding and confronting our mistakes: the epidemiology of error in radiology and strategies for error reduction. *Radiographics.* 2015;35(6):1668-1676.

27. Which of the following should be reported to the National
    Practitioner's Data Base (NPDB)?
    A. Medical malpractice payments
    B. Adverse clinical privilege actions
    C. Adverse professional society membership actions
    D. All of the above

27. **D, All of the above.** According to the following table from the NPDB HRSA website (Table 9-1), all of the actions in this question and the previous question should be reported to the NPDB.

Reference:
National Practitioner Data Bank. What you must report to the NPDB. <http://www.npdb.hrsa.gov/hcorg/whatYouMustReportToTheDataBank.jsp#reportableActions>.

Table 9-1 ACTIONS REPORTABLE TO THE NPDB

Legislation	Who Reports	What Information Is Reported	Who Is Reported
Title IV	Medical malpractice payers, including self-insured hospitals and other health care entities	Medical malpractice payments made for the benefit of a health care practitioner resulting from a written claim or judgment. *(Reports must be submitted to the NPDB and appropriate State Licensing Board within 30 days of a payment)*	Practitioners
	State medical and dental boards	Certain adverse licensure actions related to professional competence or conduct. (Medical and dental boards that meet their reporting requirements for Section 1921, described below, will also meet their requirements to report under Title IV.) *(Reports must be submitted to the NPDB within 30 days of the action)*	Physicians and dentists
	Hospitals Other health care entities with formal peer review	Professional review actions based on reasons related to professional competence or conduct adversely affecting clinical privileges for a period longer than 30 days. Voluntary surrender or restriction of clinical privileges while under, or to avoid, an investigation. *(Reports must be submitted to the NPDB and appropriate State Licensing Board within 30 days of the action)*	• Physicians and dentists • Other practitioners (optional)
	Professional societies with formal peer review	Professional review actions, based on reasons relating to professional competence or conduct, adversely affecting membership. *(Reports must be submitted to the NPDB and appropriate State Licensing Board within 30 days of the action)*	• Physicians and dentists • Other practitioners (optional)
	Drug Enforcement Administration (DEA)	DEA controlled substance registration actions* *(Reports must be submitted to the NPDB within 30 days of the action)*	Practitioners
	Department of Health and Human Services (HHS) Office of Inspector General	Exclusions from participation in Medicare, Medicaid, and other federal health care programs* *(Exclusions are reported to the NPDB monthly)*	Practitioners
Section 1921	Peer review organizations	Negative actions or findings by peer review organizations *(Reports must be submitted to the NPDB and appropriate State Licensing or Certification Authority within 30 days of the action)*	Practitioners
	Private accreditation organizations	Negative actions or findings by private accreditation organizations *(Reports must be submitted to the NPDB and appropriate State Licensing or Certification Authority within 30 days of the action)*	Health care entities, providers, suppliers
	State Licensing and Certification Authorities	State licensure and certification actions (resulting from formal proceeding) • Adverse actions (including but not limited to revocation, suspension, reprimand, censure, probation) • Any dismissal or closure of the proceedings by reason of surrendering the license or certification agreement or contract for participation in a government health care program or leaving the state or jurisdiction • Any other loss of or loss of the right to apply for or renew a license or certification agreement or contract for participation in a government health care program • Any publicly available negative action or finding *(Reports must be submitted to the NPDB within 30 days of the action)*	Practitioners, health care entities, providers, suppliers
	• State law enforcement agencies** • State Medicaid Fraud Control Units** • State agencies administering or supervising the administration of a state health care program**	• Exclusions from participation in a state health care program • Health care-related civil judgments in state court • Health care-related state criminal convictions • Other adjudicated actions or decisions (related to the payment, provision, or delivery of a health care item or service) *(Reports must be submitted to the NPDB within 30 days of the action)*	Practitioners, providers, suppliers
Section 1128E	• Federal government agencies • Health plans	• Federal licensure and certification actions*** • Formal or official actions (including but not limited to revocation, suspension, reprimand, censure, or probation) • Any dismissal or closure of the proceedings by reason of surrendering the license or certification agreement or contract for participation in a government health care program or leaving the state or jurisdiction • Any other loss of—or loss of the right to apply for or renew—a license or certification agreement or contract for participation in a government health care program • Any publicly available negative action or finding • Health care-related civil judgments in federal or state court • Health care-related criminal convictions in federal or state court*** • Exclusions from participation in a federal health care program*** • Other adjudicated actions or decisions (related to the payment, provision, or delivery of a health care item or service) *(Reports must be submitted to the NPDB within 30 days of the action)*	Practitioners, providers, suppliers

*This information is reported to the NPDB under Title IV based on a federal cooperative agreement.
**The NPDB regulations define "state law or fraud enforcement agency" to include but not be limited to these entities. The information that is reported by each entity may differ by state depending on the state structure.
***Reported only by federal government agencies.

28. Which of the following should be reported to the National Practitioner's Data Base (NPDB)?
    A. State licensure and certification actions
    B. Federal licensure and certification actions
    C. Negative actions or findings by a peer review organization
    D. All of the above

29. Who may NOT gain access to the NPDB?
    A. Hospital credentialing committees
    B. Physicians (for themselves)
    C. Medical malpractice defense lawyers
    D. State licensing and certification authorities

30. A medical malpractice case is decided by the principle of:
    A. More likely than not
    B. Clear and convincing evidence
    C. Beyond a doubt
    D. None of the above

31. The statute of limitations:
    A. Is a national standard
    B. Varies from state to state
    C. Starts ticking from the time the breach in the standard of care occurs
    D. All of the above

32. When a radiologist inadvertently leaves a piece of a catheter in a 6-year-old patient, he may be liable:
    A. For 7 years
    B. Until the patient is 18 years of age
    C. Until the patient is 21 years of age
    D. For an unlimited length of time

33. In late 2001 a patient has a percutaneous appendectomy. The surgeon inadvertently leaves a gauze in the abdomen. In early 2002, the patient begins to have severe pain underlying the endoscopy site, which requires her to take opiate medication. Because medical visits are not covered by her insurance, she delays seeing the surgeon again until late 2004, at which time she has become medication dependent. He does a CT scan January 2, 2005, and an abscess and the retained gauze are discovered. The patient decides to sue. At what time point does the statute of limitations begin to run in this case?
    A. 2001
    B. 2002
    C. 2004
    D. 2005

28. **D, All of the above.** Please see Table 9-1 from the NPDB site. All are to be reported.

Reference:
National Practitioner Data Bank. What you must report to the NPDB. <http://www.npdb.hrsa.gov/hcorg/whatYouMustReportToTheDataBank.jsp#reportableActions>.

29. **C, Medical malpractice defense lawyers.** According to the NPDB website, a plaintiff's attorney or a plaintiff representing himself is allowed to obtain information from the NPDB (1) if a medical malpractice action or claim has been filed by the plaintiff against a hospital, (2) the practitioner on whom the information is requested must be named in the action or claim, (3) if the information obtained is used only in the litigation against the hospital and not against the practitioner, and (4) if evidence has been submitted to the Department of Health and Human Services demonstrating that the hospital failed to submit a mandatory query to the NPDB on the practitioner named in the action. Medical malpractice defense lawyers do not have access to the NPDB because practitioners can request a self-query if they want it. Peer review organizations and private accreditation bodies also cannot query the NPDB.

Reference:
National Practitioner Data Bank. *How to get started for organizations.* <http://www.npdb.hrsa.gov/hcorg/howToGetStarted.jsp>.

30. **A, More likely than not.** In a criminal case each element of the case must be proven "beyond a reasonable doubt." Medical malpractice cases are civil cases and therefore have a lower burden of proof: "more likely than not." "More likely than not" assumes "a preponderance of evidence," which means the jury favors the case of the plaintiff by as much as 51%. Is it more likely than not that the plaintiff's case is true (compared to the defendant's case)?

Reference:
Wood C. The misplace of litigation in medical practice. *Aust N Z J Obstet Gynaecol.* 1998;38(4):365-376.

31. **B, Varies from state to state.** The statute of limitations defines the time frame in which a lawsuit must be filed if a person is seeking damages. For the statute of limitations, counting begins at the time of injury and ends at a time determined by each statute and state. Thus, the statute of limitations on perforation of a bowel during a barium enema in the state of Maryland runs 3 years from the date of discovery, but in Florida the statute is for only 2 years after discovery. Most states say 2 years. Only a few say one year (Kentucky, Louisiana, Nebraska, Tennessee, Washington, Wisconsin).

Reference:
<http://www.ncsl.org/research/financial-services-and-commerce/medical-liability-malpractice-statutes-of-limitation.aspx>.

32. **D, For an unlimited length of time.** In most states, there is a specific statute of limitations in place for medical malpractice claims. Part of the reason for this is it may not be obvious when a potential claim arises. It may be months or even years before a person who received substandard medical care becomes aware that he/she was actually harmed by it, and that he/she may have a valid medical malpractice claim. For example, if a person has surgery and a piece of sponge or a fragment of an instrument is left behind, it may not be immediately obvious. There may be no pain in the area right away, and the patient may not exhibit any symptoms for quite a while after the surgical error was actually committed. Each state has different rules in this regard. The issues here revolve around the patient being a minor. Some states begin the statute of limitations at the age of majority; some do not. The second issue is the retained object exception. Twenty-two states have special provisions about negligence suits and foreign objects. As an example, Arkansas stipulates the statute of limitations is:

Two years from date of injury. Foreign objects: one year from discovery if not reasonably discovered in original two year requirement. Minors: before age 9, until age 11, unless injury isn't reasonably discovered before 11th birthday, then two years after injury discovered or minor's 19th birthday, whichever is earlier. Maryland, on the other hand states: Five years from act or three years from discovery. Minors under age 11: the time limitations shall commence when the claimant reaches the age of 11. In an action for an injury (i) to the reproductive system of the claimant; or (ii) caused by a foreign object negligently left in the claimant's body, if the claimant was under the age of 16 years at the time the injury was committed, the time limitations shall commence when the claimant reaches the age of 16 years.

Texas law states: Two years from occurrence, no more than 10 years. Minors under age 12: until age 14th birthday to file.

References:
<https://www.law.uh.edu/healthlaw/perspectives/2009/(RB)%20Sponges.pdf>.
<http://www.ncsl.org/research/financial-services-and-commerce/medical-liability-malpractice-statutes-of-limitation.aspx>.

33. **B, 2002.** The statute of limitations begins to run at the point the person should have discovered the injury, that is, the date the person began experiencing severe pain. Thus she should have known in 2002. Given a 3-year statute of limitations the case must start by 2005. When a person dies or is killed due to the negligence of a physician, the surviving members of the victim's family may sue for "wrongful death." If medical malpractice results in a wrongful death, an action may be brought by the decedent's dependents within 3 years of the family member's death under a state's limitation on wrongful death cases. This clock starts at death, not the occurrence of negligence.

References:
<https://www.law.uh.edu/healthlaw/perspectives/2009/(RB)%20Sponges.pdf>.
<http://www.ncsl.org/research/financial-services-and-commerce/medical-liability-malpractice-statutes-of-limitation.aspx>.

34. The tenet that the statute of limitations does not begin to run until a person realizes that he or she has been injured is called:
    A. Standard of care
    B. Statute of limitations
    C. Discovery rule
    D. Tenet of reasonableness

35. As of 2010, what percentage of radiologists surveyed had been sued at least once?
    A. 0% to 20%
    B. 21% to 40%
    C. 41% to 60%
    D. >60%

36. With regard to the demographics of malpractice suits:
    A. Men are sued more frequently as a percentage than women
    B. Women overall are sued more frequently than men
    C. Women and men are sued equally frequently
    D. Adjusting for prevalence of women and men in radiology, there is no difference

37. By age 60, what percentage of radiologists have been sued (see Figure 9-1)?
    A. 0% to 20%
    B. 21% to 40%
    C. 41% to 60%
    D. >60%

38. Which of the following practitioner specialties is sued more commonly than radiologists?
    A. Emergency physicians
    B. Obstetricians
    C. Neurosurgeons
    D. All of the above

39. Which of the following practitioner specialties is sued less commonly than radiologists?
    A. Pediatrics
    B. Anesthesiology
    C. Internal medicine
    D. All of the above

40. Of radiologists who have been named in suits, what percentage have been named more than once?
    A. 0% to 20%
    B. 21% to 40%
    C. 41% to 60%
    D. >60%

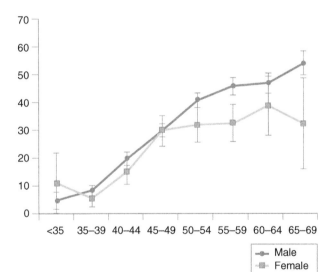

Figure 9-1 The demography of medical malpractice suits against radiologists. (From Baker SR, Whang JS, Luk L, Clarkin KS, Castro A 3rd, Patel R. The demography of medical malpractice suits against radiologists. *Radiology* 2013;266(2):539-547.)

34. **C, Discovery rule.** The statute of limitations defines the time frame in which a lawsuit must be filed if a person is seeking damages. For a statute of limitations, counting begins at the time of injury and ends at a time determined by the statute. Thus, the perforation of a bowel during a barium enema in the state of Maryland runs 5 years from the date of injury.

The delayed discovery rule suspends the running of the statutes of limitations (typically 1 to 3 years in most states) during periods of time in which the plaintiff did not discover, or despite reasonable diligence could not have discovered, the negligence of the physician and the injuries that negligence caused. Thus, the perforation of a bowel during a barium enema in the state of Maryland runs 3 years from the date that the perforation is discovered based on Maryland's delayed discovery rule. Proceedings § 5-109, the Maryland statute that addresses limitations in medical malpractice cases, states that the limitation is 5 years from the time the injury was committed or 3 years from the date the injury was discovered, whichever is shorter.

The statute of repose takes effect when an action is completed, such as when excessive radiation has been mistakenly delivered to a patient, not on the date that the patient developed leukemia many years later. Like statutes of limitations, statutes of repose vary from state to state. In Maryland it is 5 years.

Reference:
AIA Government & Community Relations Statute of Repose State Statute Compendium. <http://www.aia.org/aiaucmp/groups/aia/documents/pdf/aias078872.pdf>; January 2011.

35. **B, 21% to 40%.** In Baker's study, 31.5% of all radiologists surveyed had been sued. The rate increases from about 8% of 35- to 39-year-olds to 18% of 40- to 44-year-olds to 30% of 45- to 49-year-olds. The ten states with the highest rates of sued radiologists were New York, Utah, Indiana, New Jersey, Kansas, Pennsylvania, Florida, Arizona, Nevada, and Ohio. The states with the lowest rates of suits are Alabama, North Carolina, Virginia, Mississippi, Nebraska, Wisconsin, Oklahoma, Arkansas, Illinois, and Texas.

Reference:
Baker SR, Whang JS, Luk L, et al. The demography of medical malpractice suits against radiologists. *Radiology.* 2013;266(2):539-547. doi:10.1148/radiol.12110971. Epub 2012 Nov 28.

36. **A, Men are sued more frequently as a percentage than women.** Male radiologists, as a percentage of total suits, are sued more frequently than women at every age. The odds of ever being a defendant in a case are 1.4 times greater for men than for women. For neuroradiologists, this risk of being sued being more frequent in men than women holds as well. Overall rates per 100 practice years are 2.76 for men and 2.13 for women.

Reference:
Baker SR, Whang JS, Luk L, et al. The demography of medical malpractice suits against radiologists. *Radiology.* 2013;266(2):539-547. doi:10.1148/radiol.12110971. Epub 2012 Nov 28.

37. **C, 41% to 60%.** More men than women are sued as a percentage in radiology. The number of cumulative suits obviously increases with increasing age. As seen in the following graph from Baker's article (Figure 9-1), at age 60 around 47% of radiologists have been sued. The ratio of cases settled to those proceeding to trial was about 23 to 1. 44.4% of cases going to trial were settled in favor of the plaintiff. Payouts were, on average, $411,112, but in 52% of cases there was no payout from the radiologist. The average payment made on behalf of the radiologist when the cases were settled out of court was $295,993.

Reference:
Baker SR, Whang JS, Luk L, et al. The demography of medical malpractice suits against radiologists. *Radiology.* 2013;266(2):539-547. doi:10.1148/radiol.12110971. Epub 2012 Nov 28.

38. **D, All of the above.** The ten most frequently sued specialties according to the NEJM article cited below are:
   1. Neurosurgery
   2. Cardiovascular-thoracic surgery
   3. General surgery
   4. Orthopedic surgery
   5. Plastic surgery
   6. Gastroenterology
   7. Obstetrics and gynecology
   8. Urology
   9. Pulmonary medicine
   10. Oncology

Radiology ranks eighteenth on the list and is actually below the average for all physicians at about a 7% annual rate of being sued. The median payment was about $100,000 and the mean payment about $250,000 per claim. Of specialties that had to pay out >$1 million in awards, the most were in obstetrics and gynecology (11), pathology (10), anesthesiology (7), and pediatrics (7). Although radiologists were classified in a low risk group, the authors still found that by the age of 65 years, 75% of physicians in low risk specialties and 99% of those in high risk specialties were likely to have been sued.

Reference:
Jena AB, Seabury S, Lakdawalla D, et al. Malpractice risk according to physician specialty. *N Engl J Med.* 2011;365(7):629-636. <http://www.nejm.org/doi/full/10.1056/NEJMsa1012370#t=articleTop>.

39. **A, Pediatrics.** The ten least frequently sued specialties according to the NEJM article cited below are (1 = least):
   1. Psychiatry
   2. Pediatrics
   3. Family general practice
   4. Dermatology
   5. Pathology
   6. Nephrology
   7. Ophthalmology
   8. Radiology
   9. Anesthesiology
   10. Emergency medicine

Interestingly, although claims leading to indemnity payments ranged from 1% to 5% across all specialties, this compared with five times that many claims submitted. This means that only one-fourth or one-fifth of all malpractice suits filed resulted in an indemnity payment.

Reference:
Jena AB, Seabury S, Lakdawalla D, et al. Malpractice risk according to physician specialty. *N Engl J Med.* 2011;365(7):629-636.

40. **C, 41% to 60% (1085/2600 = 41.7%).** When Baker et al looked at all radiologists who had been sued, they found that 1085/2600 (41.7%) of these had been sued multiple times. The same finding held true in Pereira's article on neuroradiologists: 180 (44.9%) of the 401 neuroradiologists who answered the question said they had been sued once, 114 (28.4%) had been sued twice, 60 (15.0%) had been sued three times, and 47 (11.7%) had been sued more than three times. More than half of the 401 respondents who had been sued had been sued two or more times.

References:
Baker SR, Whang JS, Luk L, et al. The demography of medical malpractice suits against radiologists. *Radiology.* 2013;266(2):539-547. doi:10.1148/radiol.12110971. Epub 2012 Nov 28.
Pereira NP, Lewin JS, Yousem KP, et al. Attitudes about medical malpractice: An ASNR survey. *AJNR Am J Neuroradiol.* 2014;35(4):638-643. doi:10.3174/ajnr.A3730. Epub 2013 Dec 12.

QUESTIONS

1. What is the current mnemonic for cardiopulmonary resuscitation?
   A. ABC: airway, breathing, compression
   B. ABC: airway, breathing, cardioversion
   C. CAB: compressions, airway, breathing
   D. CAB: cardioversion, airway, breathing

2. What is wrong with this demonstration of CPR (Figure 10-1)?
   A. Position of hands is too low
   B. Position of hands is too high
   C. Left hand should be on top of right hand
   D. Fingers should be interleaved

3. What is wrong with this figure (Figure 10-2)?
   A. Hand position
   B. Ventilator mask position
   C. Head position
   D. Compression to breaths ratio

4. Jaw thrust is used for:
   A. Opening an airway in a person suspected of neck injury
   B. Opening an airway in a child
   C. In lieu of a barrier mask
   D. Airway maintenance as the default step

5. Rescue breathing rate is:
   A. One breath every 3 seconds in adults
   B. One breath every 5 seconds in infants
   C. One breath given over 1 second
   D. One breath given over 3 seconds

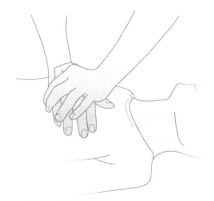

Figure 10-1 Incorrect chest compressions

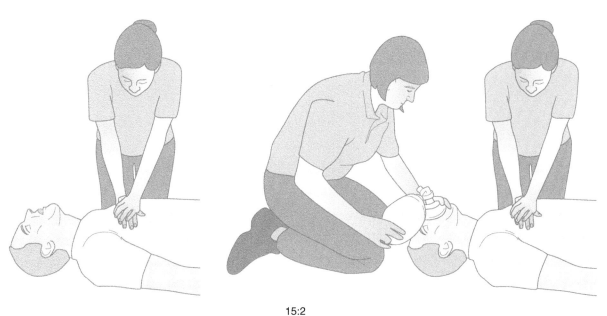

15:2
Figure 10-2 Incorrect CPR

1. **C, CAB: Compressions, airway, breathing.** The 2010 adult basic life support (BLS) guidelines introduced key changes compared to the 2005 BLS guidelines. One of the most important changes was the sequence of actions. Chest compression in the recent version precedes breathing rescue for adults, children, and infants. So, it is now **CAB** indicating Compression → Airway → Breathing, rather than **ABC** as in the prior version (Airway → Breathing → Compression).

   The reason behind that change was that the highest survival rates from cardiac arrest were reported in cases with ventricular fibrillation and pulseless ventricular tachycardia, which are usually managed with emphasis on chest compression and defibrillator.

   References:
   Berg R, et al. 2010 American Heart Association guidelines for cardiopulmonary resuscitation and emergency cardiovascular care science. Part 5: Adult basic life support. *Circulation.* 2010;122:5685-5705.
   Highlights of the 2010 American Heart Association Guidelines for CPR and ECC. 2010. Available at: <http://www.heart.org/idc/groups/heart-public/@wcm/@ecc/documents/downloadable/ucm_317350.pdf>.

2. **D, Fingers should be interleaved.** Because blood flow and therefore oxygen delivery to brain and myocardium are the most important task of basic life support, chest compression is a critical part of CPR. Chest compression is the application of forceful rhythmic pressure over the lower half of the sternum to increase blood flow by increasing the intrathoracic pressure and directly compressing the heart.

   The effective chest compression is essential and it is expected to compress to at least 2 inches' depth, allowing complete recoil of the chest. Both hands should be used to give chest compressions. They should be stacked on top of each other with fingers interlaced and raised so they do not touch the chest. Compression is done with the palm of the hand. In the picture the fingers are not intertwined.

   Reference:
   Berg R, et al. 2010 American Heart Association guidelines for cardiopulmonary resuscitation and emergency cardiovascular care science. Part 5: Adult basic life support. *Circulation.* 2010;122:5685-5705.

3. **D, Compression to breaths ratio.** The 2010 adult basic life support (BLS) guidelines recommend compression to ventilation ratio of 30:2 for adults whether there are one or two rescuers, emphasizing the importance of chest compression.

   References:
   Berg R, et al. 2010 American Heart Association guidelines for cardiopulmonary resuscitation and emergency cardiovascular care science. Part 5: Adult basic life support. *Circulation.* 2010;122:5685-5705.
   Highlights of the 2010 American Heart Association guidelines for CPR and ECC. 2010. Available at: <http://www.heart.org/idc/groups/heart-public/@wcm/@ecc/documents/downloadable/ucm_317350.pdf>.

4. **A, Opening an airway in a person suspected of neck injury.** Jaw thrust technique is only used to open an airway when head/neck injury is suspected. Jaw thrust is not used for airway maintenance but rather for opening the airway in order to give breaths. This should not be used in lieu of a barrier mask. Opening the airway in a child (**without** a suspected neck injury) would involve similar head-tilt/chin-lift technique as in adults.

   References:
   <https://eccguidelines.heart.org/index.php/circulation/cpr-ecc-guidelines-2/part-5-adult-basic-life-support-and-cardiopulmonary-resuscitation-quality/>.
   "CPR/AED for Professional Rescuers and Healthcare Providers" handbook. American Red Cross; 2011.

5. **C, One breath given over 1 second.** Rescue breathing (meaning the victim is not breathing normally but has a pulse) should be performed with one breath given over 1 second. One rescue breath should be given every 3 to 5 seconds in infants and every 5 to 6 seconds in adults.

   References:
   <www.eccguidelines.heart.org/index.php/circulation/cpr-ecc-guidelines-2/part-5-adult-basic-life-support-and-cardiopulmonary-resuscitation-quality/>.
   "CPR/AED for Professional Rescuers and Healthcare Providers" handbook. American Red Cross; 2011.

6. In what scenario would this diagram (Figure 10-3) be incorrect?
   A. It is incorrect as it is
   B. It would be incorrect for two person CPR
   C. It is incorrect in order
   D. It is incorrect in hand position

7. The number of recommended chest thrusts and back blows for foreign bodies in infants is:
   A. 5:2
   B. 2:5
   C. 5:5
   D. 2:2

8. The universal sign in Figure 10-4 is for:
   A. Choking
   B. Poisoning
   C. Harm
   D. Chest pain

9. Under what circumstances do you call 911 and get an automated external defibrillator before starting CPR?
   A. Adult patients
   B. Child patients
   C. Infant patients
   D. All patients

10. 100 compressions per minute is used for which patients undergoing CPR?
    A. Adult patients
    B. Child patients
    C. Infant patients
    D. All patients

11. Untrained individuals at CPR should attempt:
    A. Compressions and breathing
    B. Compressions
    C. Breathing
    D. No resuscitation techniques

12. Adult chest compressions should have a depth of:
    A. ½ inch
    B. 1 inch
    C. 1.5 inches
    D. 2 inches

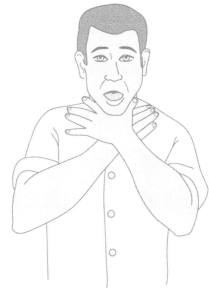

Figure 10-4 Universal sign

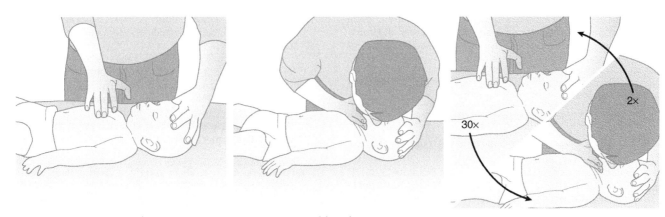

30 compressions   2 breaths

Figure 10-3 Incorrect child CPR

6. **B, It would be incorrect for two-person CPR.** According to the 2010 BLS guidelines for children and infants, the compression to breathing ratio for children and infants differs when there is one rescuer versus two. When there is one rescuer, they follow the adult ratio (30:2), but when there are two rescuers the ratio becomes 15:2.

For infants, compression on the sternum is performed with two fingers placed below the intermammary line.

Reference:
Chair MEK, et al. 2010 American Heart Association guidelines for cardiopulmonary resuscitation and emergency cardiovascular care science. Part 14: Pediatrics advanced life support. *Circulation.* 2010;122:5876-5908.

7. **C, 5:5.** More than 90% of childhood deaths from foreign body aspiration occur before the age of 5 years. Signs of foreign body airway obstruction include sudden onset respiratory distress, stridor, gagging, or wheezing. If the airway obstruction is mild the child can cough, but when it is severe the child will not be able to cough or make any sound.

When the obstruction is mild, the child should be allowed to clear the airway by coughing while the rescuer is observing for signs of severe obstruction. But when the obstruction is severe, the rescuer should interfere.

For infants, repeated cycles of 5 back blows followed by 5 chest thrusts should be delivered till the object is expelled.

References:
Vilke GM, et al. Airway obstruction in children aged less than 5 years: the prehospital experience. *Prehosp Emerg Care.* 2004;8(2):196-199.
Berg R, et al. 2010 American Heart Association guidelines for cardiopulmonary resuscitation and emergency cardiovascular care science. Part 13: Pediatric basic life support. *Circulation.* 2010;122(18 suppl 3):S862-S875.
Langhelle A, et al. Airway pressure with chest compressions versus Heimlich maneuver in recently dead adults with complete airway obstruction. *Resuscitation.* 2000;44(2):105-108.

8. **A, Choking.** Recognizing airway obstruction quickly is vital for a good outcome. Airway obstruction is a preventable cause of death, most commonly occurring in adults while they are eating. Choking adults may clutch their necks with their hands, known as the universal choking sign. Abdominal thrusts should be performed if coughing becomes silent or there is severe respiratory difficulty. Abdominal thrusts should also be performed if the patient becomes unresponsive from choking.

Reference:
American Heart Association. Part 5: Adult basic life support and cardiopulmonary resuscitation, section 9.5: Foreign-body airway obstruction. CPR-ECC guidelines. <https://eccguidelines.heart.org/index.php/circulation/cpr-ecc-guidelines-2/part-5-adult-basic-life-support-and-cardiopulmonary-resuscitation-quality/?strue=1&id=9-5>. Accessed January 3, 2016.

9. **A, Adult patients.** After checking the safety of the surrounding environment of an unresponsive adult patient, immediately activating the "Emergency Response System" (calling 911) and acquiring an automated electronic defibrillator (AED) are important steps of basic life support and are performed before confirming cardiopulmonary arrest and initiating CPR.

Ventricular fibrillation and pulseless ventricular tachycardia are arrhythmias that are treatable with cardiac defibrillation. Survivability of these arrhythmias is highest when defibrillation and CPR are delivered within 3 to 5 minutes of collapse. It is therefore reasonable for an AED to be used immediately in a witnessed cardiac arrest. In an unwitnessed arrest, the AED should be immediately applied, but CPR should be performed until the device is ready.

For infants and children, calling 911 and acquiring an AED are not performed by the lone rescuer until 2 minutes after performing high quality CPR. As opposed to adult cardiac arrest, pediatric cardiac arrest is more likely to coincide with respiratory arrest, and immediate initiation of CPR takes precedence. If a second rescuer becomes available during CPR, he or she should call 911 and obtain an AED before assisting.

Ideally, more than one rescuer will be present from the onset of attempted resuscitation of either an adult or pediatric patient, in which case one rescuer starts performing CPR and the second rescuer calls 911 and obtains an AED.

References:
Kleinman ME, Brennan EE, Goldberger ZD, et al. Part 5: Adult basic life support and cardiopulmonary resuscitation quality: 2015 American Heart Association guidelines update for cardiopulmonary resuscitation and emergency cardiovascular care. *Circulation.* 2015;132(suppl 2):S414-S435.
Atkins DL, Berger S, Duff JP, et al. Part 11: Pediatric basic life support and cardiopulmonary resuscitation quality: 2015 American Heart Association guidelines update for cardiopulmonary resuscitation and emergency cardiovascular care. *Circulation.* 2015;132(suppl 2):S519-S525.

10. **D, All patients.** In addition to hand positioning and compression depth, an appropriate rate of compression has been associated with improved survival. In an adult patient, a rate of 100 to 120 compressions per minute has been shown to be the ideal rate for chest compressions.

There is insufficient data on the pediatric population for an optimal chest compression rate. To simplify the CPR algorithms and training, the adult rate of 100 to 120 compressions per minute is used on the pediatric patient.

References:
Kleinman ME, Brennan EE, Goldberger ZD, et al. Part 5: Adult basic life support and cardiopulmonary resuscitation quality: 2015 American Heart Association guidelines update for cardiopulmonary resuscitation and emergency cardiovascular care. *Circulation.* 2015;132(suppl 2):S414-S435.
Atkins DL, Berger S, Duff JP, et al. Part 11: Pediatric basic life support and cardiopulmonary resuscitation quality: 2015 American Heart Association guidelines update for cardiopulmonary resuscitation and emergency cardiovascular care. *Circulation.* 2015;132(suppl 2):S519-S525.

11. **B, Compressions.** Untrained lay rescuers should perform compression only CPR until trained rescuers arrive, ideally with the guidance of an emergency dispatcher over the telephone. When telephone guidance is needed, compression only CPR has improved survival compared to conventional CPR.

Multiple studies have shown that there is no benefit of conventional CPR over compression only CPR in cases of out-of-hospital cardiac arrest. However, lay rescuers and medical professionals should continue to use conventional CPR, because they are more likely to provide CPR for extended periods of time, at which point the absence of ventilation may be harmful.

Reference:
Kleinman ME, Brennan EE, Goldberger ZD, et al. Part 5: Adult basic life support and cardiopulmonary resuscitation quality: 2015 American Heart Association guidelines update for cardiopulmonary resuscitation and emergency cardiovascular care. *Circulation.* 2015;132(suppl 2):S414-S435.

12. **D, 2 inches.** In the adult patient, a compression depth of 2 inches is recommended. Compression depth in the range of 1.6 to 2.2 inches is associated with higher survival. While there is insufficient evidence regarding survival for compressions that are too deep, injuries are more likely to occur when compressions exceed 2.4 inches.

Reference:
Kleinman ME, Brennan EE, Goldberger ZD, et al. Part 5: Adult basic life support and cardiopulmonary resuscitation quality: 2015 American Heart Association guidelines update for cardiopulmonary resuscitation and emergency cardiovascular care. *Circulation.* 2015;132(suppl 2):S414-S435.

13. Infant chest compressions should have a depth of:
    A. ½ inch
    B. 1 inch
    C. 1.5 inches
    D. 2 inches

14. CPR may not save the victim even when performed properly, but if started within 4 minutes of cardiac arrest, and defibrillation is provided within 10 minutes, a person has a XX% chance of survival?
    A. 5
    B. 10
    C. 20
    D. 40

15. Checking for breathing or a pulse each should take no more than:
    A. 5 seconds
    B. 10 seconds
    C. 20 seconds
    D. 0 seconds

16. To best determine if rescue breathing is effective, identify:
    A. Change in skin color
    B. Expiratory sounds after breath is given
    C. Chest rise
    D. Abdominal distention

17. For children and adults, one should check the pulse:
    A. In the arm in children but carotid in adults
    B. In the arm for both
    C. In the carotids for both
    D. In the carotid for children but arm for adults

13. **C, 1.5 inches.** There is insufficient data regarding compression depth for the pediatric population. It is reasonable to use a compression depth of one-third of the anteroposterior chest diameter, which equates to 1.5 inches for infants. For children from infancy to the onset of puberty, one-third of the anteroposterior chest distance is 2 cm, which is the same as the recommended adult chest compression depth.

Reference:

Atkins DL, Berger S, Duff JP, et al. Part 11: Pediatric basic life support and cardiopulmonary resuscitation quality: 2015 American Heart Association guidelines update for cardiopulmonary resuscitation and emergency cardiovascular care. *Circulation*. 2015;132(suppl 2):S519-S525.

14. **D, 40.** Survival for out of hospital cardiac arrest is overall poor, with only 10.8% of those with nontraumatic cardiac arrests surviving to hospital discharge, even when CPR is performed. However, for patients with witnessed ventricular fibrillation or ventricular tachycardia, close to 40% survive when they receive high quality CPR which includes cardioversion.

References:

Daya MR, Schmicker RH, Zive DM, et al. Resuscitation Outcomes Consortium Investigators. Out-of-hospital cardiac arrest survival improving over time: Results from the Resuscitation Outcomes Consortium (ROC). *Resuscitation*. 2015;91:108-115.

Kleinman ME, Brennan EE, Goldberger ZD, et al. Part 5: Adult basic life support and cardiopulmonary resuscitation quality: 2015 American Heart Association guidelines update for cardiopulmonary resuscitation and emergency cardiovascular care. *Circulation*. 2015;132(suppl 2):S414-S435.

15. **B, 10 seconds.** Checking for a pulse and breathing should occur before initiating CPR and after each shock delivered by an AED. Limiting the time to 10 seconds avoids delaying chest compressions. Ideally, checking for a pulse and checking for breathing can occur simultaneously to avoid further delay. Due to difficulty in finding a palpable pulse quickly, lay rescuers do not check for a pulse before resuming CPR.

Reference:

Kleinman ME, Brennan EE, Goldberger ZD, et al. Part 5: Adult basic life support and cardiopulmonary resuscitation quality: 2015 American Heart Association guidelines update for cardiopulmonary resuscitation and emergency cardiovascular care. *Circulation*. 2015;132(suppl 2):S414-S435.

16. **C, Chest rise.** The goal of rescue breathing is to deliver a volume of approximately 600 mL with each rescue breath. This equates to a 1-second inspiratory time and should cause a noticeable and immediate chest rise. Volumes of less than 500 mL, which may not cause a chest rise, often require supplemental oxygen to achieve adequate blood oxygenation.

Reference:

Sayre MR, Koster RW, Botha M, et al. on behalf of the Adult Basic Life Support Chapter Collaborators. Part 5: Adult basic life support: 2010 international consensus on cardiopulmonary resuscitation and emergency cardiovascular care science with treatment recommendations. *Circulation*. 2010;122(16 suppl 2):S298-S324.

17. **C, In the carotids for both.** It is recommended that a patient's pulse is checked by trained lay rescuers or medical professions before initiating CPR and after each shock delivered by an AED. Palpation of a pulse should occur quickly (10 seconds or less) to avoid delaying chest compressions, and the easiest artery to palpate should be selected. In children and adults, the carotid artery should be palpated. In infants, the brachial artery is preferred.

References:

Kleinman ME, Brennan EE, Goldberger ZD, et al. Part 5: Adult basic life support and cardiopulmonary resuscitation quality: 2015 American Heart Association Guidelines Update for Cardiopulmonary Resuscitation and Emergency Cardiovascular Care. *Circulation*. 2015;132(suppl 2):S414-S435.

Atkins DL, Berger S, Duff JP, et al. Part 11: Pediatric basic life support and cardiopulmonary resuscitation quality: 2015 American Heart Association guidelines update for cardiopulmonary resuscitation and emergency cardiovascular care. *Circulation*. 2015;132(suppl 2):S519-S525.

18. What is the grade of a reaction to contrast medium in which there is a liquid feeling in the arm as the saline flush is injected upon insertion of the intravenous catheter, which resolves immediately after the saline injection?
    A. No reaction
    B. Mild reaction
    C. Moderate reaction
    D. Severe reaction

19. What is the grade of a reaction to contrast medium in which there is chest pain?
    A. No reaction
    B. Mild reaction
    C. Moderate reaction
    D. Severe reaction

20. What is the grade of a reaction to contrast medium in which there is bronchospasm without hypoxia?
    A. No reaction
    B. Mild reaction
    C. Moderate reaction
    D. Severe reaction

21. What is the grade of a reaction to contrast medium in which there is brief vasovagal reaction that does not require intervention?
    A. No reaction
    B. Mild reaction
    C. Moderate reaction
    D. Severe reaction

22. What is the grade of a reaction to contrast medium in which there is laryngeal edema?
    A. No reaction
    B. Mild reaction
    C. Moderate reaction
    D. Severe reaction

23. What is the grade of a reaction to contrast medium in which there is contrast dye infiltration?
    A. No reaction
    B. Mild reaction
    C. Moderate reaction
    D. Severe reaction

18. **A, No reaction.** Acute reactions to either iodinated or gadolinium based intravenous contrast can be classified as either physiologic or allergic-like reactions and stratified by severity. "Allergic-like" reactions are often not associated with an IgE-mediated response and thus not considered true allergies. They encompass symptoms similar to true allergic reactions ranging from mild itching or sneezing to more severe symptoms of bronchospasm, laryngeal edema, and anaphylactic shock. Physiologic reactions are those related to the intravenous contrast itself. Physiologic reactions can also range from mild to severe. Distinction between physiologic and allergic-like acute reactions is important in the management of contrast reactions. Not only do the treatments differ, but also premedication with corticosteroids plays no role in preventing physiologic reactions. Likewise, a prior physiologic reaction is not an indication for future premedication.

Another important distinction in the management of contrast reactions is severity. Though assessment of severity is somewhat subjective, the ACR has grouped both allergic-like and physiologic reactions into three broad categories of mild, moderate, and severe reactions (see Table 10-1). The majority of acute reactions are mild and self-limited. Moderate reactions are those with more pronounced symptoms, often requiring treatment. Severe symptoms have the potential to be life threatening or cause permanent morbidity if not treated appropriately.

Many groups would consider self-limiting symptoms such as hot or cold sensation in the arm, altered taste, nausea and vomiting, anxiety, and total body warm sensation (flushing) as simple physiologic responses to injected intravenous contrast. However, the ACR contrast guidelines do list many of these symptoms as mild acute physiologic reactions including hot or cold sensation in the arm. The feeling that something is being injected in the vein is not considered a contrast reaction, especially since no contrast was administered.

Reference:
ACR Manual on Contrast Media, Version 10.1. Reston, VA: American College of Radiology; 2015.

19. **C, Moderate reaction.** Isolated chest pain is considered a moderate physiologic reaction. It is a nonspecific symptom that requires medical attention to exclude urgent/emergent causes of acute chest pain.

Reference:
ACR Manual on Contrast Media, Version 10.1. Reston, VA: American College of Radiology; 2015.

20. **C, Moderate reaction.** Even mild wheezing or bronchospasm is considered a moderate allergic-like reaction and requires medical management. If it is accompanied by significant hypoxia, the reaction is considered severe. Treatment is based on severity but includes supplemental oxygen and a beta-agonist inhaler. Epinephrine can be used in more severe cases.

Reference:
ACR Manual on Contrast Media, Version 10.1. Reston, VA: American College of Radiology; 2015.

21. **B, Mild reaction.** Vasovagal reactions are relatively common physiologic reactions characterized by hypotension and bradycardia. They can be related to anxiety and can occur at any time, including during contrast injection. Most are of the mild variety, brief and not requiring intervention. Vasovagal reactions that do require intervention but are responsive to treatment are considered moderate reactions. Rarely, vasovagal reactions can be severe and resistant to treatment.

Reference:
ACR Manual on Contrast Media, Version 10.1. Reston, VA: American College of Radiology; 2015.

22. **D, Severe reaction.** Laryngeal edema presents with stridor and/or hypoxia and is considered a severe allergic-like reaction requiring emergent treatment with supplemental oxygen and epinephrine.

Reference:
ACR Manual on Contrast Media, Version 10.1. Reston, VA: American College of Radiology; 2015.

23. **A, No reaction.** Though considered an adverse event related to the injection of intravenous contrast, contrast dye infiltration is not considered an acute contrast reaction. Extravasation of contrast material into the tissues surrounding the injection site incites an inflammatory response. Most cases do not result in any significant damage. However, rarely cases can lead to compartment syndrome, skin ulceration, or tissue necrosis.

Reference:
ACR Manual on Contrast Media, Version 10.1. Reston, VA: American College of Radiology; 2015.

Table 10-1 CATEGORIES OF ACUTE REACTIONS

	Allergic-like Reaction	Physiologic Reaction
Mild	• Limited urticaria or pruritis • Limited cutaneous edema • Limited "itchy" or "scratchy" throat • Nasal congestion • Sneezing, conjunctivitis, or rhinorrhea	• Limited nausea or vomiting • Transient flushing, warmth or chills • Headache, dizziness, anxiety, or altered taste • Mild hypertension • Vasovagal reaction that spontaneously resolves
Moderate	• Diffuse urticaria or pruritis • Diffuse erythema (stable vital signs) • Facial edema without dyspnea • Throat tightness or hoarseness without dyspnea • Wheezing or bronchospasm with mild or no hypoxia	• Protracted nausea or vomiting • Isolated chest pain • Hypertensive urgency • Vasovagal reaction that requires and is responsive to treatment
Severe	• Diffuse edema, or facial edema with dyspnea • Diffuse erythema with hypotension • Laryngeal edema with stridor and/or hypoxia • Wheezing or bronchospasm with significant hypoxia • Anaphylactic shock (hypotension + tachycardia)	• Arrhythmia • Convulsions or seizures • Hypertensive emergency • Vasovagal reaction resistant to treatment

(From *ACR Manual on Contrast Media*, Version 10.1. Reston: American College of Radiology, 2015. 103–104. http://www.acr.org/~/media/37D84428BF1D4E1B9A3A2918DA9E27A3.pdf).

24. What is the grade of a reaction to contrast medium in which there is vasovagal reaction unresponsive to therapy?
    A. No reaction
    B. Mild reaction
    C. Moderate reaction
    D. Severe reaction

25. What is the grade of a reaction to contrast medium in which there is headache with mild hypertension?
    A. No reaction
    B. Mild reaction
    C. Moderate reaction
    D. Severe reaction

26. What is the grade of a reaction to contrast medium in which there is a transient whole body flushing feeling?
    A. No reaction
    B. Mild reaction
    C. Moderate reaction
    D. Severe reaction

27. What is the grade of a reaction to contrast medium in which there is cardiopulmonary arrest?
    A. No reaction
    B. Mild reaction
    C. Moderate reaction
    D. Severe reaction

28. What is the eGFR level at which patients with chronic renal insufficiency are at risk for contrast induced nephropathy?
    A. <30 mL/min/1.73 m^2
    B. 2 g/dL
    C. 4 g/dL
    D. None

29. The overall incidence of allergic iodinated contrast dye reactions using low osmolality agents:
    A. Is 0.1% to 1% for any type of reaction
    B. Is less than 1 in 1,000,000 for an anaphylactic life-threatening reaction
    C. Increases with metformin administration
    D. Is less than that of gadolinium-based contrast agents

30. Given a previous iodinated contrast dye reaction, the risk of a subsequent allergic reaction is:
    A. No higher than baseline rate
    B. Twice the baseline likelihood rate
    C. Three times the baseline rate
    D. More than three times the baseline rate

31. Which of the following does not increase the risk of allergic reaction to iodinated contrast dye?
    A. Asthma
    B. Shellfish anaphylaxis
    C. Chronic kidney disease
    D. Peanut allergy severe reactions

24. **D, Severe reaction.** Rarely, vasovagal reactions (hypotension and bradycardia) can be severe and unresponsive to initial treatments of Trendelenburg positioning, supplemental oxygen, and IV fluids. IV atropine may be given. These cases may require emergent medical treatment.

Reference:
ACR Manual on Contrast Media, Version 10.1. Reston, VA: American College of Radiology; 2015.

25. **B, Mild reaction.** Both headaches and mild hypertension are considered mild acute physiologic reactions. In cases of mild hypertension, blood pressures would not be elevated enough to raise concerns for end-organ damage. In addition, isolated headache has not been shown to be a risk factor for end-organ central nervous system damage.

Reference:
ACR Manual on Contrast Media, Version 10.1. Reston, VA: American College of Radiology; 2015.

26. **B, Mild reaction.** A transient feeling of whole body flushing is a mild physiologic response to contrast media that is self-limited. It is thought to be related to hyperosmolality of contrast media in the vasculature leading to peripheral vasodilation.

Reference:
ACR Manual on Contrast Media, Version 10.1. Reston, VA: American College of Radiology; 2015.

27. **D, Severe reaction.** Cardiopulmonary arrest is a nonspecific end-stage result that can occur from a variety of severe reactions whether allergic or physiologic. If it is unclear what etiology caused the cardiopulmonary arrest, it may be judicious to assume that the reaction is/was an allergic-like one. Severe allergic-like reactions include:

- Diffuse edema, or facial edema with dyspnea
- Diffuse erythema with hypotension
- Laryngeal edema with stridor and/or hypoxia
- Wheezing/bronchospasm, significant hypoxia
- Anaphylactic shock (hypotension + tachycardia)
  Severe physiologic reactions include:
- Vasovagal reaction resistant to treatment
- Arrhythmia
- Convulsions, seizures
- Hypertensive emergency

Reference:
ACR Manual on Contrast Media, Version 10.1. Reston, VA: American College of Radiology; 2015.
Kessler CS, Joudeh Y. Evaluation and treatment of severe asymptomatic hypertension. *Am Fam Physician.* 2010;81(4):470-476. PMID 20148501.

28. **A, < 30 mL/min/1.73 m².** According to the *ACR Manual on Contrast Media* v.10.1, <30 mL/min/1.73 m² is the threshold with the greatest level of evidence to suggest increased risk for contrast induced nephropathy. The *ACR Manual* states the following: "At the current time, there is very little evidence that IV iodinated contrast material is an independent risk factor for AKI in patients with eGFR ≥30 mL/min/1.73 m². Therefore, if a threshold for CIN risk is used at all, 30 mL/min/1.73 m² seems to be the one with the greatest level of evidence. Any threshold put into

practice must be weighed on an individual patient level with the benefits of administering contrast material."

Reference:
Post-contrast acute kidney injury and contrast-induced nephropathy in adults. In: *ACR Manual on Contrast Media, Version 10.1.* Reston, VA: American College of Radiology; 2015:36. Print.

29. **A, is 0.1% to 1% for any type of reaction.** Incidence of allergic-type adverse events with low osmolar contrast medium intravenous iodinated contrast (LOCM) is less than 1% according to several large population studies but is higher than the 0.004% to 0.7% range incidence of allergic-type events reported with gadolinium-based intravenous contrast agents. Serious acute reactions including anaphylaxis to IV LOCM are rare at approximately 4 in 10,000 (0.04%). Metformin can increase the risk of lactic acidosis in a subset of patients with acute or chronic kidney disease but has not been documented to increase the risk of allergic-type reactions.

References:
Cochran ST, Bomyea K, Sayre JW. Trends in adverse events after IV administration of contrast media. *AJR Am J Roentgenol.* 2001;176(6):1385-1388.
Mortele KJ, Oliva MR, Ondategui S, et al. Universal use of nonionic iodinated contrast medium for CT: evaluation of safety in a large urban teaching hospital. *AJR Am J Roentgenol.* 2005;184(1):31-34.
Wang CL, Cohan RH, Ellis JH, et al. Frequency, outcome, and appropriateness of treatment of nonionic iodinated contrast media reactions. *AJR Am J Roentgenol.* 2008;191(2):409-415.
Katayama H, Yamaguchi K, Kozuka T, et al. Adverse reactions to ionic and nonionic contrast media. A report from the Japanese Committee on the Safety of Contrast Media. *Radiology.* 1990;175(3):621-628.

30. **D, More than three times the baseline rate.** Prior allergic-type reaction to iodinated intravenous contrast material is the single most substantial risk factor for development of repeat reaction. Compared with a baseline risk of less than 1% in the background population, non-premedicated patients with prior allergic-type reaction to iodinated intravenous contrast have a 10% to 35% risk of repeat reaction. Premedication decreases this risk to approximately 10%.

References:
Katayama H, Yamaguchi K, Kozuka T, et al. Adverse reactions to ionic and nonionic contrast media. A report from the Japanese Committee on the Safety of Contrast Media. *Radiology.* 1990;175(3):621-628.
ACR Manual on Contrast Media, Version 10.1. Reston, VA: American College of Radiology; 2015.

31. **C, Chronic kidney disease.** Risk factors for allergic-type reactions to intravenous iodinated contrast include atopic conditions (ie, multiple food allergies) and asthma. Chronic kidney disease does not convey an increased risk for allergic-type reactions for the administration of intravenous iodinated contrast reaction but can increase the risk for contrast induced nephropathy, as well as lactic acidosis in a subset of the population concurrently taking metformin.

References:
Meth MJ, Maibach HI. Current understanding of contrast media reactions and implications for clinical management. *Drug Saf.* 2006;29(2):133-141.
ACR Manual on Contrast Media, Version 10.1. Reston, VA: American College of Radiology; 2015.

32. The limit of iohexol allowed in the cerebrospinal fluid, based on the package insert, is:
    A. 10 cc
    B. 3 g
    C. 15 cc
    D. 1.5 g

33. The reason metformin is held after iodinated contrast administration is:
    A. Renal toxicity
    B. Delayed hepatorenal failure
    C. Lactic acidosis concurrent with renal failure
    D. All of the above

34. The most frequently used steroid premedication regimen for prophylaxis for iodinated contrast allergic reaction is:
    A. No premedication
    B. Prednisone 50 mg p.o. 24, 12, and 2 hours prior to injection
    C. Prednisone 50 mg p.o. 13, 7, and 1 hour prior to injection
    D. Prednisone 50 mg p.o., 24, 13, 7, and 1 hour prior to injection

35. The administration of steroids for premedication before iodinated contrast injection is NOT associated with:
    A. Decreased intraocular pressure
    B. Hypertension
    C. Hyperglycemia
    D. Fluid retention

36. The administration of midazolam for sedation is associated with:
    A. Increased intraocular pressure
    B. Hypertension
    C. Hyperglycemia
    D. Fluid retention

32. **B, 3 g.** The package insert for iohexol (Omnipaque) states that there is a recommended 3-gram iodine limit for scintillation intrathecally. This means that 10 cc of iohexol 300 mg/mL or 12 cc of iohexol 240 mg/mL or 17 cc of iohexol 180 mg/mL should be the maximum dosage allowed. The insertion of more than 3 grams may raise the negligible risk of seizures to an unacceptable risk level. For children that dose limit is stated as 2.7 g (usually limited to 180 mg/mL concentration). Iohexol 140 mg/mL and 350 mg/mL are not approved for intrathecal use.

The agent is to be instilled over 1 to 2 minutes. Its opacification for myelographic images degrades after 1 hour, but it is readily visible on CT scans for 3 to 4 hours. Drugs that lower the seizure threshold, especially phenothiazine derivatives, are typically held prior to myelograms. The class of MAO inhibitors and tricyclic antidepressants also should be curtailed if possible prior to these procedures. In general, all psychoactive drugs place the patient at increased risk when they are being given intrathecal injection of iodinated compounds. That said, seizures during myelography are incredibly uncommon.

Reference:
Package insert iohexol: GE Healthcare Omnipaque-Bulk-Pack-Prescribing-Information 032012.pdf.

33. **C, Lactic acidosis concurrent with renal failure.** It is well known that those patients who proceed to acute renal failure after iodinated contrast dye administration may be at risk for lactic acidosis if they are receiving metformin (Glucophage). Metformin is a biguanide prescribed in Type II diabetic patients. In those patients who do not show contrast nephropathy, such a risk is not demonstrated. However, because we cannot know who will or will not have kidney shutdown as an idiosyncratic reaction to iodinated contrast, most radiology departments hold metformin for 48 hours after contrast enhanced studies until the kidney function has been demonstrated to be normal. Note that no one is advocating holding the metformin before the study (unless the patient is in severe kidney failure, for which metformin may be contraindicated anyway). Diabetic patients are at risk because of their propensity for transient kidney effects after iodinated agents. Other hypoglycemic agents can be substituted for metformin during the period around the radiographic study.

Reference:
Rasuli PL, Hammond DI. Metformin and contrast media: where is the conflict? *Can Assoc Radiol J.* 1998;49(3):161-166.

34. **C, Prednisone 50 mg p.o. 13, 7, and 1 hour prior to injection.** The main aim of premedication prior to contrast administration is pretreatment of at-risk patients, who have higher risk for developing acute allergic-like reaction to contrast media administration.

The etiology of contrast reactions is not completely known, yet 90% of the adverse reactions are related to direct release of histamine and other mediators from basophils and eosinophil, and only 4% of patients are thought to have IgE mediated allergic reaction.

Because the risk of a few doses of oral corticosteroids are extremely low (it is more frequent with IV corticosteroids, especially succinate steroids) oral steroids are pre-

ferred to IV ones for premedication. Prednisone and methylprednisolone were found to be equally effective.

The two frequently used regimens are:

OPTION 1: Prednisone: 50 mg orally at 13, 7, and 1 hour before contrast injection + diphenhydramine (Benadryl): 50 mg (IV, IM, or orally) 1 hour before contrast injection

OPTION 2: Methylprednisolone (Medrol): 32 mg orally 12 and 2 hours before contrast injection ± diphenhydramine (Benadryl): 50 mg (IV, IM, or orally) 1 hour before contrast injection

References:
Lasser EC, et al. Pretreatment with corticosteroids to alleviate reactions to intravenous contrast material. *N Engl J Med.* 1987;317(14):845-849.
Wolf GL, Mishkin MM, Roux SG, et al. Comparison of the rates of adverse drug reactions. Ionic contrast agents, ionic contrast agents combined with steroids, and nonionic agents. *Invest Radiol.* 1991;26(5):404-410.
ACR Manual on Contrast Media, Version 10.1. Reston, VA: American College of Radiology; 2015. Available at: <http://www.acr.org/~/media/37D84428BF1D4E1B9A3A2918DA9E27A3.pdf>.

35. **A, Decreased intraocular pressure.** Steroids are associated with a spike in intraocular pressure. This has been attributed to the reduced aqueous humor outflow from the posterior chamber due to its vague influence on the canals of Schlemm in transmitting that fluid. This impact of steroids has also been associated with steroid nasal sprays and oral or intravenous administrations. The use of steroids is also associated with a higher rate of cataracts.

Steroids are known to have effects on blood pressure, glucose, and immune competency. Therefore it is wise to assess patients, before instituting systemic corticosteroid therapy, for hypertension, diabetes, glaucoma, infections (varicella, tuberculosis), osteoporosis, and peptic ulcer disease. Many medications will have reduced effectiveness in a patient receiving concomitant corticosteroids, particularly antibiotics, diuretics, and hypoglycemics. Because the course of treatment given for premedication for allergic reactions in radiology departments is so short, one rarely runs into such deleterious influences.

Reference:
Stanbury R, Graham E. Systemic corticosteroid therapy—side effects and their management. *Br J Ophthalmol.* 1998;82(6):704-708.

36. **A, Increased intraocular pressure.** Midazolam (trade name Versed) is a frequently used agent for its sedative and amnestic qualities because it is a well-tolerated rapid onset agent with a short half-life. It is a benzodiazepine and as such can increase intraocular pressure through its fluid retention properties, particularly in those patients with acute narrow angle glaucoma. Midazolam may lead to forward movement of the lens-iris diaphragm that can further obstruct the flow of aqueous humor and increase the pressure in the posterior chamber of the globe. Cholinergic agents, serotonin reuptake inhibitors, H2 receptor agonists, adrenergic agonists, and oral steroids may also be contraindicated in patients with volatile open and closed angle glaucoma.

Reference:
Carter K, Faberowski LK, Sherwood MB, et al. A randomized trial of the effect of midazolam on intraocular pressure. *J Glaucoma.* 1999;8(3):204-207. <http://www.ncbi.nlm.nih.gov/pubmedhealth/PMHT0011217/?report=details>.

37. Precautions should be taken in patients sedated with fentanyl who:
    A. Are diabetic
    B. Are taking MAO inhibitors
    C. Have open angle glaucoma
    D. Ate over 24 hours prior to sedation

38. When comparing the topical anesthetics of the ester group (benzocaine, procaine, tetracaine, oxybuprocaine, chlorprocaine, and butoform) versus the amide group (lidocaine, mepivacaine, prilocaine, bupivacaine, etidocaine, ropivacaine, and dibucaine):
    A. The ester group has a higher rate of allergic reactions than the amide group
    B. The ester group has a lower rate of allergic reactions than the amide group
    C. The ester group has the same rate of allergic reactions as the amide group
    D. None of the above

39. If a patient is allergic to an ester group topical anesthetic agent:
    A. He/She will also cross-react with local anesthetics in the amide group
    B. He/She will cross-react with other agents in the ester group
    C. He/She will cross-react with both ester and amide agents
    D. He/She usually do not cross-react at all

40. Anaphylaxis to povidone-iodine (Betadine):
    A. Predisposes to a higher rate of reaction to iodinated contrast media
    B. Predisposes to a lower rate of reaction to iodinated contrast media
    C. Shows no impact on the rate of reaction to iodinated contrast media
    D. All of the above

41. The most frequently used antihistamine premedication regimen for prophylaxis for iodinated contrast allergic reaction is:
    A. No premedication
    B. Diphenhydramine 50 mg 1 hour prior to injection
    C. Diphenhydramine 50 mg 1/2 hour prior to injection
    D. Loratadine 50 mg 1 hour prior to injection

37. **B, Are taking MAO inhibitors.** Monoamine oxidase inhibitors (MAOIs) are often prescribed as part of treatment for depression. These medications in combination with serotonin reuptake inhibitors (SRIs) can lead to a dramatic surge in serotonin levels, leading to hyperreflexia/tremor/clonus, autonomic hyperactivity/fever/tachycardia/tachypnea, and anxiety/agitation/confusion. Some opioid anesthetics like fentanyl, which are used because of their rapid onset of action and short duration, ideal for sedation during imaging studies, may also lead to upticks in serotonin levels. When the serotonin surge occurs, it does so rapidly and soon after the combination of drugs cross-react. In the patients on MAOI and/or SRIs, one may consider morphine for sedation/analgesia because it does not cause the same level of potential toxicity.

Reference:
Gillman PK. Monoamine oxidase inhibitors, opioid analgesics and serotonin toxicity. *Br J Anaesth*. 2005;95(4):434-441.

38. **A, The ester group has a higher rate of allergic reactions than the amide group.** The ester group of local anesthetics has a higher rate of allergic reactions than the amide group. The metabolite para-aminobenzoic acid (PABA) is implicated for triggering the allergic reaction and is characteristic of ester but not amide agent synthesis. The allergen in the amide agent reactivity is the methylparaben preservative. In addition to causing such reactions, methylparabens have been found in breast tissue of patients with breast cancer. Although the link between parabens and cancer is still unresolved, consumers are demanding that many hair and skin care products (cosmetics, lip balms, and shampoos and conditioners) remove these agents from their ingredients. Preservative free amide local anesthetics have been created that address the allergy risk.

Reference:
Eggleston ST1, Lush LW. Understanding allergic reactions to local anesthetics. *Ann Pharmacother*. 1996;30(7-8):851-857.

39. **B, They will cross-react with other agents in the ester group.** The topical anesthetics in the ester group have a higher rate of allergic reactions compared to the amide group. These ester group anesthetics include benzocaine, procaine, and tetracaine. The metabolite para-aminobenzoic acid (PABA) is the agent usually triggering the IgE mediated allergic reaction. Because of those allergic reactions, most institutions have switched to the amide group of local anesthetics such as lidocaine, bupivacaine, and etidocaine. In the event of an allergic reaction to an ester group anesthetic it is appropriate to switch to an amide group anesthetic.

Reference:
González-Delgado P, Antón R, Soriano V, et al. Cross-reactivity among amide-type local anesthetics in a case of allergy to mepivacaine. *J Investig Allergol Clin Immunol*. 2006;16(5):311-313.

40. **C, Shows no impact on the rate of reaction to iodinated contrast media.** Betadine is a combination of polyvinylpyrrolidone (povidone, PVP) and elemental iodine (Purdue Frederick, Norwalk, CT) as is Povidine (Alpharma, Baltimore, MD). Diatomic iodine is the bactericidal agent of these compounds. There is no known cross-reactivity of these topical antiseptics and the iodine administered for contrast studies in radiology. Similiarly, the "shellfish allergy" that used to be a source of concern in administering iodinated contrast agents has been debunked as a risk factor because the antigen is believed to be the fish equivalent of the muscle protein tropomyosin. That said, any atopic history or allergic reactions leads to an increased risk of an allergic reaction to iodinated contrast; it's just that seafood allergy and betadine allergy do not confer any higher risk.

Reference:
Schabelman E, Witting M. The relationship of radiocontrast, iodine, and seafood allergies: a medical myth exposed. *J Emerg Med*. 2010;39(5):701-707. <http://www.dermnetnz.org/treatments/iodine.html>.

41. **B, Diphenhydramine 50 mg 1 hour prior to injection.** Osmolality, size, and complexity of contrast agents are all contributing factors in the risk of contrast reactions. Hyperosmolality has been associated with histamine release stimulation from mast cells and basophils. Non-ionic monomers are also associated with histamine release. The regimen commonly used is adding 50 mg diphenhydramine (IV, IM or PO) to the steroids (prednisone or methylprednisolone) one hour prior to contrast injection.

References
Peachell PT, Morcos SK. Effect of radiographic contrast media on histamine release from human mast cells and basophils. *Br J Radiol*. 1998;71(841):24-30.
ACR Manual on Contrast Media, Version 10.1. Reston, VA: American College of Radiology; 2015 Available at <http://www.acr.org/~/media/37D84428BF1D4E1B9A3A2918DA9E27A3.pdf>.

QUESTIONS

1. The Choosing Wisely program is an initiative of:
   A. The Joint Commission
   B. The American Board of Radiology
   C. The American Board of Internal Medicine (ABIM)
   D. The American College of Radiology

2. The principles of the Choosing Wisely campaign are to:
   A. Eliminate redundancy
   B. Do no harm
   C. Decide through evidence-based medicine
   D. All of the above

3. Which of the following is an Image Wisely recommendation by the American College of Radiology?
   A. Don't recommend follow-up imaging for clinically inconsequential adnexal cysts
   B. Don't do computed tomography (CT) for the evaluation of suspected appendicitis in children until after ultrasound has been considered as an option
   C. Avoid admission or preoperative chest x-rays for ambulatory patients with unremarkable history and physical exam
   D. All of the above

4. Which of the following is an Image Wisely recommendation by the American College of Radiology?
   A. Don't image for suspected pulmonary embolism (PE) without high pretest probability of PE and positive D-dimers
   B. Don't do imaging for uncomplicated headache
   C. Don't do imaging for migraine headaches even if there is pupil dilatation
   D. MR should precede CT for appendicitis in children

5. Which of the following is a recommendation of the Society of Nuclear Medicine and Molecular Imaging for the Image Wisely campaign?
   A. Don't use PET imaging in the evaluation of patients with dementia unless the patient has been assessed by a specialist in this field
   B. Avoid using a computed tomography angiogram to diagnose pulmonary embolism in young women with a normal chest radiograph; consider a radionuclide lung study ("V/Q study") instead
   C. Don't perform routine annual stress testing after coronary artery revascularization
   D. All of the above

6. Which of the following is a recommendation of the Society of Nuclear Medicine and Molecular Imaging for the Image Wisely campaign?
   A. Don't use nuclear medicine thyroid scans to evaluate thyroid nodules in patients with hyperthyroidism
   B. Don't use nuclear medicine thyroid scans to evaluate thyroid nodules in patients with hypothyroidism
   C. Don't use PET/CT for cancer screening in healthy individuals
   D. All of the above

1. **C, The American Board of Internal Medicine (ABIM).** The Choosing Wisely campaign is an initiative of the American Board of Internal Medicine Foundation which partnered with Consumer Reports in 2012. The ABIM solicited Top Five lists from a variety of specialty societies for making correct choices in medicine, leading to over 70 societies providing their recommendations to the program. The goal of the program is to engage physicians and patients in conversations designed to reduce wasteful, unnecessary tests and procedures. Consumer Reports has participated by translating the medical terminology into common English and encouraging patients to question their physicians about such unnecessary testing. In 2012 the American College of Radiology provided its top 5 list.

Reference:
Wolfson D, Santa J, Slass L. Engaging physicians and consumers in conversations about treatment overuse and waste: a short history of the Choosing Wisely campaign. *Acad Med.* 2014;89(7):990-995.

2. **D, All of the above.** According to the Choosing Wisely website, the principles they follow are to provide care that is:
   1. Supported by evidence
   2. Not duplicative of other tests or procedures already received
   3. Free from harm
   4. Truly necessary

   The charter provides for the primacy of patient welfare, patient autonomy, and social justice. The charter emphasizes managing conflicts of interest, improving the quality of care, improving access to care, and promoting the just distribution of finite resources.

References:
Medical Professionalism Project: American Board of Internal Medicine Foundation, American College of Physicians–American Society of Internal Medicine Foundation, and European Federation of Internal Medicine. Medical professionalism in the new millennium: A physicians' charter. *Lancet.* 2002;359: 520-522.
<http://www.choosingwisely.org/wp-content/uploads/2015/04/About -Choosing-Wisely.pdf>.

3. **D, All of the above.** Strangely enough, the Image Wisely campaign is an initiative of the American Board of Internal Medicine (ABIM) foundation, which solicited support from various societies. The ACR in 2012 provided five initial guidelines for imaging wisely on their website. These are:
   1. Don't do imaging for uncomplicated headache.
   2. Don't image for suspected pulmonary embolism (PE) without moderate or high pretest probability of PE.
   3. Avoid admission or preoperative chest x-rays for ambulatory patients with unremarkable history and physical exam.
   4. Don't do computed tomography (CT) for the evaluation of suspected appendicitis in children until after ultrasound has been considered as an option.
   5. Don't recommend follow-up imaging for clinically inconsequential adnexal cysts.

Reference:
<http://www.choosingwisely.org/societies/american-college-of-radiology/>.

4. **B, Don't do imaging for uncomplicated headache.** The ACR 2012 Image Wisely statement about imaging of uncomplicated headaches says:

Don't do imaging for uncomplicated headache.

Imaging headache patients absent specific risk factors for structural disease is not likely to change management or improve outcome. Those patients with a significant likelihood of structural disease requiring immediate attention are detected by clinical screens that have been validated in many settings. Many studies and clinical practice guidelines concur. Also, incidental findings lead to additional medical procedures and expense that do not improve patient well-being.

The American Headache Society has a slightly different take on this: "Don't perform neuroimaging studies in patients with stable headaches that meet criteria for migraine."

Clinical guidelines state that imaging for headaches is typically not needed and most underlying causes can be adequately diagnosed through clinical examination, though special consideration is warranted in the following instances: headaches with sudden onset and maximum severity; presence of neurological symptoms indicating a secondary cause; signs suggesting a systemic disorder; headaches that are worsened by exertion; or headaches that are new or different from a patient's typical pattern of headaches, especially for individuals aged 50 and over.

Reference:
<http://www.choosingwisely.org/societies/american-college-of-radiology/>.
<http://www.choosingwisely.org/wp-content/uploads/2015/05/ICER _Headache.pdf>.

5. **D, All of the above.** The SNMMI has put out their recommendation about PET and dementia: If no dementia, the benefit of PET does not justify the radiation. Even with dementia, PET may not point to a specific cause of the dementia, so clinical evaluation is critical to make a reliable diagnosis and to plan care. For β-amyloid PET imaging, a positive PET result in a patient without cognitive impairment is of unknown value.

References:
<http://www.choosingwisely.org/wp-content/uploads/2015/02/SNMMI -Choosing-Wisely-List.pdf>.
<http://www.choosingwisely.org/clinician-lists/society-nuclear -medicine-molecular-imaging-pet-imaging-to-evaluate-dementia>.

6. **C, Don't use PET/CT for cancer screening in healthy individuals.** The Society of Nuclear Medicine does not believe that screening healthy adults for cancer should be performed by PET-CT. One would hope that any type of whole body screening would be deemed inappropriate for the general public. For those entrepreneurs setting up such enterprises for those wealthy individuals paying out of pocket for screening (executive VIP screenings), one might consider whole body MR/MRA instead or with a combination of MR and Doppler US to reduce the radiation exposure that would otherwise predispose that person to subsequent cancer development.

Reference:
<http://www.imagewisely.org/imaging-modalities/nuclear-medicine/articles/ clinical-aspects>.

7. The Step Lightly campaign principles do not include:
   A. Consider ultrasound instead of CT for appendicitis evaluation in children
   B. Take time out: stop and child-size the technique
   C. Step lightly on the fluoroscopy pedal and limit fluoroscopic time as much as possible
   D. Consider ultrasound or, when applicable, MRI guidance for procedures

8. To reduce radiation exposure the most beneficial step is:
   A. Use last image hold whenever possible instead of exposures
   B. Use ultrasound
   C. Use pulse rather than continuous fluoroscopy when possible and with as low a pulse as possible
   D. Minimize use of electronic magnification; use digital zoom whenever possible

9. Which of the following would increase exposure during fluoroscopy?
   A. Using digital zoom instead of electronic magnification
   B. Lowering the frame rate from 8 to 4 per second
   C. Moving the table toward the x-ray tube and the patient away from the detectors
   D. None of the above

10. When physicians at a hospital are evaluated annually by a compliance committee for their competency it is termed:
    A. Peer review
    B. Ongoing professional practice evaluation (OPPE)
    C. Focused provider practice evaluation (FPPE)
    D. Credentialing

11. OPPE and FPPE are mandated by:
    A. ABR
    B. TJC
    C. ACR
    D. ACGME

7. **A, Consider ultrasound instead of CT for appendicitis evaluation in children.** Because the Step Lightly campaign pertains to radiation safety in pediatric interventional radiology (fluoroscopic) studies, it would not have an opinion between CT and ultrasound in the diagnostic noninterventional domain of appendicitis. However, the ALARA principles would lead one to consider ultrasound instead of CT for appendicitis evaluation in children. The Step Lightly initiative may suggest substituting non-radiation-producing modalities for guiding interventional procedures (ultrasound guided) to drain an appendiceal abscess over those that generate x-rays (fluoroscopic/CT guidance).

Reference:
Sidhu M, Goske MJ, Connolly B, et al. Image Gently, Step Lightly: promoting radiation safety in pediatric interventional radiology. *AJR Am J Roentgenol.* 2010;195(4):W299-W301.

8. **B, Use ultrasound.** The concept of radiation exposure reduction begins with appropriate substitutes that do not generate any radiation. Therefore ultrasound is a very good option for the evaluation of many clinical problems, despite the fact that Americans tend to underutilize that modality compared to the rest of the world. Certainly there are many entities in the head and neck, including lymph nodes, salivary glands, parathyroid glands, and deep neck masses, that are imaged primarily with CT in daily practice that can be easily imaged with ultrasound even before MR for cost bases. When dealing with children, these are the best substitutes to "image gently." Sometimes there is a trade-off between having to sedate a child for an MR procedure versus performing an MDCT (incurring radiation) without sedation. The risk/benefit discussion should be held between the radiologist, the clinician, and the patient/guardian, factoring in the likelihood of making a definitive diagnosis.

Reference:
<http://www.imagegently.org/Portals/6/Procedures/ImGen_StpLight_Chcklst.pdf>.

9. **C, Moving the table toward the x-ray tube and the patient away from the detectors.** One way of increasing patient exposure during a fluoroscopic procedure is to move the patient toward the x-ray tube. In so doing, the anatomy may be magnified by having the patient farther away from the detectors. Magnification can be reduced by bringing the detectors in closer to the patient, and this may lead to a reduction in energy needed to adequately view the anatomy. Bringing the tube and detectors closer to the patient has the added benefit of reduced scatter.

The inverse square law describes the degree of radiation exposure reduction caused by divergence:

$$Xa = Xb \times (Db/Da)^2$$

where Xa is the radiation exposure rate at distance Da, and Xb is the radiation exposure rate at distance Db. This relationship indicates that decreasing the distance from a radiation source by half increases radiation exposure fourfold (Figure 11-1).

If the detector receives more radiation, by moving the x-ray source and the patient closer to it, the automatic brightness control on the fluoroscopic unit will compensate by generating fewer x-rays (which decreases radiation exposure) and/or making them less penetrating by reducing their energy.

Reference:
<http://www.crcpd.org/Pubs/QC-Docs/QC-Vol3-Web.pdf>.

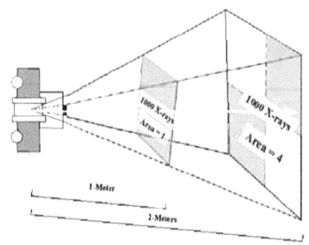

Figure 11-1 Radiation exposure, magnification, and detector distances

10. **B, Ongoing professional practice evaluation (OPPE).** Peer review is a general term describing continuous, systematic evaluation of physician performance using structured procedures. Ongoing professional practice evaluation (OPPE) and focused professional practice evaluation (FPPE) are specific quality assurance standards mandated by The Joint Commission. OPPE is a routine monitoring of competency of current physicians, whereas FFPE is the follow-up process to determine the validity of any concerns found through OPPE. FPPE is also used for new providers requesting privileges or existing providers requesting expanded privileges. Credentialing refers to the process applied by hospitals to verify a practitioner's current licensure, relevant education and training, and competence to perform the privileges requested.

Reference:
Steele JR, Hovsepian DM, Schomer DF. The Joint Commission practice performance evaluation: a primer for radiologists. *J Am Coll Radiol.* 2010;7(6):425-430.

11. **B, TJC.** The Joint Commission (TJC) mandates continuous data-based evaluation and monitoring of physician practice performance through ongoing professional practice evaluation (OPPE) and focused professional practice evaluation (FPPE). OPPE is a process whereby health care organizations are required to review data that reflect competence, not just procedure volume or lack of complications. Each department determines the scope of that review for specific privileges, but there cannot be different standards of care for different departments within the same hospital. FPPE is a locally predefined process whereby a hospital evaluates the competency of a single provider. It is used for new providers requesting privileges, existing providers requesting expanded privileges, or existing providers with whom there is concern about the quality of their practice.

Reference:
Steele JR, Hovsepian DM, Schomer DF. The Joint Commission practice performance evaluation: a primer for radiologists. *J Am Coll Radiol.* 2010;7(6):425-430.

12. Peer review data are:
    A. Subject to subpoena
    B. Discoverable
    C. Not discoverable
    D. Publicly available

13. With regard to continuing medical education, the ABR recommends:
    A. A minimum of 500 credit hours of Accreditation Council for Continuing Medical Education (ACCME) approved Category 1 training over the 10-year cycle
    B. A minimum of 70% of credit hours be in specialty-specific or related areas
    C. Twenty-four self-assessment modules must be completed over the 10-year cycle
    D. At least 25 CME credit hours should be accumulated every year

14. Which of the following qualifies as Category 1 credit?
    A. Attending medical meetings, lectures, and courses that are not designated for Category 1 credit
    B. Teaching medical students, residents, and other graduate physicians or health care professionals
    C. Study of authoritative literature
    D. Test item writing for ACCME

15. Which of the following is not considered Category 2 credit?
    A. Creating a teaching file for oneself
    B. Preceptorships
    C. Medical writing
    D. Self-assessment activities

16. Which of the following is not part of the MOC process?
    A. Lifelong learning and self-assessment
    B. ACR accreditation of your facility
    C. Cognitive expertise
    D. Practice quality improvement

17. Without licensure documentation, your MOC status is:
    A. Out of compliance
    B. Limited unless you are retired
    C. Good for the 10-year cycle
    D. Contingent on fulfilling the other components of MOC

18. The ACR appropriateness criteria are based on scientific evidence and when insufficient data are available:
    A. No recommendations are made
    B. All options are given equal weighting
    C. Expert consensus is used
    D. All of the above

19. The ACR appropriateness criteria are mainly geared to:
    A. Reducing radiation dose
    B. Optimizing profit
    C. Patient safety
    D. Optimizing limited health care resources

20. ACR appropriateness criteria rely first and foremost on:
    A. Expert opinions
    B. Evidence-based medicine
    C. Consensus statements of societies
    D. Radiation dose calculations

12. **C, Not discoverable.** Peer review data are generally not discoverable in subsequent legal action. To encourage free participation in quality improvement measures in the interest of public health, federal and state laws hold that all materials related to such proceedings must remain confidential and privileged. Actions undertaken by a peer review committee must meet certain standards to qualify for immunity from legal claims brought by physicians who have been corrected or disciplined after making a gross error. Those being reviewed are protected from abuses of peer review proceedings resulting either from malice or ulterior motives. In addition, letters, emails, discussions between physicians and hospital administrators, and incident reports may well, under certain circumstances, not meet the criteria for privilege mandated by the courts.

Reference:
Berlin L. Performance improvement and peer-review activities: are they immune from legal discovery? *AJR Am J Roentgenol.* 2003;181(3):649-653.

13. **B, A minimum of 70% of credit hours be in specialty-specific or related areas.** Maintenance of certification (MOC) requires that at least 75 AMA Category 1 CME credits are obtained every 3 years. The ABR recommends that at least 70% of these credit hours be in diagnostic radiology or related areas. The remaining 30% of credit hours should be in clinically related areas or other relevant topics such as risk assessment, ethics, statistics, processes of continuous quality improvement, and methodologies of outcome measurement, among others. Furthermore, at least 25 of the 75 Category 1 CME credits must be in self-assessment CME.

Reference:
<http://www.theabr.org/moc-dr-faq-iv-requirements#one>.

14. **D, Test item writing for ACCME.** The American Medical Association (AMA) defines Category 1 CME credit as any activity that is expected to "serve to maintain, develop, or increase the knowledge, skills, and professional performance and relationships that a physician uses to provide services for patients, the public, or the profession." Category 1 CME activities include attendance-based learning at ACCME-accredited courses; CME activities in journals; CME enduring materials; presentations at conferences; publication in peer-reviewed journals; and test item writing.

References:
<http://www.acr.org/~/media/FBCDC94E0E25448DAD5EE9147370A8D1.pdf>.
<http://csms.org/wp-content/uploads/2014/03/physician-faq1.pdf>.

15. **A, Creating a teaching file for oneself.** AMA Category 2 CME credits are self-designated and claimed by the physician for participation in worthwhile educational activities that do not meet criteria for Category 1 credits. Examples of Category 2 CME credits include attending medical meetings, lectures, and courses that are not designated for Category 1 credit; teaching medical students, residents, and other graduate physicians or health care professionals; study of authoritative literature; unstructured learning and online searches; participation in peer review and quality assurance activities; participation on medical and related scientific panels and committees; research; preceptorships; medical writing; self-assessment activities; and consultation with peers and medical experts.

References:
<http://www.acr.org/~/media/FBCDC94E0E25448DAD5EE9147370A8D1.pdf>.
<http://csms.org/wp-content/uploads/2014/03/physician-faq1.pdf>.

16. **B, ACR accreditation of your facility.** The MOC program seeks to continuously evaluate six essential competencies, which are defined by the Accreditation Council on Graduate Medical Education (ACGME) and the American Board of Medical Specialties (ABMS). The six essential competencies are medical knowledge, patient care and procedural skills, interpersonal and communication skills, professionalism, practice-based learning and improvement, and systems-based practice. The MOC process evaluates the six competencies by assessing professional standing, lifelong learning and self-assessment, cognitive expertise, and practice quality improvement (PQI).

Reference:
<http://www.theabr.org/moc-gen-landing>.

17. **A, Out of compliance.** MOC requires maintaining valid, unrestricted licensure to practice medicine in all states in which the diplomate holds an active license. Without licensure documentation, the diplomate's MOC status will be out of compliance. In addition, if any disciplinary action is taken against a diplomate's state medical license, the diplomate must inform the ABR of the disciplinary action within 60 days.

Reference:
<http://www.theabr.org/moc-dr-faq-iv-requirements#one>.

18. **C, Expert consensus is used.** Comment (from ACR website):

The American College of Radiology (ACR) Appropriateness Criteria (AC) methodology is based on the RAND Appropriateness Method. The appropriateness ratings for each of the procedures or treatments included in the AC topics are determined using a modified Delphi method. A series of surveys are conducted to elicit each panelist's expert interpretation of the evidence, based on the available data, regarding the appropriateness of an imaging or therapeutic procedure for a specific clinical scenario. The expert panel members review the evidence presented and assess the risks or harms of doing the procedure balanced with the benefits of performing the procedure. The direct or indirect costs of a procedure are not considered as a risk or harm when determining appropriateness. When the evidence for a specific topic and variant is uncertain or incomplete, expert opinion may supplement the available evidence or may be the sole source for assessing the appropriateness.

Reference:
<https://www.guideline.gov/content.aspx?id=49074&search=radiology>.

19. **D, Optimizing limited health care resources.** ACR appropriateness criteria are mainly geared to optimizing limited health care resources. They are evidence-based guidelines assisting providers to make the most appropriate imaging decisions for a specific clinical condition, including topics in diagnostic radiology, interventional radiology, and radiation oncology.

Reference:
<http://www.acr.org/Quality-Safety/Appropriateness-Criteria/About-AC>.

20. **B, Evidence-based medicine.** ACR appropriateness criteria guidelines are the most comprehensive guidelines for selection of diagnostic imaging, radiotherapy protocols, and image-guided interventional procedures, and they rely first and foremost on evidence-based medicine. When the scientific data in the literature are insufficient, then the decisions for given patient clinical conditions are managed by expert consensus. In addition to radiologists, physicians from other medical specialties are also represented in the expert panel.

Reference:
<http://www.acr.org/Quality-Safety/Appropriateness-Criteria/About-AC>.

21. ACR appropriateness criteria are currently being employed in:
    A. Physician decision support order entry
    B. Medicolegal scenarios
    C. ACR practice parameter guidelines
    D. NIH study protocols

22. In the ACR's view of peer review the gold standard is:
    A. Pathology proof
    B. Clinical impression (i.e., discharge diagnosis)
    C. Peer consensus
    D. An expert adjudicator

23. Why is the peer review term *discrepancy* used rather than *error*?
    A. Pathology proof is required
    B. There is rarely a reliable gold standard available
    C. Reading of imaging is subjective
    D. For medicolegal purposes

24. The guidelines of all specialties in medicine are distributed on what website?
    A. AMA's Guidelines of Specialties
    B. National Guideline Clearinghouse of the Agency for Healthcare Research and Quality
    C. Health Resources and Services Administration
    D. Center for Medicare Services (CMS)

25. The modified Delphi technique for ACR appropriateness criteria refers to :
    A. Using an indirect, anonymous, iterative method to achieve consensus among experts by serial rounds of voting
    B. Using sequential voting to eliminate outliers from consideration first and then rank ordering procedures
    C. Having less authoritative rankers provide initial listings with experts revising the initial assessments through the process of elimination
    D. Using open discussion and voting to arrive at consensus rankings of studies

26. Relative radiation risk is assessed in the ACR appropriateness criteria based on:
    A. An adult effective dose from 0 mSv to 100 mSv
    B. An estimated adult effective dose from 1 rad to 5 rad
    C. None to minimal to moderate to marked
    D. None of the above

21. **A, Physician decision support order entry.** ACR appropriateness criteria are currently being employed in physician decision support order entry as ACR Select™, which is a licensed product of the ACR, ready to incorporate into computerized ordering systems to guide providers when ordering medical imaging scans. Whenever the exam seems to be inappropriate, appropriateness feedback appears with alternative exams.

Reference:
<http://www.acr.org/~/media/ACR/Documents/AppCriteria/Misc/ACRSelect_CPOE.pdf>.

22. **C, Peer consensus.** In the ACR's view of peer review, the gold standard is peer consensus. Confirmation with pathology is not always available and, if available, still relies on the interpretation of a pathologist. Clinical follow-up may not be 100% accurate and is subject to change if new labs or studies become available. A single expert adjudicator may be prone to bias and/or subjectivity. The peer review process should strive to be as fair as possible and minimize bias.

Reference:
Borgstede JP, Lewis RS, Bhargavan M, et al. RADPEER quality assurance program: a multifacility study of interpretive disagreement rates. *J Am Coll Radiol.* 2004;1(1):59-65.

23. **B, There is rarely a reliable gold standard available.** The peer review term *discrepancy* is used rather than *error* because there is rarely a reliable gold standard available. In an ideal scenario, a quality evaluation process would assess the accuracy of a report rather than a discrepancy among different radiologists. However, that level of assessment would necessitate confirmation with pathology or operative findings, which might be available only in a limited number of cases. Further, these "gold standards" may not always be 100% reliable and would need to be independently verified.

Reference:
Larson PA, Pyatt RS Jr, Grimes CK, et al. Getting the most out of RADPEER™. *J Am Coll Radiol.* 2011;8(8):543-548.

24. **B, National Guideline Clearinghouse of the Agency for Healthcare Research and Quality.** The National Guideline Clearinghouse of the Agency for Healthcare Research and Quality uses expert panels and a vetting process for literature reliability to arrive at its guidelines. The guidelines for multiple specialties can be found on this website. ACR appropriateness criteria can be found there by searching on keyword *radiology*.

The strength of the evidence is graded as follows:

Rating Scheme for the Strength of the Evidence
Study Quality Category Definitions
Category 1: The study is well-designed and accounts for common biases.
Category 2: The study is moderately well-designed and accounts for most common biases.Category 3: There are important study design limitations.
Category 4: The study is not useful as primary evidence. The article may not be a clinical study or the study design is invalid, or conclusions are based on expert consensus. For example:
  1. The study does not meet the criteria for or is not a hypothesis-based clinical study (eg, a book chapter or case report or case series description).
  2. The study may synthesize and draw conclusions about several studies such as a literature review article or book chapter but is not primary evidence.
  3. The study is an expert opinion or consensus document.

With respect to the ACR appropriateness guidelines, the ACR uses an ordinal scale of integers from 1 to 9, grouped into three categories: 1, 2, or 3 are in the category "usually not appropriate," where the harms of doing the procedure outweigh the benefits; and 7, 8, or 9 are in the category "usually appropriate," where the benefits of doing a procedure outweigh the harms or risks. The middle category, designated "may be appropriate," is represented by 4, 5, or 6 on the scale. The middle category is when the risks and benefits are equivocal or unclear, the dispersion of the individual ratings from the group median rating is too large (ie, disagreement), the evidence is contradictory or unclear, or there are special circumstances or subpopulations that could influence the risks or benefits that are embedded in the variant.

Reference:
<https://www.guideline.gov/content.aspx?id=49074&search=radiology>.

25. **A, Using an indirect, anonymous, iterative process to achieve consensus among experts by serial rounds of voting.** The modified Delphi process is a method for developing consensus that combines evidence-based medicine, supported by systematic literature reviews, with the Delphi process. The Delphi process employs multiple rounds of anonymous voting to promote change of views from a previously held position without embarrassment, together with controlled feedback regulated by a nonvoting chairperson. Evidence-based medicine reviews are delivered to the voting members so that the process shifts from mere clinical opinions to methodologically sound evidence. Multiple iterations of the votes, and finally the consensus statements, are floated before a group decision is achieved.

The process may look like this:
1. Open ended questionnaire
2. Collect responses
3. Convert questionnaire to a more specific target question
4. Provide literature review to voters
5. Second round of survey data collected
6. Rank order options with rationale for rankings
7. Share responses with group
8. Additional rounds as needed

References:
<http://www.ncbi.nlm.nih.gov/pmc/articles/PMC2563522/>.
Hsu CC, Sandford BA. The Delphi technique: making sense of consensus. *Pract Assess Res Eval.* 2007;12(10):1531-7714.

26. **A, An adult effective dose from 0 mSv to 100 mSv.** Based on the BEIR VII report on the risks of cancer and leukemia in patients exposed to medical procedures, the adult effective dose range between 0 mSv and 100 mSv is provided. This is graded on a 0 to 5 radiation shield scale to demonstrate the degree of radiation dose from various radiologic procedures. Because exact numbers vary due to patient habitus and scanning parameters used, the qualitative scale is generally preferred.

Reference:
<http://www.acr.org/~/media/a27a29133302408bb86888eafd460a1f.pdf>.

27. According to the ACR appropriateness criteria for relative radiation dose level, an abdomen CT without and with contrast has the same score for radiation risk as:
    A. A nuclear medicine bone scan
    B. Transjugular intrahepatic portosystemic shunt placement
    C. Whole body PET
    D. 20 hand radiographs

28. Residency milestones in diagnostic health care economics include:
    A. Describes the mechanisms for reimbursement, including types of payers
    B. States relative costs of common procedures
    C. Describes measurements of physician productivity and performance (eg, relative value units)
    D. All of the above

29. Ultrasound accreditation by the American College of Radiology is limited to:
    A. Radiology departments
    B. Radiology and obstetrics departments
    C. Radiology, obstetrics, and emergency medicine departments
    D. It is not limited to any specific departments

30. To maintain ultrasound accreditation a physician must interpret a minimum of how many cases in a 24-month period?
    A. 240
    B. 480
    C. 960
    D. None of the above

27. **C, Whole body PET.** According to the ACR Relative Radiation Risk Document, Table 11-1 shows dose equivalency of common studies in radiology. Based on this algorithm, the 4 radiation shield emblem study equivalent in radiation dosage to abdominal CT with and without contrast is a whole body PET.

Reference:
<http://www.acr.org/~/media/a27a29133302408bb86888eafd460a1f.pdf>.

28. **D, All of the above.** From the Radiology Milestone project, Table 11-2 shows the expectations and parameters.

Reference:
The Diagnostic Radiology Milestone Project. A joint initiative of the Accreditation Council for Graduate Medical Education and the American Board of Radiology. <https://www.acgme.org/acgmeweb/Portals/0/PDFs/Milestones/DiagnosticRadiologyMilestones.pdf>.

29. **D, It is not limited to any specific departments.** Ultrasound accreditation refers to the equipment and expertise that are used and "approved" by the ACR. Physicians who are in emergency medicine and obstetrics and gynecology can be accredited by the ACR if they meet the same criteria and submit the requisite quality clinical images. Nonetheless, the ACR Practice Parameter for performing and interpreting ultrasound (2014) states:

Physicians not board certified in radiology or not trained in a diagnostic radiology residency program,

and who assume these responsibilities for sonographic imaging exclusively in a specific anatomical area should meet the following criteria: Completion of an ACGME approved residency program in specialty practice plus 200 hours of Category I CME in the subspecialty where ultrasound reading occurs; and supervision and/or performance, interpretation, and reporting of 500 cases relative to each subspecialty area interpreted (eg, pelvic, obstetrical, breast, thyroid, vascular) during the past 36 months in a supervised situation.

Reference:
<http://www.acr.org/~/media/ACR/Documents/Accreditation/US/USFAQ.pdf>.

30. **D, None of the above.** The physician seeking accreditation in ultrasonography must have (1) earned at least 15 CME in ultrasound (half of which must be Category 1) over the prior 36-month period, and (2) interpreted a minimum average of 9 examinations per month over a 24-month period. To be accredited in vascular ultrasound, the physician must specify (along with the cases submitted) the diagnostic criteria the physician uses to characterize the studies as normal vs abnormal, including velocity tables for duplex carotid exams.

Reference:
<http://www.acr.org/~/media/ACR/Documents/Accreditation/US/USFAQ.pdf>.

Table 11-1 RELATIVE RADIATION LEVEL DESIGNATIONS ALONG WITH COMMON EXAMPLE EXAMINATIONS FOR EACH CLASSIFICATION

Relative Radiation Level*	Adult Effective Dose Estimate Range	Pediatric Effective Dose Estimate Range	Example Examinations
0	0	0 mSv	Ultrasound; MRI
☢	<0.1 mSv	<0.03 mSv	Chest radiographs; hand radiographs
☢☢	0.1-1 mSv	0.03-0.3 mSv	Pelvis radiographs; mammography
☢☢☢	1-10 mSv	0.3-3 mSv	Abdomen CT, nuclear medicine bone scan
☢☢☢☢	10-30 mSv	3-10 mSv	Abdomen CT without and with contrast; whole body PET
☢☢☢☢☢	30-100 mSv	10-30 mSv	CTA chest abdomen and pelvis with contrast; transjugular intrahepatic portosystemic shunt placement

*The RRL assignments for some of the examinations cannot be made, because the actual patient doses in these procedures vary as a function of a number of factors (eg, the region of the body exposed to ionizing radiation, the imaging guidance that is used, etc.). The RRLs for these examinations are designated as "Varies." (From http://www.acr.org/~/media/A27A29133302408BB86888EAFD460A1F.pdf.)

Table 11-2 SYSTEMS-BASED PRACTICE (SBP2)

SBP2: Health Care Economics					
Has not achieved Level 1	Level 1	Level 2	Level 3	Level 4	Level 5
	Describes the mechanisms for reimbursement, including types of payors	States relative cost of common procedures	Describes the technical and professional components of imaging costs	Describes measurements of productivity (eg, RVUs)	Describes the radiology revenue cycle

31. The Dose Index Registry pertains to:
    A. CT
    B. Radiography
    C. Nuclear medicine
    D. All of the above

32. Compliance and monitoring through the Dose Index Registry fulfills The Joint Commission requirement for:
    A. Root cause analysis
    B. Practice quality improvement
    C. Meaningful use
    D. Value modifier

33. The national mammography database (NMD) provides data on which of the following parameters?
    A. Cancer detection rates
    B. Positive predictive value rates
    C. Recall rates
    D. All of the above

34. When the NMD provides its data it does so for:
    A. Physicians
    B. Facilities
    C. Groups
    D. All of the above

31. A, CT. The Dose Index Registry is a site where facilities can compare their CT measures of radiation dose output of a CT scanner. Parameters may include median, 25th, and 75th percentile values of (1) normalized size specific dose estimate (SSDE), (2) CTDIvol = CTDIw/pitch, or (3) dose length product (DLP) assessed as CTDIvol × scan length.

Dose indices for all CT exams are collected, anonymized, transmitted to the ACR, and stored in a database. The ACR provides facilities with feedback comparing their radiation doses by body part and exam type to the national data.

The ACR specifies that dose indices for head exams are normalized to a 16-cm phantom, and dose indices for body exams are normalized to a 32-cm phantom for comparison.

For exams involving the head region using a phantom size 32, the normalized CTDIvol is obtained by multiplying the mean CTDIvol, and normalized DLP is obtained by multiplying the DLP by the conversion factor of 2.3. For head exams using a 16-cm phantom, the normalized CTDIvol and DLP are the same as the original CTDIvol and DLP.

For body exams not done with a phantom size 16, normalized CTDIvol and DLP are calculated by dividing the mean CTDIvol and DLP by a conversion factor of 2.3. For body exams using a 32-cm phantom, the normalized CTDIvol and DLP are the same as the original CTDIvol and DLP.

References:
<http://www.acr.org/~/media/ACR/Documents/PDF/QualitySafety/NRDR/DIR/DIR%20Measures.pdf>.
<http://www.acr.org/Quality-Safety/National-Radiology-Data-Registry/Dose-Index-Registry>.

32. B, Practice quality improvement. This is yet another ACR-generated idea for a practice quality improvement initiative for fulfillment of certification purposes. Also in 2015, the ACR National Radiology Data Registry was approved as a Qualified Clinical Data Registry (QCDR) for the CMS Physician Quality Reporting System (PQRS). CMS states that one must report (1) at least 9 measures covering three National Quality Strategy (NQS) domains for at least 50% of applicable patients (all patients, not just Medicare) seen during the 2015 participation period and (2) at least two outcome measures. If two outcome measures are not available, then report on at least one outcome measure and one of the additional measures listed: resource use, patient experience of care, efficiency appropriate use, or another patient safety measure.

Reference:
<http://www.acr.org/Quality-Safety/National-Radiology-Data-Registry>.

33. D, All of the above. The NMD provides assessments of physicians, groups, and facilities as far as the entity's cancer detection, positive predictive value, and recall rates in semi-annual reports. National benchmark data are provided by the NCI-funded Breast Cancer Surveillance Consortium, which is a research resource for studies designed to assess the delivery and quality of breast cancer screening and related patient outcomes in the United States. It is funded in part by the National Cancer Institute. The goal is to assess the impact of breast cancer screening on stage at diagnosis, survival, and/or breast cancer mortality.

Reference:
http://www.acr.org/Quality-Safety/National-Radiology-Data-Registry/National-Mammography-DB.

34. D, All of the above. The goal of the National Mammography Database is to provide comparable data for national and regional benchmarking. Participation serves as fulfilling a practice quality improvement initiative as part of the ABR's MOC program. It also fulfills the practice-based learning and improvement goal of the Core Competencies.

Reference:
<http://www.acr.org/Quality-Safety/National-Radiology-Data-Registry/National-Mammography-DB>.

CHAPTER 12 Quality Improvement Tools and Concepts

QUESTIONS

1. The type of diagram depicted in Figure 12-1 is called a:
   A. Pareto diagram
   B. Cause and effect diagram
   C. Scatter plot diagram
   D. Gantt chart diagram

2. The type of diagram depicted in Figure 12-2 is called a:
   A. Pareto diagram
   B. Fishbone diagram
   C. Flow chart diagram
   D. Gantt chart diagram

3. The type of diagram depicted in Figure 12-3 is called a(n):
   A. Pareto chart
   B. Pie chart
   C. Exploded pie chart
   D. Gantt chart

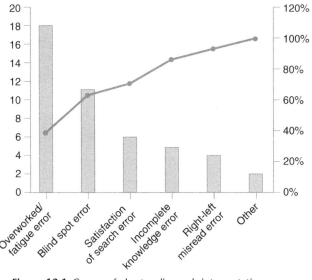

Figure 12-1 Causes of chest radiograph interpretation errors

Figure 12-3 Sales in 2017

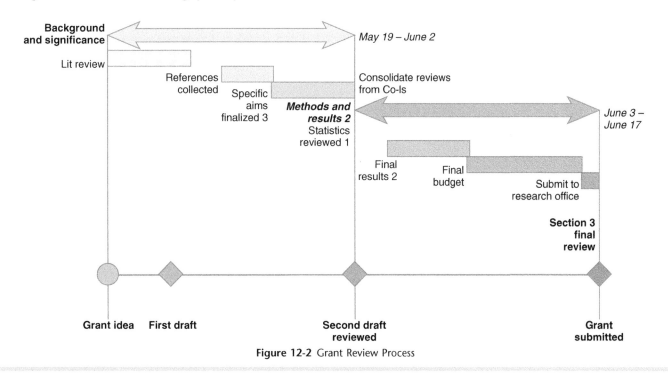

Figure 12-2 Grant Review Process

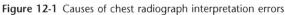

1. **A, Pareto diagram.** A Pareto diagram or chart is a bar graph that is used to analyze data about the frequency or causes of a problem (see Figure 12-1). When there are many causes for a problem, the most cost-effective way to improve the quality is to focus on the most significant causes and address them first. The lengths of the bars represent frequency or cost (time or money) and are arranged with the longest bars on the left and the shortest to the right. In this way the chart visually depicts which situations are more significant. The percentage for each category is calculated, such as 38% for the "over-worked-fatigue" category as in Figure 12-1. Then, the cumulative sum is calculated and drawn on the graph as a line (ie, purple line in the figure). The cumulative sum line should reach 100% on the right scale.

Reference:
<http://asq.org/learn-about-quality/cause-analysis-tools/overview/pareto.html>.

2. **D, Gantt chart diagram.** A Gantt chart is commonly used in project management to display activities against time (see Figure 12-2). It illustrates what needs to be done and when. Different activities or tasks are listed on the left of the chart and a suitable time scale is seen along the activity bar or on the top of the chart. The length of the bar represents the start date, duration, and end date of the activity. Figure 12-2 depicts different activities for a grant submission. The time scale of each activity is mentioned and short-term goals for each subcategory of activities are defined. Gantt charts illustrate the start and finish dates of the terminal elements and summary elements of a project. Modern Gantt charts also show the dependency (ie, precedence network) relationships between activities. Gantt charts can be used to show current schedule status using percent-complete shadings and a vertical "TODAY" line as shown in the figure.

Reference:
<http://www.gantt.com>.

3. **C, Exploded pie chart.** A pie chart (or a circle chart) is a circular statistical graphic that is divided into slices to illustrate numerical proportion (see Figure 12-3). In a pie chart, the arc length of each slice (and consequently its central angle and area), is proportional to the quantity it represents. Although it is named for its resemblance to a pie that has been sliced, there are variations on the way it can be presented. An exploding pie chart is used to emphasize an individual slice or multiple slices of a pie chart; you can move it back from the rest of the pie chart and you can fit it back in. 3D pie chart effects and exploding slices can produce optical effects that make it easier (or harder) to compare different categories.

Reference:
<http://www2.le.ac.uk/offices/ld/resources/numerical-data/pie-charts>.

4. Dr. Jones is asked to review the previous 100 misses in mammography. He looks at all the cases retrospectively and determines that one of the issues is that the flat plate screen used had a defect at the 3 o'clock location of the detector, leading to misses in that area. This is an example of:
   A. Quality control analysis
   B. Quality improvement analysis
   C. Quality assurance analysis
   D. Total quality management

5. Having completed his retrospective analysis, Dr. Jones begins to review each mammogram prospectively for homogeneity across the digital screen detector. He implements a new screen scanner that each morning (8 AM), afternoon (1 PM), and evening (5 PM) scans to detect heterogeneous luminance. This is an example of:
   A. Quality control analysis
   B. Quality improvement analysis
   C. Quality assurance analysis
   D. Peer review analysis

6. Dr. Jones' chief mammography technician employs a process whereby she screens each case to ensure that medial and lateral markers are placed just to the lateral edge of the study to ensure peripheral cancers are not missed. If a marker is misplaced she has the tech repeat the study. This is an example of:
   A. Quality control analysis
   B. Quality improvement analysis
   C. Quality assurance analysis
   D. Total quality management

7. Dr. Ames looks up the RVU numbers for a musculoskeletal radiologist in academic medicine on the AAARAD and ACR sites. She then sets goals for her MSK division to achieve. This is an example of:
   A. Dashboarding
   B. Credentialing
   C. Certifying
   D. Benchmarking

8. The letters PDSA in quality improvement refer to:
   A. Plan-Do-Study-Act
   B. Prospective Delivery System Activity
   C. Propose Diagnose Survey Actual
   D. Perform Deliberate Suggest Action-plan

9. The difference between Lean Process Improvement and Six Sigma process improvement is:
   A. The degree of detail provided
   B. Lean comes after Six Sigma
   C. One is Toyota based and the other is General Electric based
   D. Lean is continuous; Six Sigma is for resolving a problem

10. The Five S Tool Kit refers to which of the following?
   A. Sorting, straightening, sweeping, standardizing, sustaining
   B. Strategizing, sorting, streamlining, standardizing, sustaining
   C. Sorting, streamlining, systemic cleaning, standardizing, sustaining
   D. Sorting, straightening, systemic cleaning, standardizing, sustaining

4. **C, Quality assurance analysis.** This is an example of quality assurance (QA). QA was a common term for a number of years. Quality improvement (QI) is a more recent phenomenon in health care and has replaced QA. QA can be considered reactive, generally retrospective, occasionally involving policing, and in many ways punitive or finger pointing. It often involves determining who was at fault after a medical error.

Reference:
<http://www.hrsa.aquilentprojects.com/healthit/toolbox/HealthITAdoption-toolbox/QualityImprovement/whatarediffbtwqinqa.html>.

5. **B, Quality improvement analysis.** This is an example of quality improvement (QI). QI is a more recent phenomenon than quality assurance in health care and involves both prospective and retrospective reviews. It is aimed at improvement—measuring where you are and figuring out ways to make things better. It specifically attempts to avoid attributing blame and to create systems that prevent errors from happening. It is a continuous process (also known as continuous quality improvement, or CQI) that must occur consistently in an ongoing fashion, unlike QA, which is static. QI activities can be very helpful in improving how things work. Trying to locate the "defect" in the system and determining new ways to do things can be challenging and fun. It's a great opportunity to "think outside the box."

The following chart explains the difference between QA and QI:

	Quality Assurance	Quality Improvement
Motivation	Measuring compliance with standards	Continuously improving processes to meet standards
Means	Inspection	Prevention
Attitude	Required, defensive	Chosen, proactive
Focus	Outliers: *"bad apples"* Individuals	Processes Systems
Scope	Medical provider	Patient care
Responsibility	Few	All

(From http://www.hrsa.aquilentprojects.com/healthit/toolbox/HealthITAdoptiontoolbox/QualityImprovement/whatarediffbtwqinqa.html)

6. **C, Quality assurance analysis.** This is an example of quality assurance. It relies on inspection and focuses on the noncompliant individuals. It is reactive, generally retrospective, punitive, and involves policing. It often involves determining who was at fault after a medical error (see preceding chart).

Reference:
<http://www.hrsa.aquilentprojects.com/healthit/toolbox/HealthITAdoption-toolbox/QualityImprovement/whatarediffbtwqinqa.html>.

7. **D, Benchmarking.** Benchmarking is measurement of the quality of an organization's policies, products, programs, strategies, and their comparison with standard measurements or similar measurements of its peers. The objectives of benchmarking are (1) to determine what and where improvements are called for, (2) to analyze how other organizations achieve their high performance levels, and (3) to use this information to improve performance.

Dashboarding is not the correct answer. A dashboard is a visual display of the most important information needed to achieve one or more objectives, consolidated and arranged on a single screen so the information can be monitored at a glance.

Credentialing is the process whereby one gains admission to a medical staff, in the case of a hospital, or to a panel of health care providers, in the case of an insurance company or other institution. This is essentially a verification process or background check conducted through a formal application process.

Reference:
<http://bizbench.com/dashboarding-vs-benchmarking/>.

8. **A, Plan-Do-Study-Act.** The PDSA (Plan-Do-Study-Act) cycle is a four-step process commonly used for continuous quality improvement. This simple but powerful tool may serve as the basis for an action-oriented iterative process by linking multiple PDSA cycles repeated in sequence. An initial cycle is performed to obtain baseline data, followed by subsequent cycles applied to assess the effects of quality improvement initiatives.

In recent years PDSA has replaced the PDCA acronym (the Study process has replaced the Checking step). W. Edwards Deming, considered the father of modern quality improvement efforts, initially used PDCA to imply more straightforward quality improvement projects, and PDSA was to be applied in more complex scenarios that required more introspection. Thus Deming recommended converting from PDCA to PDSA to emphasize the importance of reflecting on the meaning of the metrics you've checked. Deming emphasized using the PDSA cycle lessons to better understand the product or process being improved.

Reference:
<http://www.valuebasedmanagement.net/methods_demingcycle.html>.

9. **D, Lean is continuous, Six Sigma is for resolving a problem.** Lean is a continuous process of improvement first developed by Toyota, designed to eliminate waste. Lean has five essential elements: identify value, identify value stream, flow, pull, and perfection. Six Sigma is a method designed to resolve a specific problem by reducing variation, and can be remembered by the acronym DMAIC: **D**-define, **M**-measure, **A**-analyze, **I**-improve, **C**-control.

Reference:
Nave D. How to Compare Six Sigma, Lean and the Theory of Constraints. *Quality Prog.* 2002;35(3):73-78. <http://www.lean.org/Search/Documents/242.pdf>.

10. **D, Sorting, straightening, systemic cleaning, standardizing, sustaining.** 5S comes from the Japanese process of Lean and is designed to help build a quality physical work environment. The 5S condition of a workplace is critical to employee morale and customer first impressions. The 5S's are: sort (eliminate nonessential items), straighten (organize whatever remains), systemic cleaning or shine (clean the work area), standardize (schedule regular cleaning and maintain), sustain (make 5S a way of life).

Reference:
Five S (5S) Tutorial. <http://asq.org/learn-about-quality/lean/overview/five-s-tutorial.html>.

11. Dr. Elfert maintains very few aneurysm coils in house because he fears they will expire due to his low volume of cases. Instead, he orders his coils the day before his elective aneurysm procedures to ensure lack of waste. This process is called:
    A. Inventory management
    B. Pull system management
    C. Optimal product quotient preparedness
    D. Lean inventory

12. Dr. Francis was performing a series of 24 RF ablations of mouse liver tumors, one after the other, during a research day when he realized that the burn magnitude on the ablater had been set too high on mouse 19. To immediately address the issue he should:
    A. Call a code
    B. "Stop the line"
    C. Demand a Six Sigma analysis
    D. Ask for a root cause analysis

13. The Six Sigma process uses the acronym *DMAIC*, which stands for:
    A. Design, manipulate, adapt, invent, collaborate
    B. Delegate, measure, analyze, improvise, coordinate
    C. Design, measure, analyze, improve, control
    D. Designate, manipulate, align, interrogate, collect

14. Six Sigma refers to:
    A. The first six versions of the 1.5T GE Sigma MR scanner
    B. The six system tools defined by the Japanese words *seiri, seiton, seiso, seiketsu, shitsuke, saison*
    C. 3.4 defects per million occurrences
    D. 6.66666 defects per million attempts

15. Two Sigma refers to the equivalent of:
    A. P value < 0.05
    B. 2 errors per million occurrences
    C. Two Lean Sigma studies
    D. *Seiri* and *seiton*

16. Which is not a scenario where Six Sigma would apply?
    A. Wrong site surgery
    B. Plane takeoffs and landings
    C. Epi-pen functionality
    D. Perioperative infections

17. The key performance indicators that Dr. James Thrall of Harvard Medical School likely has established for his department might reasonably be:
    A. Total NIH grant value, patient satisfaction, RSNA awards
    B. Report turnaround times, physician salary ranks, ROI on capital equipment
    C. Manuscripts, NIH grant dollars, faculty on editorial boards
    D. Resident evaluations, teaching awards, medical students taking radiology rotations

18. A dashboard is useful for:
    A. Preventing damage from random errors
    B. Assessing the "state of the state"
    C. Identifying root cause analyses
    D. Selecting the best employees

19. The kind of flow chart that optimally shows how two parallel and intermingling processes work together (ie, preparing a fibula for myocutaneous graft reconstruction of an oral cavity cancer at the same time as the resection of the oral cavity cancer and mandible) is a:
    A. Value stream diagram
    B. Spaghetti diagram
    C. Pareto diagram
    D. Swim lane diagram

20. A map of the location of a specimen after an ultrasound guided biopsy as it proceeds to pathology would best be depicted with a:
    A. Value stream diagram
    B. Spaghetti diagram
    C. Pareto diagram
    D. Swim lane diagram

11. **B, Pull system management.** Pull system management is one of the five essential steps of Lean thinking. The steps of the Lean process are: (1) identify which features create value, (2) identify the sequence of activities (called the value stream), (3) make the activities flow, (4) let the customer pull product or service through the process, and (5) perfect the process. By using this inventory management strategy, Dr. Elfert is best able to manage his inventory costs. The other answer choices are not part of the Lean methodology.

Reference:
Nave D. How to Compare Six Sigma, Lean and the Theory of Constraints. *Quality Prog.* 2002;35(3):73-78. <http://www.lean.org/Search/Documents/242.pdf>.

12. **B, "Stop the Line."** In this case, Dr. Francis must "stop the line" and adjust the ablater settings. "Stop the line" is a Lean concept originating from Toyota where any factory worker was capable of stopping the assembly line if he/she noticed a defect. In this application of "stop the line" to health care, Dr. Francis immediately stops his procedure and searches for the root cause of the problem.

Reference:
Stop the line manufacturing and continuous integration. Available at: <https://leanbuilds.wordpress.com/tag/stop-the-line/>.

13. **C, Design, measure, analyze, improve, control.** DMAIC is the acronym to help remember the essential processes of Six Sigma, **D**-define, **M**-measure, **A**-analyze, **I**-improve, **C**-control. The first step in Six Sigma is to define the process: who the customers are, what their problems are, what is important to them, and what the current process elements are. Next, the process is measured and data are collected and then analyzed for problems or causes of defects. Then solutions to the process are developed and implemented to improve the process. Finally, if the process is performing as desired it is "put under control" and monitored for unexpected changes.

Reference:
Nave D. How to Compare Six Sigma, Lean and the Theory of Constraints. *Quality Prog.* 2002;35(3):73-78. <http://www.lean.org/Search/Documents/242.pdf>.

14. **C, 3.4 defects per million occurrences.** Six Sigma is a methodology for eliminating defects and minimizing variability from a process using data. The goal is to achieve six standard deviations from the mean and the nearest specification limit, which comes out to be no more than 3.4 defects per million opportunities, with a defect being anything outside of specifications, and the opportunity being the total number of chances for a defect. Answer B is part of the Five S tool that focuses on standardization of work areas.

Reference:
<http://howardgitlow.com/definitionsofsixsigma.htm>.

15. **A, P value <0.05.** As Sigma represents standard deviation from the mean (Six Sigma being 6 standard deviations), Two Sigma stands for 2 standard deviations from the mean (95%), which corresponds to a P value of <0.05. One standard deviation is 68%, and 3 is 99.7%.

Reference:
<http://howardgitlow.com/definitionsofsixsigma.htm>.

16. **D, Perioperative infections.** Six Sigma performance has a target rate of defect of 3.4 per million opportunities. Answers A through C all represent scenarios in which this target rate of defect is acceptable. Perioperative infections, however, are far more common than 3.4 per million opportunities, and therefore fall far below Six Sigma level of performance.

Reference:
<https://www.psqh.com/julsep04/pextonyoung.html>.

17. **A, Total NIH grant value, patient satisfaction, RSNA awards.** A key performance indicator is any measure that is selected to evaluate the success of an organization. These can be financial, quality, or both. Indicators should be established by each organization, meaning they are not universal, and all indicators should have the ability to be reproducibly measured. In this example, option B focuses entirely on financials, option C focuses entirely on research, and option D focuses entirely on education. Option A offers the most well rounded KPI for an academic institution.

Reference:
Abujudeh HH, Kaewlai R, Asfaw BA, et al. Quality initiatives: Key performance indicators for measuring and improving radiology department performance. *Radiographics.* 2010;30(3):571-580.

18. **B, Assessing the "state of the state."** A dashboard is a display of important information on one screen so information can be monitored efficiently in the effort to achieve an objective. Some examples of items that could be measured are case volumes throughout the day, turnaround time, RVUs.

Reference:
<http://bizbench.com/dashboarding-vs-benchmarking/>.

19. **D, Swim lane diagram.** Swim lane flow charts separate processes or decisions into two lanes, divided by a parallel line. The sequence of events in the overall process occurs in order in the longitudinal direction with each step falling into one of the subprocesses in one of the lanes. Arrows extend between the subprocesses indicating how materials or information is transferred between the steps.

Reference:
<https://www.mindtools.com/pages/article/newTMC_89.htm>.

20. **B, Spaghetti diagram.** Spaghetti diagrams track the path of a specific item as it travels through the process of an organization. This can be used to map the motion of information, patients, or, as in this case, materials. This differs from a value stream map in that a value stream map is a customer-centered process that uses data elements to assess flow of materials and information to deliver a product or service to a customer. Pareto diagrams assess problems under the principle that a small number of processes contribute to a majority of problems. These processes are stacked in a column in descending order, with the highest occurrence being on top and/or to the left in the diagram. As it descends, the cumulative percentage can be used to determine the 20% of items that contribute to 80% of the problem.

Reference:
<http://asq.org/learn-about-quality/process-analysis-tools/overview/spaghetti-diagram.html>.

21. The saying that "20% of the people cause 80% of the problems" is a reflection of the:
    A. Lean Sigma principle
    B. Deming principle
    C. Kaizan principle
    D. Pareto principle

22. Dr. Frommer lists the 25 most common mistakes in mammographic misdiagnosis on the board. She tells her 12 faculty that they will collectively do peer review projects on three of them. She asks each faculty member to select five mistakes they are most susceptible to in order to identify the three that have the highest number of votes to focus on. This is an example of:
    A. Multivoting
    B. The process of elimination
    C. Supermajority selection
    D. Prioritization matrix

23. This shape (Figure 12-4) in a flow chart represents:
    A. The start or the end of a process
    B. A step in the process
    C. A decision point with no particular preference
    D. Data in the flow chart

24. This shape (Figure 12-5) in a flow chart means:
    A. The start or the end of a process
    B. A step in the process
    C. A decision point with no particular preference
    D. A variable in the flow chart

25. This shape (Figure 12-6) in a flow chart represents:
    A. The start or the end of a process
    B. A step in the process
    C. A decision point with no particular preference
    D. Data in the flow chart

26. This shape (Figure 12-7) in a flow chart represents:
    A. The start or the end of a process
    B. A step in the process
    C. A decision point with no particular preference
    D. A variable in the flow chart

27. This shape (Figure 12-8) in a flow chart represents:
    A. A jumping off point in the flow chart (for inspection)
    B. A step in the process
    C. A yes or no decision point in the process
    D. A delay in the flow chart

28. A line with an arrowhead in a flow chart shows:
    A. Two decision points
    B. The direction of the flow in the process
    C. The possibilities at a decision tree
    D. A delay in the flow

29. This shape (Figure 12-9) in a flow chart represents:
    A. A jumping off point in the flow chart (for inspection)
    B. A step in the process
    C. A yes or no decision point in the process
    D. A delay in the flow chart

Figure 12-4 Shape used in a flow chart

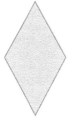

Figure 12-5 Shape used in a flow chart

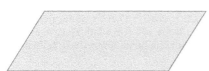

Figure 12-6 Shape used in a flow chart

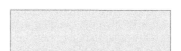

Figure 12-7 Shape used in a flow chart

Figure 12-8 Shape used in a flow chart

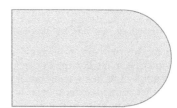

Figure 12-9 Shape used in a flow chart

149

21. **D, Pareto principle.** As was discussed in previous questions, Pareto diagrams assess problems under the principle that a small number of processes contribute to a majority of problems. These processes are stacked in a column in descending order, with the highest occurrence being on top and/or to the left in the diagram. As it descends, the cumulative percentage can be used to determine the 20% of items that contribute to 80% of the problem. Lean principles focus on (1) elimination of waste and (2) forging long-term relationships between and within the organization and customers based on respect, trust, and continuous improvement. Lean Sigma combines principles of Six Sigma with Lean to both remove waste and focus on quality by removing variation. The Deming principle is a set of 14 principles of management to improve effectiveness of an organization. The Kaizen principle is a method of continual improvement by incremental change in which all workers contribute.

References:
The Deming Institute. <https://www.deming.org/theman/theories/fourteen points>.
Adama HG, Aurora S. *Total Quality in Radiology: A Guide to Implementation.* Boca Raton, FL: CRC Press; 1994.
Saleem M, Khan N, Hameed S, et al. An analysis of relationships between total quality management and kaizen. *Life Sci J.* 2012;9(3):31-40.

22. **A, Multivoting.** Multivoting is a process in which a large list of possibilities is narrowed to a smaller list by asking people to vote for several items that they feel are the highest priority. The items receiving the most votes are then focused on. Supermajority selection requires votes received on an issue to be higher than the typical >50% required for a majority in an effort to help protect those in the minority on a nearly split issue. For example, this could be a three-to-five or two-to-three consensus. A prioritization matrix involves creating a matrix of criteria important to the organization to help rank issues with the most highly ranked issue being addressed first. The value of multivoting is that it narrows a large list of possibilities down to a few and the chooses the "best" based on allowing the item that is favored by all, but not the top choice of any, to rise to the top.

Reference:
<http://asq.org/learn-about-quality/decision-making-tools/overview/multivoting.html>.

23. **A, The start or the end of a process.** An oval or rounded rectangle shape represents the terminal or terminator symbol in a flow chart (see Figure 12-4). The terminal symbol denotes the start or end of a process. This shape usually contains the word "start" or "end," or another word signaling the start or end of a process. A flow chart usually has one starting point but can have as many ending points as needed.

Reference:
Stockhoff BA. Core tools to design, control, and improve performance. In: Juran JM, De Feo JA, eds. *Juran's Quality Handbook: The Complete Guide to Performance Excellence.* 6th ed. New York, NY: McGraw-Hill; 2010:541-582.

24. **B, A step in the process.** A diamond shape represents the decision symbol in a flow chart (see Figure 12-5). The decision symbol indicates a decision or branch point in the process that contains a question to be answered, commonly yes/no or true/false questions. The answer to the question determines which path to follow out of the decision shape. There may be two or more exit points depending on the complexity of the situation.

Reference:
Stockhoff BA. Core tools to design, control, and improve performance. In: Juran JM, De Feo JA, eds. *Juran's Quality Handbook: The Complete Guide to Performance Excellence.* 6th ed. New York, NY: McGraw-Hill; 2010:541-582.

25. **D, Data in the flow chart.** A parallelogram shape represents the data symbol, also called the input/output (I/O) symbol because it indicates inputs to and outputs from a process (see Figure 12-6). Examples of input are receiving data or getting an order. Examples of output are generating a report or faxing a message. One can only move in one direction from input to output and not vice versa.

Reference:
Langabeer JR, Helton J. Quality management. In: *Health Care Operations Management: A Systems Perspective.* 2nd ed. Burlington, MA: Jones & Bartlett Learning; 2016:75-96.

26. **B, A step in the process.** A rectangle shape represents the process symbol in a flow chart (see Figure 12-7). In most flow charts, the rectangle is the most common shape. The process symbol represents a single step in the process, such as an action, task, or operation. The text in the rectangle typically includes a verb.

Reference:
Stockhoff BA. Core tools to design, control, and improve performance. In: Juran JM, De Feo JA, eds. *Juran's Quality Handbook: The Complete Guide to Performance Excellence.* 6th ed. New York, NY: McGraw-Hill; 2010:541-582.

27. **A, A jumping off point in the flow chart (for inspection).** A circle shape represents the connector symbol in a flow chart. The connector is used to show a jump from one point in the process flow to another area on the same page (see Figure 12-8). Connectors are typically labeled with capital letters (A, B, C) to show matching jump points. These symbols are particularly useful in large, complex flow charts for avoiding flow lines that cross other shapes and flow lines. In process mapping, the circle represents an inspection point. At an inspection, the quality of the product is evaluated. The flow only continues if the product is approved.

Reference:
Stockhoff BA. Core tools to design, control, and improve performance. In: Juran JM, De Feo JA, eds. *Juran's Quality Handbook: The Complete Guide to Performance Excellence.* 6th ed. New York, NY: McGraw-Hill; 2010:541-582.

28. **B, The direction of the flow in the process.** Flow charts are maps or graphical representations of a process. A line with an arrowhead indicates the direction of the flow in the process. The flow line connects the elements of the system. The line for the arrow can be solid or dashed. The meaning of the arrow with dashed line may differ from one flow chart to another and can be defined in the legend.

Reference:
Stockhoff BA. Core tools to design, control, and improve performance. In: Juran JM, De Feo JA, eds. *Juran's Quality Handbook: The Complete Guide to Performance Excellence.* 6th ed. New York, NY: McGraw-Hill; 2010:541-582.

29. **D, A delay in the flow chart.** This shape represents the delay symbol in a flow chart (see Figure 12-9). The delay symbol depicts any downtime or waiting period when there is no activity. These waiting periods must be carefully measured and recorded. Delays should be analyzed to see if they can be minimized or eliminated to streamline the process.

Reference:
Nelson EC, Batalden PB, Godfrey MM. Process mapping. In: *Quality By Design: A Clinical Microsystems Approach.* 1st ed. San Francisco, CA: Wiley; 2007:296-307.

30. This shape (Figure 12-10) in a flow chart represents:
    A. Three potential routes to the flow
    B. Documents in the flow chart (for inspection)
    C. A yes or no or unknown decision point in the process
    D. A delay in the flow chart

31. To improve the diagnostic process shown in Figure 12-11, the Institute of Medicine did NOT recommend:
    A. More physicians and physician extenders
    B. Improved communication
    C. Better education and training
    D. Developing a system to learn from errors and near misses

32. What is the role of the Patient-Centered Outcomes Research Institute (PCORI)?
    A. To detect diagnostic errors
    B. To fund comparative clinical effectiveness research
    C. To determine actuarial data on death rates and infant mortality rates
    D. To reduce animal research for human applications

33. PCORI stresses what type of research?
    A. Case control subjects
    B. Evidence-based medicine
    C. Randomized blinded control trials using animal models
    D. It does not fund research

34. Under which of the Lean Sigma principles of DMAIC falls the act of observing physician behavior and counting the mistakes that are made in reading a mammogram?
    A. Define
    B. Measure
    C. Analyze
    D. Improve

35. Under which of the Lean Sigma principles of DMAIC falls the intervention to examine whether CAD reading of mammograms is better than human reading of mammograms?
    A. Define
    B. Measure
    C. Analyze
    D. Improve

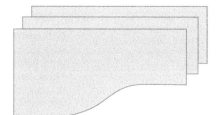

Figure 12-10 Shape used in a flow chart

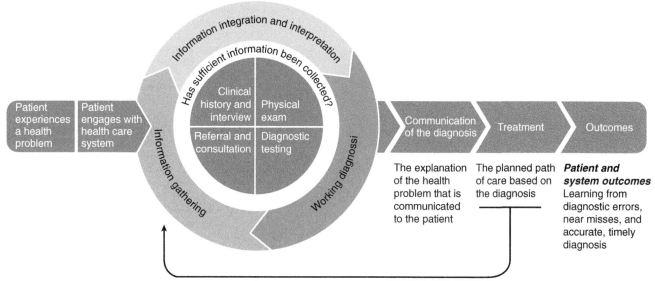

Figure 12-11 Diagnostic process.

30. **B, Documents in the flow chart (for inspection).** A rectangle with a curved bottom represents the document symbol in a flow chart (see Figure 12-10). Multiple overlapping document symbols represent multiple documents. The title or description of the document is typically shown inside the symbol. The other options are incorrect because potential routes to the flow would be depicted by lines with arrows, a decision point in the process would be depicted by a diamond shape, and a delay in the flow chart would be depicted by a rectangle with one rounded side.

Reference:
Stockhoff BA. Core tools to design, control, and improve performance. In: Juran JM, De Feo JA, eds. *Juran's Quality Handbook: The Complete Guide to Performance Excellence.* 6th ed. New York, NY: McGraw-Hill; 2010:541-582.

31. **A, More physicians and physician extenders.** Diagnostic errors, which have been largely unappreciated, persist throughout all settings of care and continue to harm an unacceptable number of patients (see Figure 12-11). Diagnostic errors stem from such sources as inadequate collaboration and communication among clinicians, patients, and their families; a health care work system that is not well designed to support the diagnostic process; limited feedback to clinicians about diagnostic performance; and a culture that discourages transparency and disclosure of diagnostic errors. The National Academies of Sciences, Engineering, and Medicine convened an expert committee to synthesize what is known about diagnostic error and propose recommendations to improve diagnosis. The expert committee outlined eight goals to reduce diagnostic error and improve diagnosis, including:

1. Facilitate more effective teamwork in the process among health care professionals, patients, and their families.
2. Enhance health care professional education and training in the diagnostic process.
3. Ensure that health information technologies (IT) support patients and health care professionals in the diagnostic process.
4. Develop and deploy approaches to identify, learn from, and reduce diagnostic errors and near misses in clinical practice.
5. Establish a work system and culture that supports the diagnostic process and improvements in diagnostic performance.
6. Develop a reporting environment and medical liability system that facilitates improved diagnosis through learning from diagnostic errors and near misses.
7. Design a payment and care delivery environment that supports the diagnostic process.
8. Provide dedicated funding for research on the diagnostic process and diagnostic errors.

Reference:
<http://iom.nationalacademies.org/~/media/Files/Report%20Files/2015/Improving-Diagnosis/DiagnosticError_ReportBrief.pdf>. Accessed December 13, 2015.

32. **B, To fund comparative clinical effectiveness research.** Traditional medical research hasn't been able to answer many of the questions that patients and their clinicians face daily when it comes to addressing their health and health care concerns. When reliable information does exist, it is not always available to patients and their caretakers in ways they can understand or use most effectively.

PCORI was established to close these gaps in evidence needed to improve key health outcomes by:
1. Identifying critical research questions
2. Funding patient-centered comparative clinical effectiveness research (CER)
3. Disseminating the results in ways that the end-users of healthcare work will find useful and valuable

Reference:
<http://www.pcori.org/>. Accessed December 13, 2015.

33. **B, Evidence-based medicine.** PCORI uses a framework to guide the funding of comparative clinical effectiveness research that will give patients and those who care for them a better ability to make informed health decisions. The priorities of the framework include:

1. Assessment of prevention, diagnosis, and treatment options
2. Improving health care systems
3. Communication and dissemination research
4. Addressing disparities
5. Accelerating patient-centered outcomes research and methodological research

Reference:
<http://www.pcori.org/about-us/what-we-do>.

34. **B, Measure.** The measure stage of Six Sigma is where the data are collected. Usually there is a stage of data collection before the improvement/intervention is initiated. These data are analyzed and a change is proposed, but a second stage of measuring is then required to see if the expected results actually occur. One of the most difficult parts of the measure process is deciding what are the key performance indicators to measure. In the example above, do you measure mistakes based on pathology, based on senior partner discrepancy rate, based on CAD readings? What is the gold standard and what if you do not get a gold standard quality answer on every one (not all negative mammograms go on to biopsy). And what should you measure related to physician behavior? Time it takes to report the mammogram? Eye tracking scanning plots? Distractions? Words in the report? BIRADS missteps? As the old tailor's expression goes, "measure twice, cut once"—but that assumes you are measuring the right things!

Reference:
<http://www.isixsigma.com/new-to-six-sigma/dmaic/six-sigma-dmaic-quick-reference/>.

35. **D, Improve.** The improvement process is the intervention/change that is implemented. What is the action plan for the way forward, and how, when, and by whom will it be applied? The suggested solutions are optimized for implementation, and the human and financial resources for the action plan are allocated. Eliminate the root causes of any failure. The goal in the improve process is to generate possible solutions, select the best solutions, and design an implementation plan for success.

Reference:
<http://www.isixsigma.com/new-to-six-sigma/dmaic/six-sigma-dmaic-roadmap/>.

36. Under which of the Lean Sigma principles of DMAIC falls the act of meeting with the breast imaging team to announce a performance improvement project and select a champion?
    A. Define
    B. Measure
    C. Analyze
    D. Control

37. Under which of the Lean Sigma principles of DMAIC falls the act of establishing that all mammograms in patients of highest risk automatically get CAD readings in addition to breast imager readings?
    A. Define
    B. Measure
    C. Analyze
    D. Control

38. Under which of the Lean Sigma principles of DMAIC falls the act of testing between double reading mammograms by humans versus readings by one human and one CAD for the detection of breast cancer nodal metastases?
    A. Define
    B. Measure
    C. Analyze
    D. Improve

39. Between Lean Sigma and Six Sigma, the former focuses on _____ whereas the latter focuses on _____?
    A. Lean on speed, Six on errors
    B. Lean on accuracy, Six on precision
    C. Lean on errors, Six on speed
    D. Lean on precision, Six on accuracy

40. Figure 12-12 represents a:
    A. Whisker diagram
    B. Anzai-Minoshima diagram
    C. Fishbone diagram
    D. Data flow diagram

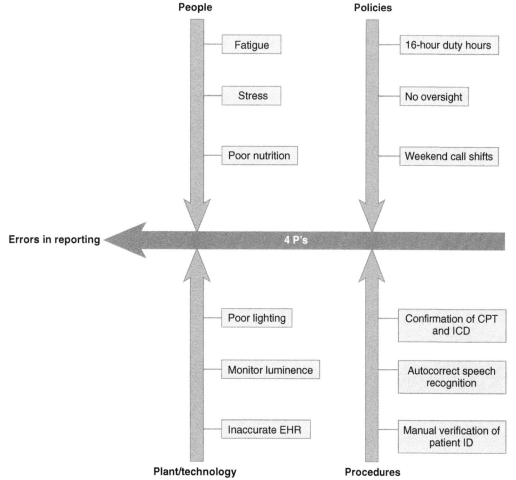

Figure 12-12 Causes of radiologists' errors in reporting

36. **A, Define.** The first part of any process improvement initiative is to define the problem. Set the goal or at least clarify what is the issue to be addressed. What are the constraints to what will be included within the domain of the improvement plan? Who are the customers and their requirements, what are the tools and resources available to manage the transition, and who is on the project team? Metrics for success, financials, stakeholders, and plan of attack are established.

Reference:
George ML, Rowlands D, Price M, et al. *Lean Six Sigma Pocket Toolbook.* New York: McGraw Hill; 2003.

37. **D, Control.** Under the control process of Six Sigma improvements are monitored to ensure sustained success. Create a control plan where surveillance for compliance with processes and maintaining good results are guaranteed. Adjust and adapt as needed.

Reference:
<http://asq.org/quality-progress/2012/11/back-to-basics/to-dmaic-or-not-to-dmaic.html>.

38. **C, Analyze.** In the analyze process of Lean Six Sigma, data are scrutinized to determine any causes of defects. The tools used include identifying (1) gaps between current performance and goal performance, (2) process inputs that affect the process outputs, (3) potential opportunities to improve, and (4) sources of variation. In the example provided, testing different techniques of reviewing mammograms would be part of the analyze function.

Reference:
<http://asq.org/quality-progress/2012/11/back-to-basics/to-dmaic-or-not-to-dmaic.html>.

39. **A, Lean on speed, Six on errors.** Lean Sigma focuses on speed and Six Sigma focuses on errors (or variability).

The main difference between Lean and Six Sigma is that Lean emphasizes eliminating unnecessary steps in the work process that do not lead to added value and for which a customer is NOT willing to pay extra. Lean cuts out wasteful steps in the production process. If something does not add value it is removed, which allows a streamlined and efficient workplace.

Six Sigma emphasizes the variability in a work process that leads to waste. Six Sigma seeks to eliminate defects by streamlining and improving business processes by emphasizing the reduction in the number of errors in a process. It focuses on the variations in the types of data inputs, and addresses the source of errors.

Reference:
<http://smallbusiness.chron.com/difference-between-lean-six-sigma-six-sigma-40621.html>.

40. **C, Fishbone diagram.** The fishbone, Ishikawa, or cause and effect diagram identifies many possible causes for an effect or problem (see Figure 12-12). It is used to sort ideas into useful categories to structure a brainstorming session. When evaluating a problem's root cause, there are often many ideas and opinions about the cause. The problem or the questions will be placed in the head of the fishbone. One main line is drawn across the page, attached to the head. Several oblique or vertical lines come out of the main line, representing different categories or "bones" such as "people," "policies," "procedures," and "plant/technology" as illustrated in Figure 12-12.

References:
<http://asq.org/learn-about-quality/cause-analysis-tools/overview/fishbone.html>.
<http://www.isixsigma.com/tools-templates/cause-effect/cause-and-effect-aka-fishbone-diagram/>.

QUESTIONS

1. According to National Council on Radiation Protection & Measurements (NCRP) report 160, the radiation exposure from CT contributes to nearly how much of all the radiation exposure from medical procedures to the U.S. population?
   A. 25%
   B. 50%
   C. 75%
   D. >90%

2. According to the IAEA the occupational exposure dose limits are:
   A. An effective dose of 20 mSv per year averaged over 5 consecutive years (100 mSv in 5 years) and of 50 mSv in any single year
   B. An equivalent dose to the lens of the eye of 20 mSv per year averaged over 5 consecutive years (100 mSv in 5 years) and of 50 mSv in any single year
   C. An equivalent dose to the extremities (hands and feet) or to the skin of 500 mSv in a year
   D. All of the above

3. For the public, the IAEA recommends dose limits of:
   A. 1 mSv in a year
   B. An equivalent dose to the lens of the eye of 25 mSv in a year
   C. An equivalent dose to the skin of 100 mSv in a year
   D. All of the above

4. The BEIR VII committee concluded that:
   A. There is no threshold value above which radiation begins to show risk in the development of cancer
   B. There is a threshold value above which radiation begins to show risk in the development of cancer but that threshold is very low
   C. There is a linear-quadratic shape to the curve defining radiation dosage and risk of cancer
   D. None of the above

5. The BEIR VII committee opined that medical radiation >100 mSv above background accounts for what percent of solid cancers or leukemia?
   A. 1% to 2%
   B. 2% to 3%
   C. 3% to 4%
   D. >4%

6. Which is not a risk factor for development of radiation induced cancer?
   A. Age at exposure
   B. Dosage
   C. Type of radiation
   D. Lifespan

7. As of 2006, what percentage of medical radiation dosage was attributable to radiographic and fluoroscopic studies?
   A. 0% to 20%
   B. 21% to 40%
   C. 41% to 60%
   D. >60%

8. As of 2006, what percentage of medical radiation dosage was attributable to nuclear medicine studies?
   A. 0% to 20%
   B. 21% to 40%
   C. 41% to 60%
   D. >60%

9. As of 2006, what percentage of medical radiation dosage was attributable to interventional studies?
   A. 0% to 20%
   B. 21% to 40%
   C. 41% to 60%
   D. >60%

10. Which of the following is considered a correct CT reference value by the ACR?
    A. CTDI for CT of the head = 60 mGy
    B. CTDI for CT of the abdomen = 40 mGy
    C. CTDI for CT of the abdomen in children = 20 mGy
    D. All are correct

1. **B, 50%.** According to the National Council on Radiation Protection and Measurements (NCRP) Report No. 160, the average annual per capita effective dose from radiation exposure in the United States in 2006 was 6.2 millisievert (mSv). Medical imaging contributed to approximately half (48%, or 3.0 mSv) of this dose. While CT imaging only accounted for 17% of all medical imaging procedures utilizing radiation, it is the source of 49% of radiation exposure from medical imaging to the U.S. population.

Reference:
National Council on Radiation Protection and Measurements. *Ionizing radiation exposure of the population of the United States*. NCRP Report No. 160. Bethesda, MD: National Council on Radiation Protection and Measurements; 2009.

2. **D, All of the above.** All of the above statements are correct related to dose limits for occupational exposure of workers older than 18 years of age.

Reference:
International Atomic Energy Agency. *Radiation protection and safety of radiation sources: international basic safety standards*. Interim ed Safety Standards Series No. GSR Part 3 (interim). Vienna: IAEA; 2011 <http://www-pub.iaea.org/MTCD/Publications/PDF/Pub1578_web-57265295.pdf>.

3. **A, 1 mSv in a year.** For public exposure, the dose limits include (a) an effective dose of 1 mSv in a year; (b) an equivalent dose to the lens of the eye of 15 mSv in a year; and (c) an equivalent dose to the skin of 50 mSv in a year (4).

Reference:
International Atomic Energy Agency. *Radiation protection and safety of radiation sources: international basic safety standards*. Interim ed Safety Standards Series No. GSR Part 3 (interim). Vienna: IAEA; 2011 <http://www-pub.iaea.org/MTCD/Publications/PDF/Pub1578_web-57265295.pdf>.

4. **A, There is no threshold value above which radiation begins to show risk in the development of cancer.** An important task of the BEIR VII committee was to develop "risk models" for estimating the relationship between exposure to low levels of low-linear energy transfer ionizing radiation and harmful health effects. The committee judged that the linear no-threshold model (LNT) provided the most reasonable description of the relation between low-dose exposure to ionizing radiation and the incidence of solid cancers that are induced by ionizing radiation.

Reference:
Public Summary. *Health Risks from Exposure to Low Levels of Ionizing Radiation BEIR VII, Phase 2*. Washington, DC: National Academies; 2006:6. Print.

5. **B, 2% to 3%.** On average, assuming a sex and age distribution similar to that of the entire U.S. population, the BEIR VII lifetime risk model predicts that approximately 1 person in 100 would be expected to develop cancer (solid cancer or leukemia) from a dose of 0.1 Sv (100 mSv) above background, while approximately 42 of the 100 individuals would be expected to develop solid cancer or leukemia from other causes. This means that 1/42 = 2.4%, making B the correct answer.

Reference:
Public Summary. *Health Risks from Exposure to Low Levels of Ionizing Radiation BEIR VII, Phase 2*. Washington, DC: National Academies; 2006:7-8. Print.

6. **C, Type of radiation.** Risk estimates are subject to several sources of uncertainty due to inherent limitations in epidemiologic data and in our understanding of exactly how radiation exposure increases the risk of cancer. In addition to statistical uncertainty, the populations and exposures for which risk estimates are needed nearly always differ from those for which epidemiologic data are available. This means that assumptions are required, many of which involve considerable uncertainty. Risk may depend on the type of cancer, the magnitude of the dose, the quality of the radiation, the dose-rate, the age and sex of the person exposed, exposure to other carcinogens such as tobacco, and other characteristics of the exposed individual. Despite the abundance of epidemiologic and experimental data on the health effects of exposure to radiation, data are not adequate to quantify these dependencies precisely.

In addition, lifespan is a risk factor for the development of radiation-induced cancer. "There is clear evidence that, for thyroid cancer, the age of exposure markedly influences the risk of developing cancer in later life. Individuals exposed as adults showed no demonstrable dose response, whereas there was a clear dose-response relationship for individuals exposed as children."

References:
Public Summary. *Health Risks from Exposure to Low Levels of Ionizing Radiation BEIR VII, Phase 2*. Washington, DC: National Academies; 2006:267. Print.
Shah DJ, Sachs RK, Wilson DJ. Radiation-induced cancer: a modern view. *Br J Radiol*. 2012;85:e1166-e1173.
Ionizing Radiation Exposure of the Population of the United States. Bethesda, MD: National Council on Radiation Protection and Measurements; 2009. NCRP report 160.

7. **A, 0% to 20%.** According to NCRP Report No. 160 *Ionizing Radiation Exposure of the Population of the United States*, in 2006, approximately 11% of the total medical radiation dose was attributable to radiographic/fluoroscopic studies, even though they made up 74% of all imaging procedures.

References:
Bolus NE. NCRP Report 160 and what it means for medical imaging and nuclear medicine. *J Nucl Med Technol*. 2013;41(1):257-258. Print.
Ionizing Radiation Exposure of the Population of the United States. Bethesda, MD: National Council on Radiation Protection and Measurements; 2009. NCRP report 160.

8. **B, 21% to 40%.** According to NCRP Report No. 160, *Ionizing Radiation Exposure of the Population of the United States*, in 2006, approximately 26% of the total medical radiation dose was attributable to nuclear medicine studies, while they made up only 5% of all imaging procedures.

Reference:
Ionizing Radiation Exposure of the Population of the United States. Bethesda, MD: National Council on Radiation Protection and Measurements; 2009. NCRP report 160.

9. **A, 0% to 20%.** According to NCRP Report No. 160 *Ionizing Radiation Exposure of the Population of the United States*, in 2006, approximately 14% of the total medical radiation dose was attributable to interventional radiology, while they made up only 4% of all imaging procedures.

Reference:
Ionizing Radiation Exposure of the Population of the United States. Bethesda, MD: National Council on Radiation Protection and Measurements; 2009. NCRP report 160.

10. **C, CTDI for Children CT of the abdomen = 20 mGy.** In 2008, the ACR established three diagnostic CT reference values from data collected for its CT accreditation program. These include $CTDI_{vol}$ values of 75 mGy for CT head, 25 mGy for CT adult abdomen, and 20 mGy for CT pediatric abdomen.

References:
ACR Practice Guideline for Diagnostic Reference Levels in Medical X-Ray Imaging; 2008.
McCollough C, et al. Diagnostic reference levels from the ACR CT Accreditation Program. *J Am Coll Radiol*. 2011;8(1):795-803.

11. What is the correct ACR established reference value for CT of the head?
    A. 60 mGy
    B. 70 mGy
    C. 80 mGy
    D. None of the above

12. In nuclear medicine, the dosage of radiotracers is based on:
    A. Glucose metabolism
    B. BMI
    C. Weight
    D. Age

13. The stochastic model of radiation exposure suggests:
    A. There is a threshold level of radiation above which the risk of development of radiation induced cancer begins.
    B. Cancer does not derive from radiation exposure.
    C. There is a lower limit of radiation below which radiation has a beneficial effect.
    D. There is no lower limit threshold below which radiation may not induce cancer.

14. An example of a nonstochastic (deterministic) effect of radiation is:
    A. Cataracts
    B. Skin burns
    C. Sterility
    D. All of the above

15. Radiation dosimetry badges are effectively:
    A. Geiger counters
    B. Radiation intensity monitors
    C. Radiation sensitive film
    D. Radiation exposure devices that are specific for x-rays

16. Ablation of the hematopoietic system by radiation occurs at a dose on the order of:
    A. 0 to 50 rads
    B. 51 to 100 rads
    C. 101 to 150 rads
    D. >150 rads

17. Skin erythema from radiation exposure varies based on:
    A. Site of exposure
    B. Skin pigmentation
    C. Smoking history
    D. All of the above

18. The typical skin dose threshold for erythema is
    A. 200 rads
    B. 300 rads
    C. 400 rads
    D. 500 rads

11. **D, None of the above.** The correct ACR established reference value for CT of the head is 75 mGy.

References:
ACR Practice Guidelines for Diagnostic Reference Levels in Medical X-Ray Imaging; 2008.
McCollough C, et al. Diagnostic reference levels from the ACR CT Accreditation Program. *J Am Coll Radiol.* 2011;8(1):795-803.

12. **C, Weight.** When performing nuclear medicine studies for patients, the appropriate radiopharmaceutical dose is most often determined by body weight (based on the North American Consensus Guidelines for Pediatric Radiopharmaceutical Administered Doses). Weight is also an important factor in adult patients, given the obesity epidemic. The standard activity of radiopharmaceuticals in adults is based on the ideal standard weight of a patient, 70 kg. In overweight and obese patients, image quality can be significantly degraded by increased soft tissue attenuation. Thus, obtaining acceptable image quality in an obese patient frequently requires use of an activity higher than used in a patient of ideal weight.

References:
Ghanem M. Impact of obesity on nuclear medicine imaging. *J Nuc Med Technol.* 2011;39:1.
Guidelines and Standards Committee of the ACR Commission on Nuclear Medicine in collaboration with the SPR. *ACR-SPR Practice Guideline for the Performance of Adult and Pediatric Skeletal Scintigraphy (Bone Scan).* American College of Radiology and Society of Pediatric Radiology; 2012 <www.acr.org/~/media/ACR/Documents/PGTS/guidelines/Skeletal_Scintigraphy.pdf>.
<www.imagegently.org/Portals/6/Nuclear%20Medicine/NA%20Guidelines%202014%20Update%20-%20Poster.pdf>.
<http://imagewisely.org/~/media/ImageWisely%20Files/NucMed/Clinical%20Aspects%20of%20General%20Nuclear%20Medicine.pdf>.

13. **D, There is no lower limit threshold below which radiation may not induce cancer.** The biologic effects of radiation can be classified as stochastic or deterministic. Stochastic effects include radiation-induced cancer and hereditary effects. Stochastic effects have no dose threshold, and the probability of occurrence of a stochastic effect increases with radiation dose. For instance, a larger absorbed radiation dose increases the risk of radiation-induced leukemia, but there will be no difference in the severity of the disease if it occurs. Stochastic effects are considered the principal health risk from low-dose radiation exposure, including diagnostic imaging procedures.

Reference:
Bushberg JT, Seibert JA, Leidholdt EM, et al. *The Essential Physics of Medical Imaging.* 3rd ed. Philadelphia, PA: Lippincott Williams & Wilkins; 2012:752.

14. **D, All of the above.** Cataracts, skin erythema, sterility, and hematopoietic syndrome are examples of deterministic effects. Increasing radiation dose will increase the severity of injury in deterministic effects (rather than the probability of occurrence as is the case with stochastic effects). Deterministic effects have a threshold dose below which the effect does not occur or is subclinical. There is significant individual variability in response to radiation, and the threshold is just an approximate dose that will likely result in the specified effect. Deterministic effects are unlikely to occur as a result of diagnostic imaging procedures, with the exception of lengthy fluoroscopically guided procedures.

Reference:
Bushberg JT, Seibert JA, Leidholdt EM, et al. *The Essential Physics of Medical Imaging.* 3rd ed. Philadelphia, PA: Lippincott Williams & Wilkins; 2012:752.

15. **C, Radiation sensitive film.** There are three main types of individual radiation recording devices used in radiology and nuclear medicine: (1) film badges, (2) dosimeters using storage phosphors (thermoluminescent dosimeters), and (3) pocket dosimeters.

A film badge is a small sealed packet of radiation sensitive film inside a plastic holder. Radiation arriving at the badge will darken the developed film. Increasing absorbed dose increases film darkening, which is measured with a densitometer.

Reference:
Bushberg JT, Seibert JA, Leidholdt EM, et al. *The Essential Physics of Medical Imaging.* 3rd ed. Philadelphia, PA: Lippincott, Williams & Wilkins; 2012: 843-848.

16. **D, >150 rads (actually >400 rads).** Hematopoietic stem cells are very radiosensitive, and damage to the hematopoietic system is maximized with posterior radiation, because the majority of hematopoietic marrow is in the spine, the posterior ribs, and the pelvis. Hematopoietic syndrome occurs after an acute radiation dose of approximately 200 rads (2 Gy). Healthy adults with proper medical care will recover after a smaller radiation dose, whereas a dose greater than 8 Gy is usually fatal unless advanced medical therapies, such as colony-stimulating factors or bone marrow transplantation, are successful.

Reference:
Bushberg JT, Seibert JA, Leidholdt EM, et al. *The Essential Physics of Medical Imaging.* 3rd ed. Philadelphia, PA: Lippincott Williams & Wilkins; 2012:787.

17. **D, All of the above.** Erythema is attributed to early change in vascular permeability and accumulation of lymphocytes in the layers of the skin caused by the effects of cell death. Acute exposure to radiation with a skin dose exceeding 2 gray (Gy) from x-ray or a skin dose of 6 to 8 Gy with 200 kV is required for erythema to occur after radiation therapy. The erythema may vary depending on site of exposure, skin pigmentation, and smoking history (affecting vascularity). Diseases such as collagen vascular diseases and diabetes mellitus make patients more susceptible to radiation induced skin injury. Previous radiation exposure also is a risk factor.

References:
<http://emergency.cdc.gov/radiation/criphysicianfactsheet.asp#2>.
Hall EJ, Giaccia AJ. *Radiobiology for the Radiologist.* 6th ed. Philadelphia, PA: Lippincott Williams & Wilkins; 2006:205.

18. **A, 200 rads.** Cutaneous radiation injury (CRI) can occur with radiation doses as low as 2 Gray (Gy) or 200 rads. Early signs and symptoms of CRI are transient erythema, itching, tingling, or edema without a history of exposure to heat or caustic chemicals. These will frequently begin within hours of exposure. Erythema is attributed to early change in vascular permeability.

Skin symptoms can occur even in the absence of more significant toxicities such as acute radiation syndrome (ARS). This is especially true among patients with acute exposures to beta radiation or low-energy x-rays, because beta radiation and low-energy x-rays are less penetrating and less likely to damage internal organs than gamma radiation.

References:
<http://emergency.cdc.gov/radiation/criphysicianfactsheet.asp#2>.
Hall EJ, Giaccia AJ. *Radiobiology for the Radiologist.* 6th ed. Philadelphia, PA: Lippincott Williams & Wilkins; 2006:205.

19. The typical dose threshold for epilation is
    A. 200 rads
    B. 300 rads
    C. 400 rads
    D. 500 rads

20. Does prior radiation exposure lead to variability in the dosage needed for nonstochastic effects of radiation?
    A. Yes
    B. No
    C. Sometimes
    D. All of the above

21. Which of the following may increase the entrance dose at fluoroscopy?
    A. Low intensity mode
    B. Patient obesity
    C. Pulsed fluoroscopy versus continuous
    D. All of the above

22. As of 2010, which of these was true?
    A. CTs are ordered at a rate of 40% of the population
    B. CTs account for 40% of the studies ordered through a radiology department
    C. CTs account for 40% of the radiation exposure from medical imaging
    D. None of the above

23. ALARA stands for:
    A. Allowable levels as regulations allocate
    B. As low as reasonably achievable
    C. Allowed levels as reasonable to achieve
    D. Acceptable levels or appropriate radiation alternatives

24. Lowering kVp leads to:
    A. Decreased conspicuity of iodine filled vessels
    B. No impact on visibility of iodine filled vessels
    C. Increased conspicuity of iodine filled vessels
    D. Iodine filled vessel artifacts

25. The dose length product (DLP) is the product of:
    A. MaS and pitch
    B. CT dose index volume and scanning length
    C. CT dose and focal spot size
    D. Dose per slice and scanning distance

19. **B, 300 rads.** Skin epilation, or hair loss, typically occurs at approximately 300 rads. These changes are attributed to reduction in the replicative ability of germinal cells or matrix within hair follicles. Effects usually begin about 3 weeks after exposure and can require up to 5 weeks for regrowth. Permanent epilation occurs when doses exceed 700 rads. It is no surprise that the necessary doses for toxic effect are lowest in the skin (erythema and epilation), because the skin is the organ that invariably receives the highest dose.

Reference:
Hall EJ, Giaccia AJ. *Radiobiology for the Radiologist.* 6th ed. Philadelphia, PA: Lippincott Williams & Wilkins; 2006:205.

20. **A, Yes.** Stochastic effects have been defined as those for which the probability increases with dose. However, there is no threshold at which an event will necessarily occur.

    In contrast, nonstochastic effects are those for which incidence and severity depend on dose but for which there is a threshold dose. Thus, regarding nonstochastic effects, prior radiation dose will always be relevant because it directly relates to a cumulative whole.

Reference:
Leenhouts HP, Chadwick KH. The molecular basis of stochastic and nonstochastic effects. *Health Phys.* 1989;57(suppl 1):343-348.

21. **B, Patient obesity.** With the prevalence of obesity now over one-third of the U.S. population, obesity is a major and rising health risk to the population at large. Modern fluoroscopy systems operate under automatic exposure control, with tube voltage (kV) and tube current (mA) adjusted to patient attenuation. They therefore result in a higher radiation load among obese patients. Numerous studies have demonstrated the increasing entrance doses among obese patients in a variety of fluoroscopic studies.

References:
Flegal KM, Carroll MD, Kit BK, et al. Prevalence of obesity and trends in the distribution of body mass index among US adults, 1999-2010. *JAMA.* 2012;307(5):491-497.
Hsi RS, Zamora DA, Kanal KM, et al. Severe obesity is associated with 3-fold higher radiation dose rate during ureteroscopy. *Urology.* 2013;82(4):780-785.

22. **D, None of the above.** As of 2010, CTs were ordered at a rate of 149 tests per 1000 patients, or 14% of the population (not choice A). They accounted for 12.0% of radiologic examinations (not choice B) and 67.8% of radiation exposure (not choice C)—a 4-fold increase in per capita radiation exposure from CT.

    The increase in imaging was likely driven by many factors, including improvements in the technology that have led to expansion of clinical applications, patient- and physician-generated demand, defensive medical practices, and medical uncertainty—all factors that would be expected to influence utilization across all systems of medical care.

Reference:
Smith-Bindman R, Miglioretti DL, Johnson E, et al. Use of diagnostic imaging studies and associated radiation exposure for patients enrolled in large integrated health care systems, 1996-2010. *JAMA.* 2012;307(22):2400-2409.

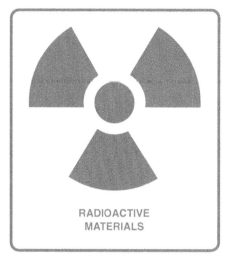

Figure 13-1 Radioactive sign

23. **B, As low as reasonably achievable.** ALARA is an acronym for As Low As Reasonably Achievable, which is a radiation safety principle for minimizing radiation doses and releases of radioactive materials (Figure 13-1) by employing all reasonable methods. It is defined in Title 10, Section 20.1003, of the Code of Federal Regulations (10 CFR 20.1003). The radiation safety officer enforces the ALARA program through management, which includes reviews of operating procedures, past dose records, inspections, and consultations with radiation safety staff.

References:
NRC library. <http://www.nrc.gov/reading-rm/basic-ref/glossary/alara.html>.
<https://www.ehs.washington.edu/manuals/rsmanual/7alara.pdf>.

24. **C, Increased conspicuity of iodine filled vessels.** A sharp increase in photoelectric absorption occurs just above the electron binding energy. Photoelectric absorption is proportional to $Z3/E3$, and there is a sharp increase in absorption when the incoming photon energy is slightly above the electron binding energy. K-edge for iodine is 33 kev, and barium is 37 kev.

References:
Hall EJ, Giaccia AJ. *Radiobiology for the Radiologist.* 6th ed. Philadelphia, PA: Lippincott Williams & Wilkins; 2006.
RSNA/AAPM. Online Physics Module: "Interactions of Radiations and Tissue."

25. **B, CT dose index volume and scanning length.** Dose length product (DLP) = $CTDI_{vol}$ × scan length. The $CTDI_{vol}$ is an index that quantifies the relative intensity of radiation incident upon a patient being scanned. The DLP can be used to quantify the total amount of radiation received by a patient during a scan. The DLP directly relates to stochastic radiation risk and has been employed to set reference values for various types of CT scans following the ALARA (as low as reasonably achievable) principle.

Reference:
Huda W, Ogden KM, Khorasani MR. Converting dose-length product to effective dose at CT. *Radiol.* 2008;248(3):995-1003.

26. The value of the Dose Index Registry is that it:
    A. Compares the radiation dosage from one part of the body to another
    B. Detects when the scanner is over-dosing
    C. Compares radiation dosage from one facility to the next
    D. Detects variations in radiation for the repetitive scans of the same body part in the same facility by the same machine and between machines

27. Which of the following is included in the five ACR recommendations for imaging wisely?
    A. Annual mammograms after age 45
    B. No imaging for uncomplicated headaches
    C. Pulmonary embolism angiography only if ventilation perfusion scans are suggestive or inconclusive
    D. Admission chest x-rays in endemic areas for pneumoconiosis

28. Based on the BEIR VII report, it is estimated that approximately 1 in 1000 individuals will develop cancer from an exposure of:
    A. 1 mSv
    B. 5 mSv
    C. 10 mSv
    D. 100 mSv

29. The annual occupational dose limit for radiologists is a total effective dose of:
    A. 5 rem
    B. 5 gray
    C. 0.5 rem
    D. 1 gray

30. The annual effective radiation occupational dose limit for a minor working in a radiology department is:
    A. 5 rem
    B. 0.5 gray
    C. 0.1 rem
    D. 0.1 gray

26. **C, Compares radiation dosage from one facility to the next.** The ACR Dose Index Registry is a data registry that allows a facility to compare its own CT dose indices to other regional and national dose values. This allows for an effective comparison of radiation dosage from one facility to the next. As part of the Dose Index Registry, institutions receive periodic feedback reports comparing their own doses from various types of CT scans to aggregate dose results. The ABR has qualified the Dose Index Registry as fulfilling criteria for practice quality improvement (PQI), one of the key components of the physician's maintenance of certification (MOC) process.

    Reference:
    <http://www.acr.org/Quality-Safety/National-Radiology-Data-Registry/Dose-Index-Registry>.

27. **B, No imaging for uncomplicated headaches.** The ACR and ABIM Choosing Wisely campaign has five key recommendations:
    1. Don't do imaging for uncomplicated headaches.
    2. Don't image for suspected pulmonary embolism (PE) without moderate or high pretest probability of PE.
    3. Avoid admission or preoperative chest x-rays for ambulatory patients with unremarkable history and physical exam.
    4. Don't do computed tomography (CT) for the evaluation of suspected appendicitis in children until after ultrasound has been considered as an option.
    5. Don't recommend follow-up imaging for clinically inconsequential adnexal cysts.

    Reference:
    <http://www.choosingwisely.org/societies/american-college-of-radiology/>.

28. **C, 10 mSv.** Biologic Effects of Ionizing Radiation VII supports the previously held notion of a "linear-no-threshold" risk model that assumes a linear relationship with even the lowest doses having the potential to cause cancer in humans without a minimum threshold. According to Beir VII, "On average, assuming a sex and age distribution similar to that of the entire U.S. population, the BEIR VII lifetime risk model predicts that approximately one individual in 100 persons would be expected to develop cancer (solid cancer or leukemia) from a dose of 100 mSv while approximately 42 of the 100 individuals would be expected to develop solid cancer or leukemia from other causes". Lower doses would produce proportionally lower risks. For example, it is predicted that approximately one individual in 1000 would develop cancer from an exposure to 10 mSv. Excess deaths from exposure to 100 mSv would occur in 410/100,000 males and 610/100,000 females from solid cancers and 70/100,000 and 50/100,000 males and females from leukemia.

    Reference:
    <http://dels.nas.edu/resources/static-assets/materials-based-on-reports/reports-in-brief/beir_vii_final.pdf>.

29. **A, 5 rem.** According to the NRC, the occupational exposure to adults should be less than either (1) the total effective dose equivalent being equal to 5 rems or (2) the sum of the deep-dose equivalent and the committed dose equivalent to any individual organ or tissue other than the lens of the eye being equal to 50 rems.

    Remember that 5 grays = 500 rads. Although we often use them interchangeably, remember the differences between the various units of radiation.

    Reference:
    <http://www.nrc.gov/reading-rm/doc-collections/cfr/part020/part020-1201.html>.

30. **C, 0.1 rem.** Although adults are allowed 5 rem per year as an occupational exposure, that rate is reduced for children because of their increased risk of developing cancers by virtue of their age at exposure and higher rate of cell turnover. The NRC says that the occupational exposure to minors, defined as an individual less than 18 years of age, should be 10% that of adults, or 0.5 rem, according to the Nuclear Regulatory Commission; however, the Department of Energy specifies 0.1 rem as specified in 10 CFR 835 (Table 13-1) and DOE O 458.1. D.

    References:
    <http://energy.gov/sites/prod/files/2014/06/f16/A_Basic_Overview_of_Occupational_Radiation_Exposure.pdf>.
    <http://energy.gov/sites/prod/files/2015/11/f27/2014_Occupational_Radiation_Exposure_Report.pdf>.

Table 13-1 DOE DOSE LIMITS FROM 10 CFR 835

Personnel Category	Section of 10 CFR 835	Type of Exposure	Acronym	Annual Limit
General employees	835.202	Total effective dose. The sum of the effective dose (for external exposures) and the committed effective dose	TED	5 rems
		The sum of the equivalent dose to the whole body for external exposures and the committed equivalent dose to any organ or tissue other than the skin or the lens of the eye	EqD-WB + CEqD (TOD)	50 rems
		Equivalent dose to the lens of the eye	EqD-Eye	15 rems
		The sum of the equivalent dose to the skin or any extremity for external exposures and the committed equivalent dose to the skin or any extremity	EqD-SkWB + CEqD-SK and EqD to the maximally exposed extremity + CEqD-SK	50 rems
Declared pregnant workers*	835.206	Total equivalent dose	TEqD	0.5 rem per gestation period
Minors	835.207	Total effective dose	TED	0.1 rem
Members of the public in a controlled area	835.208	Total effective dose	TED	0.1 rem

*Limit applies to the embryo/fetus.

31. Individual monitoring results of radiation exposure must be recorded **at least**:
    A. Monthly
    B. Quarterly
    C. Biannually
    D. Annually

32. In Figure 13-2 from 2006 on the contributions to public radiation exposure, the shaded grey represents:
    A. Medical procedures
    B. Occupational exposure
    C. Background environmental exposure
    D. Nuclear reactor exposure

33. In the same figure, the blue represents:
    A. Medical procedures
    B. Occupational exposure
    C. Background environmental exposure
    D. Nuclear reactor exposure

34. Which of the following has the same radiation weighting factor as x-rays?
    A. Alpha particles
    B. Beta particles
    C. Neutrons
    D. Protons

35. Different types of non-lead aprons are compared using what measuring unit?
    A. Rem
    B. Absorbed dose
    C. Lead-equivalent thickness
    D. Dispersion equivalent

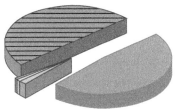

Figure 13-2 Contributions to public radiation exposure (2006 data)

31. **D, Annually.** Although many institutions in medicine provide monthly or quarterly radiation dosage metrics, the governmental requirement is only annually. This is likely because they are fixing regulations across the entire governmental realm, which includes the Department of Energy (nuclear plants), Department of Defense (nuclear warheads), and TSA (screening x-rays) where a more frequent surveillance program requirement would be burdensome. The Nuclear Regulatory Commission sets the rules for the United States.

Certainly, no one would be happy about being overexposed for 12 months by a faulty breast tomosynthesis unit and hence the more frequent review of radiation dosimetry badges in radiology departments. Radiation safety badges detect high-energy beta, gamma, and x-ray radiation but not low-energy beta radiation from some isotopes including carbon-14, tritium (H-3), or sulfur-35.

References:
<http://www.ncrppublications.org/Reports/122>.
<http://www.epa.gov/sites/production/files/2015-05/documents/fgr14-2014.pdf>.
<http://www.nrc.gov/reading-rm/doc-collections/cfr/part020/part020-2106.html>.

32. **C, Background environmental exposure (50%).** In 2006, the effective radiation exposure dose per individual in the United States was 620 mrem, about one-eighth of the allowable annual occupational exposure of a radiologist. The sources of the background radiation include radon, cosmic rays (mostly from the sun), other earth elements such as C14 and K40, and radioactive material that we consume in nature. The point is that nearly half of the exposure of the U.S. population is from "natural sources." Occupational exposure (the green sliver) and consumer products (the purple sliver) are tiny contributors to public exposures.

Reference:
<http://energy.gov/sites/prod/files/2014/06/f16/A_Basic_Overview_of_Occupational_Radiation_Exposure.pdf>.

33. **A, Medical procedures (48%).** If one were to look at such a pie chart of radiation exposure in 1987 (Figure 13-3), one would find a very small contribution of x-rays (11%) and nuclear medicine (4%) compared to such things as radon (55%) and other natural sources at that time. The explosion of medical imaging and CT scan use—in particular in the 1970s through 1990s—has led to the appearance of the pie chart shown in Figure 13-2, where medical procedures account for nearly half of the radiation exposure.

References:
<http://www.atsdr.cdc.gov/toxprofiles/tp149-c6.pdf>.
Agency for Toxic Substances and Disease Registry. <http://energy.gov/sites/prod/files/2014/06/f16/A_Basic_Overview_of_Occupational_Radiation_Exposure.pdf>.

34. **B, Beta particles.** As noted in the following chart, the radiation weighting factor of x-rays and beta particles is 1:

Type and Energy Range	Radiation Weighting Factor, WR
Gamma rays and x-rays	1
Beta particles	1
Neutrons	5–20 (depending on keV energy of Neutron)
Alpha particles	20

Alpha, beta, and gamma radiation is emitted by radioactive agents. The energy of the radiation produced may be described in Joules or ion electronvolts:

6200 billion MeV = 1 joule and 1 joule per second = 1 watt

Reference:
<http://www.ccohs.ca/oshanswers/phys_agents/ionizing.html>.

35. **C, Lead equivalent thickness.** The more lead used in an apron, the more the reduction in x-ray transmission. However, the trade-off is the weight of the lead apron and its impact on the long-term health of the user with respect to musculoskeletal strain. Although 0.50-mm lead equivalent non-lead aprons are frequently employed, they weigh 10.9 kgs. A 0.25-mm lead equivalent non-lead apron weighs as little as 3.6 kg, and a 0.35-mm apron weigh about 5.4 kgs. As for the x-ray attenuation, the 0.50-mm equivalent, as advertised, had the greatest benefit to the wearer. The experimental results showed that the 0.50-mm lead equivalent non-lead apron had a lower transit dose of 0.21 mSv per month than the 0.25-mm lead apron (P < 0.01). The 0.35-mm lead apron had a lower transit dose of 0.15 mSv per month than the 0.25-mm lead equivalent non-lead apron (P < 0.01). However, the magnitude of the dose to the wearer was very small, below the recommended minimum value for occupational workers.

Reference:
Mori H, Koshida K, Ishigamori O, et al. Evaluation of the effectiveness of x-ray protective aprons in experimental and practical fields. *Radiol Phys Technol.* 2014;7(1):158-166. doi:10.1007/s12194-013-0246-x; [Epub 2013 Dec 13].

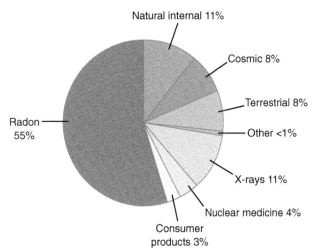

Figure 13-3 Radiation exposure to the average U.S. citizen

36. A 0.5-mm-thick lead-equivalent apron used in vascular radiology procedures has a radiation attenuation factor of approximately:
    A. 200
    B. 100
    C. 20
    D. 10

37. The purpose of placing a half apron behind the patient during an erect chest radiograph is:
    A. To reduce potential dose from tube leakage and room scatter
    B. Reduce radiation exposure to the gonads
    C. Of little value, in part due to excellent collimation
    D. All of the above

38. Most of dose to the gonads and other tissues outside the x-ray beam results from:
    A. Internal scatter
    B. Bremsstrahlung
    C. The lungs' low attenuation of radiation
    D. Compton effect

39. The Joint Commission requires lead aprons to be inspected:
    A. Annually
    B. Twice a year
    C. It does not specify
    D. Every other year

36. **A, 200.** By measuring the radiation exposure superficial to and deep to the lead apron during vascular radiology fluoroscopic and DSA examinations, Kicken and Bos were able to determine the degree of attenuation occurring with a 0.5-mm standard lead apron. Using three different techniques and procedures, the attenuation factor averaged 222 with a standard error of 30. The results were at an x-ray beam of between 60 and 110 keV (average 80 keV), which could be different if the lead apron was being used for other purposes such as nuclear medicine using higher energy agents. There is also a fudge factor depending on the number and angle/direction of the x-ray beams. Backscatter contribution to the radiation dosage was about 10%.

Reference:
Kicken PJ, Bos AJ. Effectiveness of lead aprons in vascular radiology: results of clinical measurements. Radiology. 1995 Nov;197(2):473-478.

37. **D, All of the above.** A half apron around the bottom of a patient to prevent radiation to the gonads when performing a chest radiograph has very little value, even though it is used at many institutions. Because of the outstanding collimation now done during digital radiography and the distance between the x-ray beam and the gonads, the actual amount of the incident beam accounting for radiation exposure to distant parts is minor. However, the effect of radiation bouncing off the ribs, internal organs, and body parts that may lead to scatter of the beam to affect the gonads is not truly addressed by the half apron because it occurs within the body.

A Japanese group (cited below) performed such measures and stated this in their abstract:

The influence of radiation on the absorbed dose of the gonad was mostly from scattered radiation from inside the body for the 14 × 17 inch field size, and also from the x-ray tube for the 14 × 14 inch field size. Although a certain protective effect is achieved by using the protector, the radiation dose to the gonad is only a few microGy even without a protector. ... We conclude the use of a radiation protective apron is not necessary for diagnostic chest radiography.

Reference:
Hashimoto M, Kato H, Fujibuchi T, et al. Gonad protective effect of radiation protective apron in chest radiography. *Nihon Hoshasen Gijutsu Gakkai Zasshi.* 2004;60(12):1704-1712. [Article in Japanese].

38. **A, Internal scatter.** Internal scatter is an issue that cannot be addressed by lead aprons. This is radiation that arises from the directly irradiated region of the patient, be it from a plain x-ray beam, a CT scan, an internal gamma emitter, or radiation therapy photon/proton beam. Internal scatter peripheral doses from multiple x-ray or CT beams are additive, so that their sum increases approximately in proportion with the region being imaged.

Compton scattering occurs when the incident x-ray photon is deflected from its original path by an interaction with an electron. The x-ray photon loses energy because of the interaction but continues to travel through the material but along an altered path. Compton scatter is a source of attenuation of the strength of the x-ray beam.

Reference:
Chopp M, Ewald L, Hartson M. The contribution of internal scatter to radiation dose during CT scan of the head. *Neuroradiol.* 1981;22(3):145-150.

39. **C, It does not specify.** The Joint Commission leaves it up to institutions to create a policy as to how often lead aprons should be inspected for cracks and holes. Most institutions do so at annual rates. Gloves and collars should be included in the inspection program. Folding of aprons or stacking them leads to more wear and tear than properly hanging the apron. The considerations for when to replace a lead apron revolve around (1) the area of the apron deemed flawed, (2) the site of the apron defect, and (3) the tissue/organ exposed. Lead aprons are considered an environmental chemical waste when they are disposed of.

Reference:
Michel R, Zorn MJ. Implementation of an x-ray radiation protective equipment inspection program. *Health Phys.* 2002;82(2 suppl):S51-S53.

40. For which of the following is a lead apron most effective?
    A. Tc-99m
    B. F-18
    C. I-131
    D. The lead is equally effective for all three

41. For which of the following is a lead apron least effective?
    A. Tc-99m
    B. F-18
    C. I-131
    D. The lead is equally effective for all three

42. What is the difference between a RAD and a REM?
    A. They are synonymous
    B. A REM is a unit of absorbed dose
    C. A RAD is a unit of equivalent dose
    D. None of the above

40. **A, Tc-99m.** Lead is best used for gamma radiation emitters such as Tc-99m pertechnetate, which has 140 keV. Depending on the energy of the gamma radiation, the thickness of the lead may need to be considered. It makes sense that the less time spent exposed to any radiation source the better. Also, by increasing the distance between the patient/physician and the radiation source there is better reduction in exposure. The radiation exposure decreases as you move away from the source by a factor of 1 over the distance squared. Therefore someone who is 3 feet from a source incurs nine times the exposure as someone 9 feet from the source. Step away from the isotope/image intensifier!

Reference:

Norman E. Bolus. Review of common occupational hazards and safety concerns for nuclear medicine technologists. *J Nucl Med Technol.* 2008;36(1):11-17.

41. **B, F-18.** In a nuclear medicine setting, lead aprons are most effective in reducing radiation exposure levels from a low energy gamma and pure beta emitter (83% to 99% reduction) than a mixed beta and gamma emitter such as I-131 (52.6%). Lead is least effective in blocking the radiation of a high energy gamma emitter such as F-18 (18.2%). Because alpha radiation, though high in dosage, does not penetrate very deeply, it is not generally shielded. It cannot pass through skin. Beta radiation is well shielded by using Plexiglas, glass, and plastic, materials with low Z numbers that reduce the rate of bremsstrahlung scatter of radiation. Bremsstrahlung refers to the generation of radiation when a high speed electron contacts or is deflected by an atomic nucleus. It usually leaves at a lower energy state. Lead is most effective in reducing gamma radiation emitter.

Reference:

Ahmed S, Zimmer A, McDonald N, et al. The effectiveness of lead aprons in reducing radiation exposures from specific radionuclides. *J Nucl Med.* 2007;48(suppl 2):470P.

42. **D, As seen in the table below, absorbed dose is measured in RADS whereas equivalent dose is measured in REM.**

UNITS OF RADIOACTIVITY AND RADIATION DOSE

Quantity	SI Unit and Symbol	Non-SI Unit	Conversion Factor
Radioactivity	becquerel, Bq	curie, Ci	1 Ci = 3.7 × 1010 Bq = 37 Gigabecquerels (GBq) 1 Bq = 27 picocurie (pCi)
Absorbed dose	gray, Gy	rad	1 rad = 0.01 Gy
Equivalent dose	sievert, Sv	rem	1 rem = 0.01 Sv 1 rem = 10 mSv

REM stands for Roentgen Equivalent Man and refers to the biological effect of the radiation. Radiation absorbed dosage (RAD) is what the tissue gets, but the damage varies depending upon the "Quality Factor" of the emitter, as per the table below.

Radiation	Quality Factor (Q)
Beta, Gamma and X-rays	1
Thermal Neutrons	3
Fast n, a, and protons	10
Heavy and recoil nuclei	20

Thus for the same amount of RADs, the REM of heavy nuclei radiation is much higher than X-rays.

References:

<http://www.nrc.gov/reading-rm/doc-collections/cfr/part020/part020-1201.html>.

<http://www.imagesco.com/geiger/radiation-safety.html>.

QUESTIONS

1. The Radiology Reporting Initiative:
   A. Standardizes the order of indication, technique, comparison, recommendations, and impression in reports
   B. Aims to standardize language in radiology reports to an eighth-grade level as required by Congress
   C. Is part of meaningful use legislation
   D. Creates clear and concise report templates

2. The Radiology Reporting Initiative:
   A. Is an initiative by the AMA
   B. Is being organized through the RSNA
   C. Is managed by subspecialty societies
   D. Is a mandate of The Joint Commission

3. What is the most widely used radiology lexicon?
   A. BI-RADS
   B. Urban Dictionary
   C. Merriam-Webster
   D. RadPeer

4. Radlex is one attempt at:
   A. Standardizing report formats
   B. Creating structured reports
   C. Getting all reports to a single page in length
   D. Defining the terms radiologists use

5. TI-RADS refers to:
   A. Thyroid imaging reporting lexicon
   B. Thoracic imaging reporting lexicon
   C. Tomosynthesis breast imaging reporting lexicon
   D. There is no such thing

6. Which factors are considered in the TI-RADS lexicon?
   A. Echogenicity
   B. Margins
   C. Shape
   D. All of the above

1. **D, Creates clear and concise report templates.** The Radiology Reporting Initiative is "a library of clear and consistent report templates." They are created by twelve subcommittees of subspecialty experts, with the goal of creating uniformity and improving communication with referring providers.

   Although these templates are not part of Medicare meaningful use of EHRs, they are part of other CMS pay-for-performance incentives.

   The templates are not limited to the order of sections within a report, and they also include specific information fields for data that referring physicians would be interested in, depending on the indication of the exam.

   Although the AMA previously estimated health literacy of the U.S. general public at around the eighth-grade level, Congress has not mandated an eighth-grade reading level for radiology reports.

   References:
   <www.rsna.org/Reporting_Initiative.aspx>.
   Weis BD. *Health literacy: a manual for clinicians.* Chicago, IL: American Medical Association and American Medical Foundation; 2003.
   Kahn CE, Langlotz CP, Burnside ES, et al. Towards best practices in radiology reporting. *Radiology.* 2009;252(3):852-856.

2. **B, Is being organized through the RSNA.** The Radiology Reporting Initiative was organized by the RSNA to create "a library of clear and consistent report templates." The AMA was not involved in the initiative. Although there are subcommittees composed of subspecialty experts to create the various specialty templates, the subspecialty societies are not directly involved.

   The templates that have been created by the Radiology Reporting Initiative are not mandated by The Joint Commission or any health care payers, but they may be incorporated into other CMS pay-for-performance incentives.

   References:
   Kahn CE, Langlotz CP, Burnside ES, et al. Towards best practices in radiology reporting. *Radiology.* 2009;252(3):852-856.
   <https://www.rsna.org/Reporting_Initiative.aspx>.

3. **A, BI-RADS.** The Breast Imaging Reporting and Data System (BI-RADS) is a lexicon (controlled vocabulary) developed in 1993 by the American College of Radiology to standardize mammographic reporting and reduce confusion regarding mammographic findings. Use of this lexicon was codified into law by the Mammography Quality Standards Act (MQSA) of 1997, which required that all mammograms in the United States include the BI-RADS terminology and categories of assessment.

   Urban Dictionary is a commercial website that describes itself as, "a veritable cornucopia of streetwise lingo, posted and defined by its readers." Merriam-Webster, Inc. is an American company that publishes reference books, especially dictionaries. Radpeer is a web-based program to perform cross-institution peer review. Organized by the ACR, RADPEER "allows peer review to be performed during the routine interpretation of current images."

   References:
   Liberman L, Menell JH. Breast imaging reporting and data system (BI-RADS). Radiol Clin North Am. 2002;40(3):409-430.
   MQSA Final Rule, Federal Register 62(208):55988.
   <http://www.acr.org/Quality-Safety/RADPEER>.

4. **D, Defining the terms radiologists use.** Radlex, a portmanteau term for Radiology Lexicon, is "a unified language of radiology terms for standardized indexing and retrieval of radiology information." The purpose of such a lexicon is to have a single set of terms with agreed upon meaning and minimal ambiguity that all radiologists can use.

   Standardizing reporting formats and creating structured reports is a purpose of the RSNA Radiology Reporting Initiative, which makes templates for reports created by subspecialty committees freely available to radiologists. There is no word or page limit to radiology reports endorsed by ACR or RSNA.

   References:
   <https://www.rsna.org/RadLex.aspx>.
   <http://www.acr.org/News-Publications/News/News-Articles/2013/ACR-Bulletin/201311-Setting-the-Standard>.
   Langlotz CP. RadLex: a new method for indexing online educational materials. Radio Graphics. 2006;26(6):1595-1597.

5. **A, Thyroid imaging reporting lexicon.** In 2015 the American College of Radiology proposed establishing the thyroid imaging Radiology and data system (TI-RADS) in order to standardize the reporting and terminology used for ultrasound of thyroid nodules. This standardization is analogous to the ones used for breast imaging (BI-RADS) and Liver imaging (LI-RADS) which successfully changed the way radiologists report on suspicious masses. Because so many thyroid nodules are discovered incidentally and are overwhelmingly benign, TI-RADS was thought to be justified. The terms used are derived for thyroid ultrasonography and the standardized risk stratification would be utilized to determine which nodules need to be biopsied.

   References:
   Grant EG, Tessler FN, Hoang JK, et al. Thyroid Ultrasound Reporting Lexicon: White Paper of the ACR Thyroid Imaging, Reporting and Data System (TIRADS) CommitteeJ Am Coll Radiol 2015;12:1272-1279. Copyright 2015 American College of Radiology.

6. **D, All of the above.** The TIRADS lexicon discusses the echogenicity, shape, margins, echogenic foci, size, and composition. Composition should be classified as predominantly cystic versus predominantly solid. Echogenicity should be described as hyperechoic, isoechoic, or hypo echoic or "mixed" but predominantly hyperechoic, isoechoic, or hypo echoic. Size is not scored as far as risk because of the controversy over the risk of malignancy in nodules > 1 cm. Border description uses the terms smooth, lobulated, ill-defined, halo, versus extra thyroidal extension.

   References:
   Grant EG, Tessler FN, Hoang JK, et al. Thyroid Ultrasound Reporting Lexicon: White Paper of the ACR Thyroid Imaging, Reporting and Data System (TIRADS) CommitteeJ Am Coll Radiol 2015;12:1272-1279. Copyright 2015 American College of Radiology.

7. Which of the following is an allowed PQI activity as of the September 2015 ABR ruling?
   A. Participation as a member of an institutional/departmental clinical quality and/or safety review committee
   B. Active participation in a departmental or institutional peer review process such as OPPE
   C. Invited presentation or exhibition of a peer reviewed poster at a national meeting related to quality improvement
   D. All of the above

8. The Joint Commission has specified that accredited facilities must define:
   A. Critical tests
   B. Critical results
   C. Both critical tests and critical results
   D. None of the above

9. A useful application of imaging wisely is:
   A. Radiology benefits managers
   B. Iterative reconstruction of CT studies
   C. Decision support software
   D. Computer assisted diagnosis (CAD)

7. **D, All of the above.** The ABR liberalized the potential activities that would fulfill the Part IV of the MOC program for practice quality improvement. The ABR no longer requires a project that went through the Plan Do Study Act project methodology for PQI initiatives. In addition to the three activities listed above that fulfill PQI, they allowed the following additional "participatory quality-improvement activities":

Participation as a member of a root cause analysis team evaluating a sentinel or other quality- or safety-related event

Participation in at least 25 prospective chart rounds every year (peer review of the radiation delivery plans for new cases—radiation oncology and medical physics only).

Active participation in submitting data to a national registry

Publication of a peer-reviewed journal article related to quality improvement or improved safety of the diplomate's practice content area

Regular participation (at least 10/year) in departmental or group conferences focused on patient safety

Examples include regular attendance at tumor boards, M&M conferences, diagnostic/therapeutic errors conferences, interprofessional conferences, surgical/pathology correlation conferences, etc.

Creation or active management of, or participation in, one of the elements of a quality or safety program

Examples include a department dashboard or scorecard, a daily management system to ensure quality and safety, a daily readiness assessment using a huddle system.

Local or national leadership role in a national/international quality improvement program, such as Image Gently, Image Wisely, Choosing Wisely, or other similar campaign

Local participation roles include implementation and/or maintenance of or adherence to program goals and/or requirements

Completion of a Peer Survey (quality or patient safety-focused) and resulting action plan. Survey should contain at least five quality or patient safety-related questions and have a minimum of five survey responses

Completion of a Patient Experience-of-Care (PEC) survey with individual patient feedback. Survey should contain at least five quality/patient safety-related questions and have a minimum of 30 survey responses

Active participation in applying for or maintaining accreditation by specialty accreditation programs such as those offered by ACR, ACRO, or ASTRO

Annual participation in the required Mammography Quality Standards Act (MQSA) medical audit or ACR Mammography Accreditation Program (MAP)

Completion of a Self-Directed Educational Project (SDEP) on a quality or patient safety-related topic (medical physics only)

Active participation in an NCI cooperative group clinical trial (for diagnostic radiologists, radiation oncologists, and interventional radiologists, entry of five or more patients in a year. For medical physicists, active participation in the credentialing activities)

Reference:
<http://www.theabr.org/moc-part4-activities>.

8. **C, Both critical tests and critical results.** TJC specified that accredited facilities define both critical tests and critical results as a standard aimed to improve effective communication among caregivers. A critical test is an examination that, if positive for its primary indication, would yield a critical result. A critical result is one that is significantly outside the normal range and may indicate a life-threatening situation. Further, this life-threatening situation may be averted with proper and prompt care, potentiated by effective communication.

Reference:
<http://www.jointcommission.org/assets/1/6/2015_NPSG_HAP.pdf>.

9. **C, Decision support software.** Non-ionizing imaging options are always preferable to any test with ionizing radiation, particularly in the pregnant patient. Ordering physicians may not have access to the patients' imaging or radiation dose history and/or may lack or be unaware of recommended criteria to guide their decisions, thereby potentially exposing patients to unnecessary radiation. Promotion of alternative non-ionizing imaging modalities and providing ordering clinicians with information to help better inform their image ordering decision making process can be accomplished with decision support software.

References:
<http://www.imagewisely.org/imaging-modalities/computed-tomography/medical-physicists/articles/the-pregnant-patient>.
<http://www.fda.gov/Radiation-EmittingProducts/RadiationSafety/RadiationDoseReduction/ucm199994.htm>.

10. Mr. Vandy and his family arrive in the MRI suite for his scan. He is checked in at the reception desk. They take his information and recommend he use the restroom prior to the study in the reception area. He declines. He then is escorted by the tech to a locker area in the scanner suite where his family can no longer accompany him. He puts his metallic objects in the locker and then uses the bathroom in the scanner suite. Before Mr. Vandy enters the MRI scanner, a technologist uses a wand to screen Mr. Vandy for metal. The tech finds Mr. Vandy's money clip in his patient gown pocket. She removes it from his possession and escorts Mr. Vandy into the scanner room. The bathroom in the scanner area is considered to be in which zone based on ACR designations?
    A. I
    B. II
    C. III
    D. IV

10. **B, II.** Any component of the area between the reception desk and the patient screening is designated Safety Zone II by ACR (Figure 14-1). Mr. Vandy was recommended to use the bathroom after checking in at the reception desk but before metal screening, thus the bathroom area should be designated as Safety Zone II. However, if the bathroom was located within the post-screened patient holding area it would have been designated as Safety Zone III.

Reference:
<http://www.acr.org/quality-safety/radiology-safety/mr-safety>.
Kanal E, Barkovich AJ, Bell C, et al. ACR guidance document on MR safe practices: 2013. *J Magn Reson Imaging.* 2013;37(3):501-530.

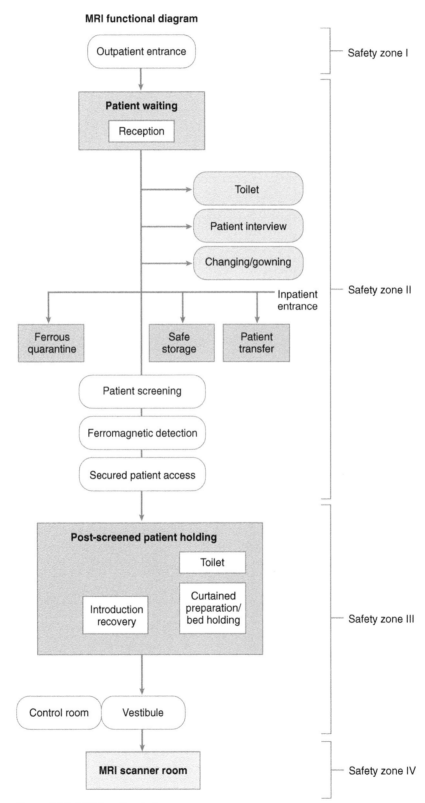

Figure 14-1 MRI Functional diagram.

11. The bathroom in the reception area is considered to be in which zone based on ACR designations?
    A. I
    B. II
    C. III
    D. IV

12. The area outside the scan room where Mr. Vandy was "wanded" for metal is considered to be in which zone based on ACR designations?
    A. I
    B. II
    C. III
    D. IV

13. The locker in the scanner area is considered to be in which zone based on ACR designations?
    A. I
    B. II
    C. III
    D. IV

14. The reception area is considered to be in which zone based on ACR designations?
    A. I
    B. II
    C. III
    D. IV

15. The scanner magnet room is considered to be in which zone based on ACR designations?
    A. I
    B. II
    C. III
    D. IV

11. **B, II.** The bathroom in the reception area is designated as Safety Zone II by ACR (see Figure 14-1).

The reference cited below states:

Zone I: This region includes all areas that are freely accessible to the general public. This area is typically outside the MR environment itself and is the area through which patients, health care personnel, and other employees of the MR site access the MR environment.

Zone II: This area is the interface between the publicly accessible, uncontrolled Zone I and the strictly controlled Zones III and IV. Typically, patients are greeted in Zone II and are not free to move throughout Zone II at will but are rather under the supervision of MR personnel. It is in Zone II that the patients are screened.

Zone III: This area is the region in which free access by unscreened non-MR personnel or ferromagnetic objects or equipment can result in serious injury or death as a result of interactions between the individuals or equipment and the MR scanner's particular environment. All access to Zone III is to be strictly restricted, with access to regions within it controlled by, and entirely under the supervision of, MR personnel.

Zone IV: This area is synonymous with the MR scanner magnet room itself, ie, the physical confines of the room within which the MR scanner is located.

References:
<http://www.acr.org/quality-safety/radiology-safety/mr-safety>.
Kanal E, Barkovich AJ, Bell C, et al. ACR guidance document on MR safe practices: 2013. *J Magn Reson Imaging*. 2013;37(3):501-530.

12. **C, III.** The area between the reception and the MRI scanner is considered Safety Zone III by ACR (Figure 14-2). Zone III: This area is the region in which free access by unscreened non-MR personnel or ferromagnetic objects or equipment can result in serious injury or death as a result of interactions between the individuals or equipment and the MR scanner's particular environment. All access to Zone III is to be strictly restricted, with access to regions within it controlled by, and entirely under the supervision of, MR personnel.

References:
<http://www.acr.org/quality-safety/radiology-safety/mr-safety>.
Kanal E, Barkovich AJ, Bell C, et al. ACR guidance document on MR safe practices: 2013. *J Magn Reson Imaging*. 2013;37(3):501-530.

13. **B, II.** The locker in the scanner area is designated as Safety Zone II by ACR. This area is the interface between the publicly accessible, uncontrolled Zone I and the strictly controlled Zones III and IV. Typically, patients are greeted in Zone II and are not free to move throughout Zone II at will but are rather under the supervision of MR personnel. It is in Zone II that the patients are screened. Rarely, one may have lockers in Zone III for patients' personal items (removable hearing aids, eyeglasses to see to get to Zone 3 from Zone 2).

References:
<http://www.acr.org/quality-safety/radiology-safety/mr-safety>.
Kanal E, Barkovich AJ, Bell C, et al. ACR guidance document on MR safe practices: 2013. *J Magn Reson Imaging*. 2013;37(3):501-530.

14. **B, II.** The reception area is designated as Safety Zone II by ACR. Zone II: This area is the interface between the publicly accessible, uncontrolled Zone I and the strictly controlled Zones III and IV. Typically, patients are greeted in Zone II and are not free to move throughout Zone II at will but are rather under the supervision of MR personnel. It is in Zone II that the patients are screened.

References:
<http://www.acr.org/quality-safety/radiology-safety/mr-safety>.
Kanal E, Barkovich AJ, Bell C, et al. ACR guidance document on MR safe practices: 2013. *J Magn Reson Imaging*. 2013;37(3):501-530.

15. **D, IV.** The scanner magnet room is designated as Safety Zone IV by ACR (Figure 14-3). Zone IV: This area is synonymous with the MR scanner magnet room itself, ie, the physical confines of the room within which the MR scanner is located.

References:
<http://www.acr.org/quality-safety/radiology-safety/mr-safety>.
Kanal E, Barkovich AJ, Bell C, et al. ACR guidance document on MR safe practices: 2013. *J Magn Reson Imaging*. 2013;37(3):501-530.

⚠ CAUTION

| **MRI ZONE III** | **Restricted Access**
 Screened MRI Patients and MRI Personnel Only |

Figure 14-2 MRI zone III.

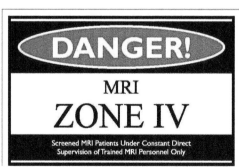

Figure 14-3 MRI zone IV.

16. The scanner control room is considered to be in which zone based on ACR designations?
   A. I
   B. II
   C. III
   D. IV

16. **C, III.** Zone III: This area is the region in which free access by unscreened non-MR personnel or ferromagnetic objects or equipment can result in serious injury or death as a result of interactions between the individuals or equipment and the MR scanner's particular environment. All access to Zone III is to be strictly restricted, with access to regions within it controlled by, and entirely under the supervision of, MR personnel.

Reference:

<http://www.acr.org/quality-safety/radiology-safety/mr-safety>.

Kanal E, Barkovich AJ, Bell C, et al. ACR guidance document on MR safe practices: 2013. *J Magn Reson Imaging*. 2013;37(3):501-530.

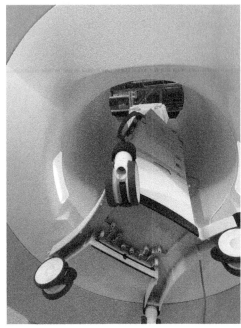

Figure 14-4 MR scanner with machine in bore.

QUESTIONS

1. The data for sick days off for a nine-member pediatric radiology group show 0, 1, 1, 1, 4, 8, 15, 17, 25 days. The mean number of sick days for the group is:
   A. 1
   B. 4
   C. 6
   D. 8

2. The data for sick days off for a nine-member pediatric radiology group show 0, 1, 1, 1, 4, 8, 15, 17, 25 days. The median number of sick days for the group is:
   A. 1
   B. 4
   C. 6
   D. 8

3. The data for sick days off for a nine-member pediatric radiology group show 0, 1, 1, 1, 4, 8, 15, 17, 25 days. The mode of sick days for the group is:
   A. 1
   B. 4
   C. 6
   D. 8

4. The data for sick days off for a nine-member pediatric radiology group show 0, 1, 1, 1, 4, 8, 15, 17, 25 days. The standard deviation of sick days for the group is approximately:
   A. 7
   B. 8
   C. 9
   D. 10

   The following are the results from a CTA study of splenic artery infarcts

Radiology Result	Pathology Proof	
	Positive	Negative
Positive	25	50
Negative	30	70

5. Based on the data above, the positive predictive value of CTA is:
   A. 33.3%
   B. 45.5%
   C. 50%
   D. 54.3%

6. Based on these data the negative predictive value of CTA is:
   A. 30%
   B. 37.5%
   C. 50%
   D. 70%

7. Based on these data the sensitivity of CTA is:
   A. 33.3%
   B. 45.5%
   C. 50%
   D. 54.3%

8. Based on these data the specificity of CTA is:
   A. 30%
   B. 41.7%
   C. 58.3%
   D. 70%

1. **D, 8.** Mean is derived by adding all the numbers in a series and dividing the sum by the total number of cases in the series. In this example, the sum is 72. This number divided by 9 entries equals 8.

References:
<http://www.theabr.org/sites/all/themes/abr media/pdf/Noninterpretive_Skills_Domain_Specification_and_Resource_Guide.pdf>.
Reid HM. *Introduction to Statistics: Fundamental Concepts and Procedures of Data Analysis.* 14th ed. Thousand Oaks, CA: Sage Publications; 2014.
Bernard R. *Descriptive Statistics. Fundamentals of Biostatistics.* 6th ed. Belmont, CA: Thomson Brooks/Cole; 2006:6-37.
Bernard R. *Probability. Fundamentals of Biostatistics.* 6th ed. Belmont, CA: Thomson Brooks/Cole; 2006:43-68.

2. **B, 4.** The median of a set of numbers can be found by ordering all numbers in ascending order. If there is an odd number of observations, then the median is the value in the middle. If there is an even number of observations, then the median is the average of the two values in the middle. In this example, the numbers are already in order (0, 1, 1, 1, 4, 8, 15, 17, 25), the number of observations is odd, and the median is 4 because it is in the middle of the list.

Reference:
Reid HM. *Introduction to Statistics: Fundamental Concepts and Procedures of Data Analysis.* 14th ed. Thousand Oaks, CA: Sage Publications; 2014.

3. **A, 1.** The mode is the value that appears most frequently in the list of numbers. In this example, the mode is 1 because it appears three times.

References:
Reid HM. *Introduction to Statistics: Fundamental Concepts and Procedures of Data Analysis.* 14th ed. Thousand Oaks, CA: Sage Publications; 2014.
Bernard R. *Descriptive Statistics. Fundamentals of Biostatistics.* 6th ed. Belmont, CA: Thomson Brooks/Cole; 2006:6-37.
Bernard R. *Probability. Fundamentals of Biostatistics.* 6th ed. Belmont, CA: Thomson Brooks/Cole; 2006:43-68.

4. **C, 9.** The standard deviation is defined as:

$$SD = \sqrt{\frac{\sum (x - \bar{x})^2}{N-1}}$$

where n is the number of observations, x_i is each observation, and $\bar{x}$ is the mean.

The mean is the sum of all observations divided by the number of observations:

$$\bar{x} = (0+1+1+1+4+8+15+17+25)/9 = 72/9 = 8$$

In this example, the standard deviation is approximately 9:

$$SD = \sqrt{\frac{\begin{array}{c}(0-8)^2 + (1-8)^2 + (1-8)^2 + (1-8)^2 \\ + (4-8)^2 + (8-8)^2 + (15-8)^2 + (17-8)^2 + (25-8)^2\end{array}}{9-1}}$$

$$= \sqrt{\frac{(-8)^2 + (-7)^2 + (-7)^2 + (-7)^2 + (-4)^2 + (0)^2 + (7)^2 + (9)^2 + (17)^2}{8}}$$

$$= \sqrt{\frac{64 + 49 + 49 + 49 + 16 + 0 + 49 + 81 + 289}{8}}$$

$$= \sqrt{\frac{646}{8}} = \sqrt{80.75} = 8.986 \approx 9$$

Reference:
Reid HM. *Introduction to Statistics: Fundamental Concepts and Procedures of Data Analysis.* 14th ed. Thousand Oaks, CA: Sage Publications; 2014.

5. **A, 33.3%.** Positive predictive value, negative predictive value, sensitivity, specificity, and accuracy can all be calculated from this 2-by-2 table:

	Disease	No Disease
Positive test	a (true positives)	b (false positives)
Negative test	c (false negatives)	d (true negatives)

Positive predictive value = a/(a + b), true positives/(true positives + false positives)

In this example, positive predictive value is 25/(25 + 50) = 0.333 = 33.3%.

References:
Bernard R. *Descriptive Statistics. Fundamentals of Biostatistics.* 6th ed. Belmont, CA: Thomson Brooks/Cole; 2006:6-37.
Bernard R. *Probability. Fundamentals of Biostatistics.* 6th ed. Belmont, CA: Thomson Brooks/Cole; 2006:43-68.

6. **D, 70%.** Positive predictive value, negative predictive value, sensitivity, specificity, and accuracy can all be calculated from this 2-by-2 table:

	Disease	No Disease
Positive test	a (true positives)	b (false positives)
Negative test	c (false negatives)	d (true negatives)

Negative predictive value = d/(c + d), true negatives/(true negatives + false negatives)

In this example, negative predictive value is 70/(70 + 30) = 0.7 = 70%.

References:
Bernard R. *Descriptive Statistics. Fundamentals of Biostatistics.* 6th ed. Belmont, CA: Thomson Brooks/Cole; 2006:6-37.
Bernard R. *Probability. Fundamentals of Biostatistics.* 6th ed. Belmont, CA: Thomson Brooks/Cole; 2006:43-68.

7. **B, 45.5%.** Positive predictive value, negative predictive value, sensitivity, specificity, and accuracy can all be calculated from this 2-by-2 table:

	Disease	No Disease
Positive test	a (true positives)	b (false positives)
Negative test	c (false negatives)	d (true negatives)

Sensitivity = a/(a + c), true positives/(true positives + false negatives)

In this example, sensitivity is 25/(25 + 30) = 0.455 = 45.5%.

References:
Bernard R. *Descriptive Statistics. Fundamentals of Biostatistics.* 6th ed. Belmont, CA: Thomson Brooks/Cole; 2006:6-37.
Bernard R. *Probability. Fundamentals of Biostatistics.* 6th ed. Belmont, CA: Thomson Brooks/Cole; 2006:43-68.

8. **C, 58.3%.** Positive predictive value, negative predictive value, sensitivity, specificity, and accuracy can all be calculated from this 2-by-2 table:

	Disease	No Disease
Positive test	a (true positives)	b (false positives)
Negative test	c (false negatives)	d (true negatives)

Specificity = d/(b + d), true negatives/(true negatives + false positives)

In this example, specificity is 70/(70 + 50) = 0.583 = 58.3%.

References:
Bernard R. *Descriptive Statistics. Fundamentals of Biostatistics.* 6th ed. Belmont, CA: Thomson Brooks/Cole; 2006:6-37.
Bernard R. *Probability. Fundamentals of Biostatistics.* 6th ed. Belmont, CA: Thomson Brooks/Cole; 2006:43-68.

9. Based on these data the accuracy of CTA is:
   A. 33.3%
   B. 45.5%
   C. 50%
   D. 54.3%

10. If the sensitivity of a study is 40%, the specificity 90%, and the prevalence of the disease in the population studied is 20%, what would be the positive predictive value?
    A. 40%
    B. 50%
    C. 66.7%
    D. 80%

11. In the scenario in question 10 (sensitivity of a study is 40%, specificity 90%), what is the accuracy of the test?
    A. 40%
    B. 50%
    C. 66.7%
    D. 80%

12. In the scenario in question 11 (specificity 90%), what is the sensitivity of the test if the prevalence increases to 50%?
    A. 40%
    B. 50%
    C. 66.7%
    D. 80%

9. **D, 54.3%.** Positive predictive value, negative predictive value, sensitivity, specificity, and accuracy can all be calculated from this 2-by-2 table:

	Disease	No Disease
Positive test	a (true positives)	b (false positives)
Negative test	c (false negatives)	d (true negatives)

Accuracy = (a + d)/(a + b + c + d), (true positives + true negatives)/ (True positives + false positives + false negatives + true negatives)

In this example, accuracy is (25 + 70)/(25 + 50 + 30 + 70) = 0.543 = 54.3%.

References:
Bernard R. *Descriptive Statistics. Fundamentals of Biostatistics.* 6th ed. Belmont, CA: Thomson Brooks/Cole; 2006:6-37.
Bernard R. *Probability. Fundamentals of Biostatistics.* 6th ed. Belmont, CA: Thomson Brooks/Cole; 2006:43-68.

10. **B, 50%.** To calculate positive predictive value and accuracy, create a 2-by-2 table matching the information provided. You may assume there are 1000 subjects (a + b + c + d = 1000). Because disease prevalence is 20%, 200 patients will have the disease (a + c = 200), and 800 patients will not (b + d = 800). Because sensitivity is 40%, the test will be positive in 80 out of the 200 patients with the disease (a = 80; c = 120). Because specificity is 90%, the test will be negative in 720 out of 800 patients without the disease (b = 80; d = 720).

	Disease	No Disease	
Positive test	a = 80	b = 80	a + b = 160
Negative test	c = 120	d = 720	c + d = 840
	a + c = 200	b + d = 800	

Therefore, positive predictive value is a/(a + b) = 80/160 = 50%.

References:
Bernard R. *Descriptive Statistics. Fundamentals of Biostatistics.* 6th ed. Belmont, CA: Thomson Brooks/Cole; 2006:6-37.
Bernard R. *Probability. Fundamentals of Biostatistics.* 6th ed. Belmont, CA: Thomson Brooks/Cole; 2006:43-68.

11. **D, 80%.** To calculate positive predictive value and accuracy, create a 2-by-2 table matching the information provided. You may assume there are 1000 subjects (a + b + c + d = 1000). Because disease prevalence is 20%, 200 patients will have the disease (a + c = 200), and 800 patients will not (b + d = 800). Because sensitivity is 40%, the test will be positive in 80 out of the 200 patients with the disease (a = 80; c = 120). Because specificity is 90%, the test will be negative in 720 out of 800 patients without the disease (b = 80; d = 720).

	Disease	No Disease	
Positive test	a = 80	b = 80	a + b = 160
Negative test	c = 120	d = 720	c + d = 840
	a + c = 200	b + d = 800	

Therefore, accuracy is (a + d)/(a + b + c + d) = (80 +720)/1000 = 80%.

References:
Bernard R. *Descriptive Statistics. Fundamentals of Biostatistics.* 6th ed. Belmont, CA: Thomson Brooks/Cole; 2006:6-37.
Bernard R. *Probability. Fundamentals of Biostatistics.* 6th ed. Belmont, CA: Thomson Brooks/Cole; 2006:43-68.

12. **A, 40%.**

Sensitivity = TP/(TP + FN)
Specificity = TN/(TN + FP)
Positive predictive value = TP/(TP + FP)
Negative predictive value = TN/(TN + FN)
TP = true positive, TN = true negative, FP = false positive, and FN = false negative

Sensitivity is a property of the test itself and does not depend on the prevalence. Hence, it will still be 40%.

The sensitivity and specificity of screening tests are characteristics of the test's performance at a given cut-off point, unaffected by the prevalence of the disease in the population that is being screened. If the prevalence of a disease is very small, 1 in 1000, a screening test may have high sensitivity and specificity at 95.0% but not be very useful unless it has high positive predictive value. If the sensitivity and specificity are 95% it means that with 20,000 people screened, you will have detected 19 out of the 20 with disease and have one false negative. However, it also means that of the 19,000 without the disease, given a specificity of 95%, 18,050 will be called negative and 950 will be called falsely positive. This would yield a positive predictive rate of 19/969 = 1.96%. If the disease prevalence is 1 in 10, and you detect 95% by the same sensitivity, then of the 2000 with disease you will detect 1900 and miss 100 (false negative). Given the same specificity, there would be 18,000 without disease, 17,100 with a negative exam, and 900 (5%) with a false positive exam. Now your positive predictive value is 1900/2800, a more respectable 67.9%. Contrast that with a test that has a 95% positive predictive rate. This means that, given a positive test in 100 people, you will have 5 people who are falsely positive. This means that, in the case of 1/1000 prevalence of a disease where you screen 20,000 people, you will have a positive test in 19 people (assuming 95% sensitivity) but, in addition, 1 will be falsely positive (with 1 false negative). Specificity will be 95%. In the case where the prevalence is 1/10 and you screen 20,000, 1900 will have a positive test (assuming 95% sensitivity) and 100 will have false positive studies. In this scenario, there will also be 100 false negative studies if you have a sensitivity of 95%. That is still better than having a 95% sensitivity and specificity.

References:
Bernard R. *Descriptive Statistics. Fundamentals of Biostatistics.* 6th ed. Belmont, CA: Thomson Brooks/Cole; 2006:6-37.
Bernard R. *Probability. Fundamentals of Biostatistics.* 6th ed. Belmont, CA: Thomson Brooks/Cole; 2006:43-68.

13. In the scenario in question 11 (sensitivity of a study is 40%, specificity 90%), what is the positive predictive value of the test if the prevalence increases to 50%?
    A. 40%
    B. 50%
    C. 66.7%
    D. 80%

14. In the scenario in question 11 (sensitivity of a study is 40%, specificity 90%), what is the accuracy of the test if the prevalence increases to 50%?
    A. 20%
    B. 40%
    C. 65%
    D. 80%

15. In the scenario in question 11 (sensitivity of a study is 40%, specificity 90%), what is the negative predictive value of the test if the prevalence increases to 50%?
    A. 40%
    B. 60%
    C. 67%
    D. 80%

16. The difference between incidence and prevalence relates to:
    A. Point in time = incidence
    B. Interval of time = prevalence
    C. Point in time = prevalence
    D. The size of the population

17. The axes on a receiver operator curve are:
    A. Sensitivity and specificity
    B. 1-Specificity and sensitivity
    C. Specificity and positive predictive value
    D. Positive predictive value and negative predictive value

18. The rate of false positives mostly affects:
    A. Sensitivity
    B. Specificity
    C. Power
    D. P values

13. **D, 80%.** Positive predictive value, accuracy, and negative predictive value depend on the prevalence. If prevalence increases to 50%, sensitivity 40% and specificity 90%, the 2-by-2 table can be adjusted as follows (using the same methods described for earlier questions):

	Disease	No Disease	
Positive test	a = 200	b = 50	a + b = 250
Negative test	c = 300	d = 450	c + d = 750
	a + c = 500	b + d = 500	

Positive predictive value is a/(a + b) = 200/250 = 80%. Of note, positive predictive value may also be calculated directly from sensitivity, specificity, and prevalence:

$$Positive\ predictive\ value = \frac{sensitivity * prevalence}{sensitivity * prevalence + (1 - specificity) * (1 - prevalence)}$$
$$= \frac{0.4 * 0.5}{0.4 * 0.5 + 0.1 * 0.5} = 0.8$$

References:
Bernard R. *Descriptive Statistics. Fundamentals of Biostatistics*. 6th ed. Belmont, CA: Thomson Brooks/Cole; 2006:6-37.
Bernard R. *Probability. Fundamentals of Biostatistics*. 6th ed. Belmont, CA: Thomson Brooks/Cole; 2006:43-68.

14. **C, 65%.** Positive predictive value, accuracy, and negative predictive value depend on the prevalence. If prevalence increases to 50%, sensitivity 40% and specificity 90%, the 2-by-2 table can be adjusted as follows (using the same methods described):

	Disease	No Disease	
Positive test	a = 200	b = 50	a + b = 250
Negative test	c = 300	d = 450	c + d = 750
	a + c = 500	b + d = 500	

Accuracy is (a + d)/(a + b + c + d) = (200 + 450)/1000 = 65%.

Of note, accuracy may also be calculated directly from sensitivity, specificity, and prevalence:

$$Accuracy = sensitivity * prevalence + specificity * (1 - prevalence)$$
$$= 0.4 * 0.5 + 0.9 * 0.5 = 0.65$$

References:
Bernard R. *Descriptive Statistics. Fundamentals of Biostatistics*. 6th ed. Belmont, CA: Thomson Brooks/Cole; 2006:6-37.
Bernard R. *Probability. Fundamentals of Biostatistics*. 6th ed. Belmont, CA: Thomson Brooks/Cole; 2006:43-68.

15. **B, 60%.** Positive predictive value, accuracy, and negative predictive value depend on the prevalence. If prevalence increases to 50%, sensitivity 40% and specificity 90%, the 2-by-2 table can be adjusted as follows (using the same methods described):

	Disease	No Disease	
Positive test	a = 200	b = 50	a + b = 250
Negative test	c = 300	d = 450	c + d = 750
	a + c = 500	b + d = 500	

Negative predictive value is d/(c + d) = 450/750 = 60%. Of note, negative predictive value may also be calculated directly from sensitivity, specificity, and prevalence:

$$Negative\ predictive\ value = \frac{specificity * (1 - prevalence)}{specificity * (1 - prevalence) + (1 - sensitivity) * prevalence}$$
$$= \frac{0.9 * 0.5}{0.9 * 0.5 + 0.6 * 0.5} = 0.6$$

References:
Bernard R. *Descriptive Statistics. Fundamentals of Biostatistics*. 6th ed. Belmont, CA: Thomson Brooks/Cole; 2006:6-37.
Bernard R. *Probability. Fundamentals of Biostatistics*. 6th ed. Belmont, CA: Thomson Brooks/Cole; 2006:43-68.

16. **C, Point in time = prevalence.** Incidence refers to the number of new cases that are generated in a given time interval (ie, the rate of disease onset over time). Prevalence refers to the number of patients afflicted by that disease in the overall population at a given time. Prevalence and incidence are related in that increasing incidence generally implies increasing prevalence. However, note that prevalence is also influenced by disease duration so that it is possible to have a relatively high disease incidence and low prevalence, for instance for diseases that are readily treated (eg, appendicitis) or those with high mortality. Conversely, diseases with low mortality and that are managed rather than cured (e.g. Crohn's disease) may have a relatively low incidence but high prevalence.

Reference:
BMJ. Epidemiology for the uninitiated, Chapter 2: Quantifying Disease Populations. <http://www.bmj.com/about-bmj/resources-readers/publications/epidemiology-uninitiated/2-quantifying-disease-populations>; Accessed November 2015.

17. **B, 1-specificity and sensitivity.** A receiver operating characteristic (ROC) curve is a plot of performance of a diagnostic test for discriminating true incidence from noise. This is classically portrayed as true positive rate (sensitivity) on the y-axis and false positive rate (1-specificity) on the x-axis.

Reference:
Alemayehu D, Zou KH. Applications of ROC analysis in medical research: recent developments and future directions. *Acad Radiol*. 2012;19(12):1457-1464.

18. **B, Specificity.** Specificity is defined as the number of healthy patients who test negative (true negatives) divided by the total number of healthy patients (true negatives plus false positives). Therefore it is most affected by false positives.

Sensitivity is defined as the number of diseased patients who test positive (true positives) divided by the total number of diseased patients (true positives plus false negatives).

Power is defined statistically as 1 − Beta, which conceptually parallels the rate of true positives as defined in a diagnostic test.

P value is the predefined threshold used to determine if a null hypothesis should be rejected.

Reference:
Sardanelli F, Di Leo G. *Biostatistics for Radiologists: Planning, Performing, and Writing a Radiologic Study*. Milan, Italy: Springer-Verlag; 2009.

19. The rate of true positives mostly affects:
    A. Positive predictive value
    B. Negative predictive value
    C. Power
    D. P values

20. The rate of false negatives mostly affects:
    A. Positive predictive value
    B. Negative predictive value
    C. Power
    D. P values

21. The rate of true negatives mostly affects:
    A. Sensitivity
    B. Specificity
    C. Power
    D. P values

22. Which of these is the better test (Figure 15-1)?
    A. Curve A
    B. Curve B
    C. Curve C
    D. They are equal

23. Curve C in Figure 15-1 shows:
    A. The ideal test value
    B. The midpoint range
    C. A test value that has equal sensitivity and specificity
    D. A test value that has equal sensitivity and 1-specificity

24. The ROC curve in Figure 15-2 shows which point on the curve to be the best value for the test?
    A. The first
    B. The second
    C. The third
    D. The fourth

25. At point two (second arrow) (see Figure 15-2):
    A. The sensitivity is 68% and the specificity is 6%.
    B. The specificity is 68% and the sensitivity is 6%.
    C. The specificity is 94% and the sensitivity is 68%.
    D. The specificity is 68% and the sensitivity is 94%.

26. The main drawback to an ROC curve is that it does not show:
    A. A P value
    B. The correlation coefficient
    C. The prevalence of disease
    D. The kappa statistic

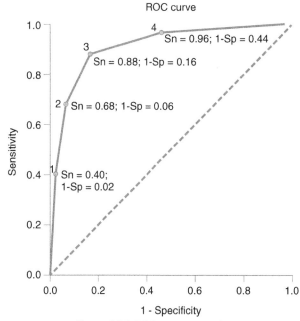

Figure 15-2 ROC curve example.

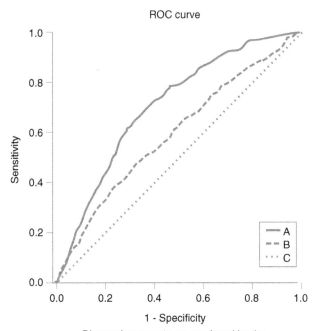

Figure 15-1 ROC curve. The area under the curve (B) for an ROC curve is a summary measure of overall diagnostic performance.

19. **A, Positive predictive value.** Positive predictive value is defined as the number of diseased patients who test positive (true positives) divided by the total number of positive tests (true positives plus false positives). Thus it is most affected by true positive rates.

Negative predictive value is defined as the number of healthy patients who test negative (true negatives) divided by the total number of negative tests (true negatives plus false negatives).

Power is defined statistically as 1 − Beta, which conceptually parallels the rate of true positives as defined in a diagnostic test.

P value is the predefined threshold used to determine if a null hypothesis should be rejected.

Reference:
Sardanelli F, Di Leo G. *Biostatistics for Radiologists: Planning, Performing, and Writing a Radiologic Study*. Milan, Italy: Springer-Verlag; 2009.

20. **B, Negative predictive value.** Negative predictive value is defined as the number of healthy patients who test negative (true negatives) divided by the total number of negative tests (true negatives plus false negatives). It is most affected by false negatives.

Positive predictive value is defined as the number of diseased patients who test positive (true positives) divided by the total number of positive tests (true positives plus false positives).

Power is defined statistically as 1 − Beta, which conceptually parallels the rate of true positives as defined in a diagnostic test.

P value is the predefined threshold used to determine if a null hypothesis should be rejected.

Reference:
Sardanelli F, Di Leo G. *Biostatistics for Radiologists: Planning, Performing, and Writing a Radiologic Study*. Milan, Italy: Springer-Verlag; 2009.

21. **B, Specificity.** Specificity is defined as the number of healthy patients who test negative (true negatives) divided by the total number of healthy patients (true negatives plus false positives). It is most affected by true negatives.

Sensitivity is defined as the number of diseased patients who test positive (true positives) divided by the total number of diseased patients (true positives plus false negatives).

Power is defined statistically as 1 − Beta, which conceptually parallels the rate of true positives as defined in a diagnostic test.

P value is the predefined threshold used to determine if a null hypothesis should be rejected.

Reference:
Sardanelli F, Di Leo G. *Biostatistics for Radiologists: Planning, Performing, and Writing a Radiologic Study*. Milan, Italy: Springer-Verlag; 2009.

22. **A, Curve A.** The area under the curve (AUC) for an ROC curve is a summary measure of overall diagnostic performance. If two ROC curves do not intersect at any point, then their AUCs can be directly compared and the curve with the larger AUC is definitively higher performance. If the curves do intersect, then there may be scenarios where an overall poorer performing test may perform better than the overall better performing test. In the provided example (see Figure 15-1), the overlap is minimal and there is no clear scenario where curve B outperforms curve A. In cases with increased complexity, regional indices have been developed for AUC analysis, but this topic is beyond the scope of this text.

Reference:
Metz CE. Receiver operating characteristic (ROC) analysis: a tool for quantitative evaluation of observer performance and imaging systems. *J Am Coll Radiol.* 2006;3(6):413-422.

23. **D, A test value that has equal sensitivity and 1-specificity.** The AUC for an ROC curve is a summary measure of overall diagnostic performance. An AUC of 1 would imply perfect performance and the curve would lie in the upper left corner of the chart. An AUC of 0.5 would imply random chance performance and the curve would diagonally bisect the chart, such as in curve C. All points along this curve would have equal sensitivity and 1-specificity by definition (see Figure 15-1).

Reference:
Metz CE. Receiver operating characteristic (ROC) analysis: a tool for quantitative evaluation of observer performance and imaging systems. *J Am Coll Radiol.* 2006;3(6):413-422.

24. **C, The third.** The highest performance point along an ROC curve would be that which lies farthest from the diagonal line that represents random chance performance (see Figure 15-2). The farther the deviation, the better the performance of the diagnostic test. Note that this type of analysis operates under the assumption that false negatives and false positives are equally undesired, which may not always be the case in clinical settings

Reference:
Riffenburgh RH. *Statistics in Medicine.* 3rd ed. Amsterdam: Elsevier Academic Press; 2012.

25. **C, The specificity is 94% and the sensitivity is 68% (see Figure 15-2).**

At point one, the specificity is 1-0.02, or 98%, and the sensitivity is 40%.

At point two, the specificity is 1-0.06, or 94%, and the sensitivity is 68%.

At point three, the specificity is 1-0.16, or 84%, and sensitivity is 88%.

At point four, the specificity is 1-0.44, or 56%, and sensitivity is 96%.

Reference:
Riffenburgh RH. *Statistics in Medicine.* 3rd ed. Amsterdam: Elsevier Academic Press; 2012.

26. **C, The prevalence of disease.** P value is the predefined threshold used to determine if a null hypothesis should be rejected and is not directly related to an ROC curve. Any clinical decision made based on an ROC curve will not relate to the P value found for a study.

Correlation coefficient is a quantitative measure of dependence of two variables on each other and is not directly related to an ROC curve. Any clinical decision made based on an ROC curve will not relate to the correlation coefficient found for a study.

Sensitivity and specificity are independent of disease prevalence. Therefore, any plot of their relationship will also be independent of disease prevalence. However, because prevalence does affect positive and negative predictive values, the "absence" of prevalence information in an ROC curve may impact actual test performance in a clinical setting (ie, accuracy). Accuracy is the proportion of true results out of all results and depends on disease prevalence (see questions 10-14). Accuracy can be calculated from sensitivity and specificity only if disease prevalence is known. An ROC curve is an estimate of test accuracy with disease prevalence.

A kappa statistic shows interobserver variability/concordance. It is not shown in an ROC curve.

Reference:
Sardanelli F, Di Leo G. *Biostatistics for Radiologists: Planning, Performing, and Writing a Radiologic Study*. Milan, Italy: Springer-Verlag; 2009.

27. Based on the ROC curve in Figure 15-3, which is correct?
    A. The sensitivity of using a 10-mm threshold for a lymph node in determining if it is malignant is over 80%.
    B. The specificity of using a 10-mm threshold for a lymph node in determining if it is malignant is less than 80%.
    C. The sensitivity of using a 15-mm threshold for a lymph node in determining if it is malignant is less than 60%.
    D. The specificity of using a 15-mm threshold for a lymph node in determining if it is malignant is less than 10%.

28. Based on the ROC curve in Figure 15-3, which is correct?
    A. The true positive rate is greater for 25 mm than for 20 mm.
    B. The specificity is greater for 25 mm than for 20 mm.
    C. The false positive rate is greater for 25 mm than for 20 mm.
    D. The size criteria are not very good.

29. Based on the ROC curve in Figure 15-3, which is correct?
    A. To maximize specificity, use 25 mm.
    B. To maximize specificity, use 10 mm.
    C. To maximize specificity, use 3 mm.
    D. To maximize 1-specificity, use 25 mm.

30. The Hawthorne effect says:
    A. As soon as you start to study something you see improvement
    B. As soon as you stop investigating something you see improvement
    C. As soon as you start studying something you see decrement
    D. None of the above

31. The complications reported in association with the use of a new flow diverter catheter for aneurysm treatment increased over the first 2 years and then declined. This is an example of:
    A. The bell-shaped curve
    B. The reversed bell-shape curve
    C. The Smortig curve
    D. The Weber effect

32. A student measures the temperature of the skin around the ear of a patient who has a gauge in it while in a 3T magnet. The readings are 102.5, 101.7, 103.1, 100.9, 100.5, and 102.2 on six different measurements. He calculates the sample mean to be 101.82. If he knows that the standard deviation for this procedure is 0.49 degrees, what is the confidence interval for the population mean at a 95% confidence level?
    A. (102.31, 101.32)
    B. (102.8, 100.84)
    C. (102.5, 100.9)
    D. None of the above

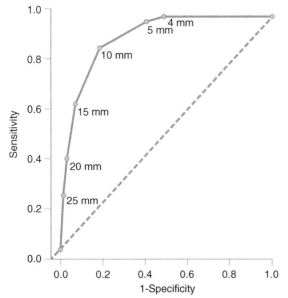

Figure 15-3 ROC curve of size of lymph node for determining malignancy.

27. **A, The sensitivity of using a 10-mm threshold for a lymph node in determining if it is malignant is over 80%.** ROC curves plot a test's false positive rate, or 1-specificity (x-axis) versus its true positive rate, or sensitivity (y-axis). Each point on the curve represents the sensitivity and false positive rate at a different decision threshold. The plotted coordinates are connected with line segments to construct an empiric ROC curve. The figure for this question (see Figure 15-3) plots the sensitivity and specificity of different size thresholds of lymph nodes for detecting malignancy. Having a small size threshold of 4 mm would result in a high sensitivity (draw a horizontal line to the y-axis from the point along the curve labeled 4 mm), but a lower specificity (drawing a vertical line to the x-axis, which is 1-specificity). Knowing that sensitivity is plotted on the y-axis allows you to correctly determine that a size of 10 mm gives you a sensitivity of just over 80%. Answer B results in a specificity of just over 80%. Answer C is incorrect because a size threshold of 15 mm corresponds to a sensitivity just over 60%. Answer D would give you a specificity of approximately 90%, not 10%. The point of highest sensitivity and specificity is in the upper left corner of the chart.

Reference:
Obuchowski NA. ROC analysis. *AJR Am J Roentgenol*. 2005;184(2):34-72.

28. **B, The specificity is greater for 25 mm than for 20 mm.** ROC curves plot a test's false positive rate, or 1-specificity (x-axis) versus its true positive rate, or sensitivity (y-axis). Each point on the curve represents the sensitivity and false positive rate at a different decision threshold. The plotted coordinates are connected with line segments to construct an empiric ROC curve. The figure for this question plots the sensitivity and specificity of different size thresholds of lymph nodes for detecting malignancy. Answer A is incorrect because the true positive rate or sensitivity increases as you go higher up the y-axis. C is incorrect because the false positive rate increases as you go farther to the right on the x-axis. D is an admittedly ambiguous statement that can be dismissed by a process of elimination. The specificity of 25 mm is greater than that of 20 mm because the x-axis on an ROC curve is 1-specificity. The fact that the value on the x-axis is smaller at 25 mm means the specificity is higher.

Reference:
Obuchowski NA. ROC analysis. *AJR Am J Roentgenol*. 2005;184(2):34-72.

29. **A, To maximize specificity, use 25 mm.** A is correct because specificity is maximized at the far left of the x-axis (see Figure 15-3). B and C are incorrect for the same reason. D is incorrect because maximizing 1-specificity is the same as maximizing the false positive rate, which would be on the far right of the x-axis.

Reference:
Obuchowski NA. ROC analysis. *AJR Am J Roentgenol*. 2005;184(2):34-72.

30. **A, As soon as you start to study something you see improvement.** People tend to change their behavior when they are aware that they are being observed. This is described as the Hawthorne effect. In many cases, this may lead to improved performance as in the case of using a video monitoring system to improve hand hygiene or radiology productivity. This increase in productivity may not always reflect a desired outcome or improvement, as seen in a study where a quality improvement initiative to decrease the incidence of falls reported an initial rise that was attributed to the Hawthorne effect.

References:
Abujudeh H, Bruno M. *Quality and Safety in Radiology*. New York: Oxford University Press; 2012.
Srigley JA, Gardam M, Fernie G, et al. Hand hygiene monitoring technology: a systematic review of efficacy. *J Hosp Infect*. 2015;89(1):51-60.
Kidwai AS, Abujudeh HH. Radiologist productivity increases with real-time monitoring: the Hawthorne effect. *J Am Coll Radiol*. 2015;12(11):1151-1154.
Abujudeh HH, Aran S, Daftari Besheli L, et al. Outpatient falls prevention program outcome: an increase, a plateau, and a decrease in incident reports. *AJR Am J Roentgenol*. 2014;203(3):620-626.

31. **D, The Weber effect.** The Weber effect describes the phenomenon of increased adverse event reporting that occurs in the first 2 years after introduction of a new agent and then peaks at the end of the second year before declining. This phenomenon was described in a recent study that evaluated the effect of abruptly substituting one gadolinium agent for another on allergic-like reactions. Bell curves describe a normal distribution of random variables as a symmetric bell-shaped graph. A reversed or inverted bell curve describes a bimodal distribution with a trough between two peaks. Answer C is a made up name for a curve. Let's hope you avoided that trap.

Reference:
Davenport MS, Dillman JR, Cohan RH, et al. Effect of abrupt substitution of gadobenate dimeglumine for gadopentetate dimeglumine on rate of allergic-like reactions. *Radiology*. 2013;266(3):773-782.

32. **B, (102.8, 100.84).** The confidence interval (CI) is a range of values calculated by statistical methods which includes the desired true population value with a probability defined in advance.

An interval can be calculated for any degree of confidence. However, the 95% confidence intervals are the most commonly utilized. Confidence interval (CI) can be calculated based on a normally distributed sample with a known standard deviation using the following formula:

$$95\% \text{ CI} = \text{Mean} \pm Z\left(\text{SD}/\sqrt{n}\right)$$

Z (standardized score) = Value of the standard normal distribution with the specific level of confidence. For a 95% CI, Z = 1.96

SD = Standard deviation

n = Sample size

For the case above, mean = 101.82, SD = 0.49, and n = 1.

Applying these to the equation:

$$95\% \text{ CI} = 101.82 \pm 1.96\left(0.49/\sqrt{1}\right)$$
$$95\% \text{ CI} = 101.82 \pm 1.96 \, 90.49)$$
$$95\% \text{ CI} = 101.82 \pm 0.96$$
$$95\% \text{ CI} = 102.8, 100.8 \text{ (rounded to one decimal place)}$$

Reference:
Medina LS, Zurakowski D. Measurement variability and confidence intervals in medicine: why should radiologists care? *Radiology*. 2003;226(2):297-301.

33. A 90% confidence interval suggests that if the measurement was repeated on multiple samples:
    A. The likelihood that the measurement would fall between the confidence intervals is 90% of the time
    B. That the mean is within the confidence interval 90% of the time
    C. That the standard deviation is within the confidence interval 90% of the time
    D. That all values within two standard deviations of the mean will fall between the confidence intervals 90% of the time

34. Type II (β) errors are:
    A. False positive
    B. False negative
    C. True negative
    D. True positive

35. Type I (α) errors are:
    A. False positive
    B. False negative
    C. True negative
    D. True positive

36. To calculate the number of subjects you need for a sample size you need to know which parameters?
    A. Effect size
    B. Alpha significance criterion (α)
    C. Statistical power (β)
    D. All of the above

37. The typical value for power (β) acceptable is:
    A. 95%
    B. 97.5%
    C. 80%
    D. 50%

38. The larger the sample size:
    A. The larger the possibility of type 1 error
    B. The larger the power
    C. The less likely you are to reject the null hypothesis
    D. The wider the confidence intervals

33. **A, The likelihood that the measurement would fall between the confidence intervals (CIs) is 90% of the time.** The CI is a range of values calculated by statistical methods that includes the desired true population value with a probability defined in advance.

In a given population, if samples are repeatedly obtained and CIs constructed for each sample, a certain percentage of the CIs will include the value of the true population and a certain percentage of them will not include that value. In statistical analysis, a confidence level of 95% is frequently selected. This means that if samples are repeatedly obtained from a population and CIs are constructed for each sample, the CI covers the true value in 95 of 100 studies performed. Hence the likelihood that the measurement would fall between the CIs is 95% of the time, while 5% of the time the measurement will fall out of the CIs. Similarly, a 90% CI suggests that if the measurement was repeated on multiple samples, the likelihood that the measurement would fall between the CIs is 90% of the time, while 10% of the time the measurement will fall out of the CIs.

References:
Prel JBD, Hommel G, Röhrig B, et al. Confidence interval or P-value? *Dtsch Arztebl Int.* 2009;106(19):335-339.
Medina LS, Zurakowski D. Measurement variability and confidence intervals in medicine: why should radiologists care? *Radiology.* 2003;226:297-301.

34. **B, False negative.** Following the completion of a study, the investigator utilizes statistical tests to try to reject the null hypothesis in favor of an alternative. Assuming that the study is free of bias, and depending on whether the null hypothesis is true or false in the target population, there are four possible outcomes. In two of the outcomes, the findings in the sample study and reality in the population are concordant. The result is that the investigator's inference will be correct. In the other two outcomes, either a type I (α) or a type II (β) error will be made. The result is that the investigator's inference will be incorrect.

A type II (β) error (false negative) is the type of error that occurs if the investigator fails to reject a null hypothesis that is actually false in the population.

Reference:
Banerjee A, Chitnis UB, Jadhav SL, et al. Hypothesis testing, type I and type II errors. *Ind Psychiatry J.* 2009;18(2):127-131.

35. **A, False positive.** Following the completion of a study, the investigator utilizes statistical tests to try to reject the null hypothesis in favor of an alternative. Assuming that the study is free of bias and depending on whether the null hypothesis is true or false in the target population, there are four possible outcomes. In two of the outcomes, the findings in the sample study and reality in the population are concordant. The result is that the investigator's inference will be correct. In the other two outcomes, either a type I (α) or a type II (β) error will be made. The result is that the investigator's inference will be incorrect.

A type I (α) error (false positive) is the type of error that occurs if an investigator rejects a null hypothesis that is actually true in the population.

Reference:
Banerjee A, Chitnis UB, Jadhav SL, et al. Hypothesis testing, type I and type II errors. *Ind Psychiatry J.* 2009;18(2):127-131.

36. **D, All of the above.** The sample size refers to the number of individuals needed in a research study. It is a very important consideration in the analysis of many clinical studies and often a question is raised as to appropriate sample size in a given study.

An appropriate sample size depends on five study design parameters, including the minimum expected difference or the effect size, the estimated measurement variability, the desired statistical power, the significance criterion, and whether a one- or two-tailed statistical analysis is planned.

The minimum expected difference, or the effect size, refers to the smallest measured difference that the investigator would like the study to detect between comparison groups. As this parameter is made smaller, the sample size needed to detect statistical significance increases.

The estimated measurement variability is the expected standard deviation in the measurements made within each comparison group. The sample size needed to detect the minimum difference increases as statistical variability increases.

The statistical power refers to the power that is desired from the study. As this parameter is increased, the sample size increases.

The significance criterion refers to the maximum P value at which a difference is to be considered statistically significant. As the significance criterion is made more strict, the sample size needed to detect the minimum difference increases. The significance criterion is customarily set to 0.05.

References:
Eng J. Sample size estimation: how many individuals should be studied? *Radiology.* 2003;227(2):309-313.
Obuchowski NA, Hillis SL. Sample size tables for computer aided detection studies. *AJR Am J Roentgenol.* 2011;197(5):W821-W828.

37. **C, 80%.** Statistical power is one of five study design parameters that affect the sample size of a clinical study. It refers to the power that is desired from a study. Although many clinical trial experts now advocate a power of 0.90, in randomized controlled trials the statistical power is usually set to a number greater than or equal to 0.80.

Reference:
Eng J. Sample size estimation: how many individuals should be studied? *Radiology.* 2003;227(2):309-313.

38. **B, The larger the power.** Statistical power is the ability of a study to allow the detection of a statistically significant difference when one truly exists. It is similar in some ways to the sensitivity of a diagnostic test. It is closely related to sample size of a population because it is one of the key parameters that determine an appropriate sample size.

An appropriate sample size for a clinical study comparing two means can be calculated using the following equation:

$$N = 4\sigma^2(Zcrit + Zpwr)^2/D^2$$

Where:
N = Sample size (the sum of the sizes of both comparison groups)
σ = The assumed SD of each group
Zcrit = Significance criterion
Zpwr = Statistical power
D = The minimum expected difference between the two means

As power increases, sample size increases and vice versa. In randomized controlled trials, the statistical power is customarily set to a number greater than or equal to 0.80.

Reference:
Eng J. Sample size estimation: how many individuals should be studied? *Radiology.* 2003;227(2):309-313.

39. The criticality index is a product of:
    A. Likelihood of failure and severity of damage
    B. Order of occurrence and likelihood of occurrence
    C. Number of downstream factors affected and impact score
    D. Severity of illness and cost of care

40. Which of the following images has high precision and high accuracy (Figure 15-4)?
    A. Image 1
    B. Image 2
    C. Image 3
    D. Image 4

41. Which of the following has low precision but high accuracy (Figure 15-4)?
    A. Image 1
    B. Image 2
    C. Image 3
    D. Image 4

42. Which of the following has low precision and low accuracy (Figure 15-4)?
    A. Image 1
    B. Image 2
    C. Image 3
    D. Image 4

43. Which of the following has high precision but low accuracy (Figure 15-4)?
    A. Image 1
    B. Image 2
    C. Image 3
    D. Image 4

44. Accuracy refers to clustering around _____ whereas precision refers to degree of _____.
    A. Each other, dispersion
    B. The target, dispersion
    C. The target, accuracy
    D. Precision, accuracy

45. Classification based on species is considered:
    A. Ordinal
    B. Nominal
    C. Noncategorical
    D. Linear

46. Minimal, moderate, and marked degrees of lumbar stenosis are classifications that are:
    A. Ordinal
    B. Nominal
    C. Noncategorical
    D. Linear

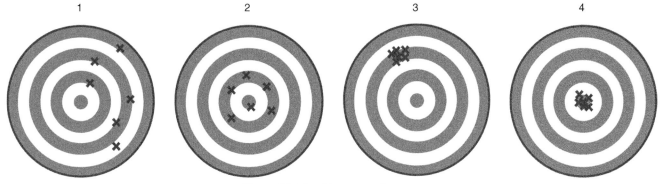

Figure 15-4 Precision versus Accuracy.

39. A, Likelihood of failure and severity of damage. The criticality index is also referred to as the risk priority number. It is a quantitative measure used to evaluate and assess a failure mode. It is a product of the probability of failure, detectability, and the severity of damage.

In a study, criticality indices are ranked to allow a triage or prioritization of the failure modes. The aim of this prioritization process is to identify the failure modes that exceed acceptable limits and need to be targeted for change. The highest criticality index identified should always be prioritized for corrective action. The lower criticality index steps should be excluded from the prioritization process because they are unlikely to affect the process.

Reference:
Thornton E, Brook OR, Mendiratta-Lala M, et al. Application of failure mode and effect analysis in a radiology department. *Radiographics.* 2011;31(1): 281-293.

40. D, Image 4. Precision can be defined as a level of measurement that produces minimum variability and consistent results when repeated. On the other hand, measurements that yield high variability are referred to as imprecise. Accuracy can be defined as a level of measurement that produces true and consistent results.

If we think of throwing darts at a dart board as in the images in the question (see Figure 15-4), the group of darts that have their center close to the bull's eye would represent the high accuracy group while the group of darts that have a small spread would represent a high precision group. An imprecise group would form a large cluster contrary to the high precision group. A tightly clustered grouping around the center of the target, as in Image 4, has high accuracy and precision.

Measurements can also be accurate but imprecise or even inaccurate but precise. Option A, Image 1, demonstrates poor precision and low accuracy. Option B, Image 2, demonstrates poor precision and intermediate accuracy. Option C, Image 3, demonstrates high/good precision and low accuracy.

Reference:
Levin SG. Understanding and using statistics in nuclear medicine. *J Nucl Med.* 1979;20(6):550-558.

41. B, Image 2. Accuracy reflects how close a measured value is to the actual (true) value. Precision is how close the measured values are to each other. In this case there are random (multifactorial) errors preventing the measurements from clustering around a specific value, but the results are equally close to the true value.

If we think of throwing darts at a dart board as in the images in the question (see Figure 15-4), the group of darts that have their center close to the bull's eye would represent the high accuracy group while the group of darts that have a small spread would represent a high precision group. An imprecise group would form a large cluster contrary to the high precision group. Option B, Image 2, demonstrates poor precision but relatively good accuracy.

Reference:
Levin SG. Understanding and using statistics in nuclear medicine. *J Nucl Med.* 1979;20(6):550-558.

42. A, Image 1. Precision can be defined as a level of measurement that produces minimum variability and consistent results when repeated. On the other hand, measurements that yield high variability are referred to as imprecise. Accuracy can be defined as a level of measurement that produces true and consistent results.

If we think of throwing darts at a dart board as in the images in the question (see Figure 15-4), the group of darts

that have their center close to the bull's eye would represent the high accuracy group while the group of darts that have a small spread would represent a high precision group. An imprecise group would form a large cluster contrary to the high precision group. Option A, Image 1, demonstrates poor precision and low accuracy.

Reference:
Levin SG. Understanding and using statistics in nuclear medicine. *J Nucl Med.* 1979;20(6):550-558.

43. C, Image 3. Precision can be defined as a level of measurement that produces minimum variability and consistent results when repeated. On the other hand, measurements that yield high variability are referred to as imprecise. Accuracy can be defined as a level of measurement that produces true and consistent results.

If we think of throwing darts at a dart board as in the images in the question (Figure 15-4), the group of darts that have their center close to the bull's eye would represent the high accuracy group while the group of darts that have a small spread would represent a high precision group. Option C, Image 3, demonstrates high/good precision and low accuracy.

Reference:
Levin SG. Understanding and using statistics in nuclear medicine. *J Nucl Med.* 1979;20(6):550-558.

44. B, The target, dispersion. *Accuracy* is a general term without a numerical expression that describes the degree of closeness of a measurement to the true value. Usually the deviation from the true value is in the same direction. It is associated with the concept of systematic error, a form of deterministic observational error that has a definite and potentially solvable cause. In target grouping the concept is represented by clustering of measurements around the center of the target (the true value). *Precision* is a general term without a numerical expression that describes the closeness of agreement among a set of repeated measurements under unchanged conditions. It is associated with the concept of random error, a form of stochastic observational error that is always present in measurements and is due to multiple factors that we cannot or do not control. In target grouping the concept is represented by clustering of measurements around each other. A precise measurement yields consistent results when repeated.

References:
JCGM 200. 2012 International vocabulary of metrology: basic and general concepts and associated errors. Published by the JCGM in the name of the BIPM, IEC, IFCC, ILAC, ISO, IUPAC, IUPAP, and OIML.
BS ISO 5725-1: Accuracy (trueness and precision) of measurement methods and results - Part 1: general principles and definitions; 1994:1.
Taylor JR. *An Introduction to Error Analysis: The Study of Uncertainties in Physical Measurements.* Sausalito, CA: University Science Books; 1999:94, §4.1.

45. B, Nominal. Nominal classification divides data into groups without relative values or order. Examples include gender, race, and occupation.

Reference:
Nick TG. Descriptive statistics. *Methods Mol Biol.* 2007;404:33-52. doi: 10.1007/978-1-59745-530-5_3. Review. PubMed PMID: 18450044.

46. A, Ordinal. Ordinal data are divided into groups that have inherent order but the interval between groups is not equal. Minimal, moderate, and marked degrees of lumbar stenosis are examples of ordinal classification.

Reference:
Nick TG. Descriptive statistics. *Methods Mol Biol.* 2007;404:33-52. doi: 10.1007/978-1-59745-530-5_3. Review. PubMed PMID: 18450044.

47. Age is a variable that is:
    A. Nominal
    B. Continuous
    C. Categorical
    D. Random

48. In a box plot (Figure 15-5), the shaded rectangular area represents:
    A. The mean plus one standard deviation
    B. The mean plus two standard deviations
    C. The area enclosing the upper and lower quartiles
    D. The mean and confidence intervals

49. On that same plot (see Figure 15-5), the thick horizontal line represents:
    A. The mean
    B. The median
    C. The mode
    D. The target value

50. The upper and lower whiskers of the box plot (see Figure 15-5) represent:
    A. The range of the mean and two standard deviations
    B. The range of the upper and lower quintiles
    C. The range of the upper and lower quartiles
    D. The range of all values

51. In this box plot (Figure 15-6), the single point located at value 12 represents:
    A. An outlier outside the range specified
    B. The target value
    C. A value beyond two standard deviations from the mean
    D. The mode

52. In a study like mammography where the most important part of the test is to rule in cancer in patients who have it, one would want:
    A. High sensitivity
    B. High specificity
    C. High positive predictive value
    D. High negative predictive value

53. In a screening test like TB skin testing where you want to make sure that you don't have to incur the cost of a lot of chest radiographs on patients to make sure they do not have TB, one would want:
    A. High sensitivity
    B. High specificity
    C. High positive predictive value
    D. High negative predictive value

54. In a study where the most important part of the test is to rule out cancer (ie, CT for lymph nodes in order to avoid an elective neck dissection), you might adjust your threshold values lower in order to have a:
    A. High sensitivity
    B. High specificity
    C. High positive predictive value
    D. High negative predictive value

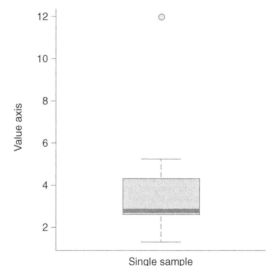

Figure 15-6 Sample Data Box Plot.

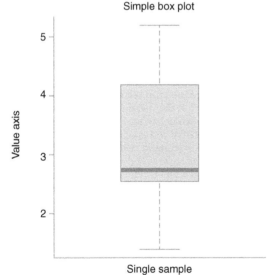

Figure 15-5 Box Plot of Data.

47. **B, Continuous.** Interval data have inherent order and the interval between values is equal. Interval data are divided into continuous data and discrete data. Continuous data are measured on a continuum where data can always be further subdivided—eg, age. Discrete data are based on counts and cannot be further subdivided—eg, the number of residents in a radiology program.

Reference:
Nick TG. Descriptive statistics. *Methods Mol Biol.* 2007;404:33-52. doi: 10.1007/978-1-59745-530-5_3. Review. PubMed PMID: 18450044.

48. **C, The area enclosing the upper and lower quartiles.** In a box plot (Figure 15-7), the shaded box represents the bounds of the lower quartile and the upper quartile and the dark horizontal line represents the median. The height of the box plot represents the interquartile range.

Reference:
Dawson B, Trapp RG. Chapter 3. Summarizing data & presenting data in tables & graphs. In: Dawson B, Trapp RG, eds. *Basic & Clinical Biostatistics.* 4th ed. New York, NY: McGraw-Hill; 2004.

49. **B, The median.** In a box plot (see Figure 15-7), the shaded box represents the bounds of the lower quartile, and the upper quartile and the dark horizontal line represent the median. The height of the box plot represents the interquartile range.

Reference:
Dawson B, Trapp RG. Chapter 3. Summarizing data & presenting data in tables & graphs. In: Dawson B, Trapp RG, eds. *Basic & Clinical Biostatistics.* 4th ed. New York, NY: McGraw-Hill; 2004.

50. **D, The range of all values.** In a box plot (see Figure 15-7), the shaded box represents the bounds of the lower quartile and the upper quartile and the dark horizontal line represents the median. The height of the box plot represents the interquartile range. Whiskers are vertical lines extending from the upper and lower bounds of the box. The whiskers indicate the spread of data. This can include the entire range, the range minus outliers, or a defined percentile. A common method calculates 1.5 times the interquartile range and the whiskers extend this length above the 75th percentile and below the 25th percentile. In this example, no data points are present outside of the whiskers, and therefore the whiskers represent the entire range of data.

Reference:
Dawson B, Trapp RG. Chapter 3. Summarizing data & presenting data in tables & graphs. In: Dawson B, Trapp RG, eds. *Basic & Clinical Biostatistics.* 4th ed. New York, NY: McGraw-Hill; 2004.

51. **A, An outlier outside the range specified.** In this example (see Figure 15-6), a single data point is seen above the upper whisker. Without more information, all that can be inferred is that this data point is outside the range specified by the researcher. Whiskers can include the entire range, the range minus outliers, or a defined percentile. A common method calculates 1.5 times the interquartile range, and the whiskers extend this length above the 75th percentile and below the 25th percentile.

Reference:
Dawson B, Trapp RG. Chapter 3. Summarizing data & presenting data in tables & graphs. In: Dawson B, Trapp RG, eds. *Basic & Clinical Biostatistics.* 4th ed. New York, NY: McGraw-Hill; 2004.

52. **A, High sensitivity.**

Sensitivity = TP/(TP + FN)
Specificity = TN/(TN + FP)
Positive predictive value = TP/(TP + FP)
Negative predictive value = TN/(TN + FN)
TP = true positive, TN = true negative, FP = false positive, and FN = false negative

Sensitivity reflects the probability that the test will be positive in patients who actually have the disorder. With a high sensitivity, there is a low number of false negatives, and therefore patients can be reassured that a negative test is accurate. In a screening test, it is most important to have a high sensitivity. If the screening test has a low positive predictive value, many more breast biopsies will be required because of a high rate of false positive readings—exams where the imaging suggests cancer but there really is no cancer.

Reference:
Dawson B, Trapp RG. Chapter 12. Methods of evidence-based medicine and decision analysis. In: Dawson B, Trapp RG, eds. *Basic & Clinical Biostatistics.* 4th ed. New York, NY: McGraw-Hill; 2004.

53. **B, High specificity.**

Sensitivity = TP/(TP + FN)
Specificity = TN/(TN + FP)
Positive predictive value = TP/(TP + FP)
Negative predictive value = TN/(TN + FN)
TP = true positive, TN = true negative, FP = false positive, and FN = false negative

The sensitivity of the test reflects the probability that the screening test will be positive among those who are diseased. In contrast, the specificity of the test reflects the probability that the screening test will be negative among those who, in fact, do not have the disease. In the case of TB, you want the test to be negative on patients without disease. If it is falsely positive and the patient does not have TB, you end up doing radiography and possibly even putting the patient on anti-TB meds for no reason.

Reference:
Dawson B, Trapp RG. Chapter 12. Methods of evidence-based medicine and decision analysis. In: Dawson B, Trapp RG, eds. *Basic & Clinical Biostatistics.* 4th ed. New York, NY: McGraw-Hill; 2004.

54. **D, High negative predictive value.**

Sensitivity = TP/(TP + FN)
Specificity = TN/(TN + FP)
Positive predictive value = TP/(TP + FP)
Negative predictive value = TN/(TN + FN)
TP = true positive, TN = true negative, FP = false positive, and FN = false negative

In this scenario, you want to make sure that the negative test rules out the presence of cancer in the neck. You are trying to avoid having to do a neck dissection, so if the test is negative and is reliable, you can feel more comfortable. In this scenario, a high negative predictive value is important because you do not want a high rate of false negatives (cases where you say the study is negative but the patient really has cancer).

Reference:
Dawson B, Trapp RG. Chapter 12. Methods of evidence-based medicine and decision analysis. In: Dawson B, Trapp RG, eds. *Basic & Clinical Biostatistics.* 4th ed. New York, NY: McGraw-Hill; 2004.

55. In a study where you do not want to make a mistake and mislabel someone with a disease who does not have the disease (ie, genetic testing for Down's syndrome in amniocentesis), you want a test that has a high:
    A. Sensitivity
    B. Specificity
    C. Positive predictive value
    D. Negative predictive value

56. In Figure 15-7, the point at A represents:
    A. The median value
    B. The mean value
    C. The mode value
    D. None of the above

57. In Figure 15-7, the values between the two "B"s are likely to represent:
    A. First quartiles
    B. Second quartiles
    C. One standard deviation from the mean
    D. Two standard deviations from the mean

58. In Figure 15-7, the values between the two "C"s are likely to represent:
    A. First quartiles
    B. Second quartiles
    C. One standard deviation from the mean
    D. Two standard deviations from the mean

59. The answers in questions 56 through 58 assume:
    A. A normal distribution
    B. An asymptotic distribution
    C. A binomial distribution
    D. Bayes, theorem applies

60. If the variance from the mean of a distribution of values is measured at 9, then the standard deviation:
    A. Cannot be determined without knowing the mean value
    B. Cannot be determined
    C. Is 81
    D. Is 3

61. The best statistical test to evaluate for interobserver variation is:
    A. McNemar
    B. Kappa
    C. Confidence intervals
    D. Variance/standard deviation

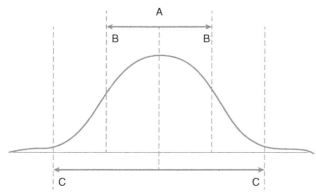

Figure 15-7 Plot of Data-Bell shaped curve.

55. C, High positive predictive value.

Sensitivity = TP/(TP + FN)
Specificity = TN/(TN + FP)
Positive predictive value = TP/(TP + FP)
Negative predictive value = TN/(TN + FN)
TP = true positive, TN = true negative, FP = false positive, and FN = false negative

If the amniocentesis test has a low positive predictive value, there would be the potential of terminating pregnancies in fetuses that did not have Down's syndrome because of a high rate of false positive tests—genetic tests where the results suggests Down's but there really is no genetic abnormality. Instead, you want to be very certain that if the genetic profile is positive for Down's the child will definitely have Down's syndrome and allow the parents to make some tough choices. Therefore a high positive predictive value is very important—few false positives (mislabeling someone with a disease who does not have the disease). Having cases where the test is falsely negative and the child is born with Down's would occur with a low sensitivity test.

Reference:
Dawson B, Trapp RG. Chapter 12. Methods of evidence-based medicine and decision analysis. In: Dawson B, Trapp RG, eds. *Basic & Clinical Biostatistics.* 4th ed. New York, NY: McGraw-Hill; 2004.

56. B, The mean value. The provided curve demonstrates a normal distribution (see Figure 15-7). Typically, the peak of the curve A, represents the mean or average, σ, of all values included in the distribution, f(x). Please note that in a perfectly normal distribution, the mean equals the mode and the median.

Reference:
<https://en.wikipedia.org/wiki/Normal_distribution>.

57. C, One standard deviation from the mean. The endpoints delineated by the points labeled B are within 1 standard deviation, σ, from the mean (see Figure 15-7). In a normal distribution, these points are inflection points delineating a slope change moving away from the central mean. Sixty-eight percent of a normal distribution lies within 1 standard deviation of the mean.

Reference:
<https://en.wikipedia.org/wiki/Normal_distribution>.

58. D, Two standard deviations from the mean. The endpoints delineated by the points labeled C are within two standard deviations, 2σ, from the mean (see Figure 15-7). Ninety-five percent of a normal distribution lies within two standard deviations of the mean.

Reference:
<https://en.wikipedia.org/wiki/Normal_distribution>.

59. A, A normal distribution. All of the preceding questions about Figure 15-7 assume a normal distribution. An asymptotic distribution has values that approach a certain number—in other words, is "limiting" toward an asymptote. An asymptotic distribution, for example, may model a cumulative distribution function with a limit of 1. A binomial distribution models the probability of a process with success or failure, without continuous variables as seen in a normal distribution. Bayes' theorem describes the conditional probability of an event and is not a required assumption of a normal distribution.

References:
<https://en.wikipedia.org/wiki/Asymptotic_distribution>.
<http://mathworld.wolfram.com/BinomialDistribution.html>.
<https://en.wikipedia.org/wiki/Bayes%27_theorem>.

60. D, Is 3 (the standard deviation is the square root of the variance). Variance and standard deviation are statistical measures of dispersion, and therefore summarize variability around the mean. Variance is calculated by the sum of the squared deviation from the mean for each value, divided by the total number of observations minus 1 (where the deviation is the value of the observation minus the mean). The standard deviation is the square root of the variance and therefore can be calculated from the variance without knowing the value of the mean. In this example, the variance is equal to $\sqrt{9} = 3$.

Reference:
Krousel-Wood MA, Chambers RB, Muntner P. Clinicians' guide to statistics for medical practice and research: Part I. *Ochsner J.* 2006;6(2):68-83. PMID: 21765796.

61. B, Kappa. Agreement between observers (interobserver agreement) when analyzing categorical data in which the response variable is classified into nominal (or possibly ordinal) multinomial categories is often reported as a kappa statistic. This provides a quantitative measure of the magnitude of agreement between observers and assesses precision (reliability). The kappa test scale is listed as:

Kappa Statistic

Value	Rate of Agreement
<0	Less than chance agreement
0.01-0.20	Slight agreement
0.21-0.40	Fair agreement
0.41-0.60	Moderate agreement
0.61-0.80	Substantial agreement
0.81-0.99	Almost perfect agreement

When the data are quantitative, tests for interobserver agreement are usually obtained from standard ANOVA mixed models or random effects models. Intraclass coefficients may also be calculated.

Reference:
Viera AJ, Garrett JM. Understanding interobserver agreement: the kappa statistic. *Fam Med.* 2005;37(5):360-363.

Page numbers followed by "*f*" indicate figures, and "*t*" indicate tables.

Printed and bound by CPI Group (UK) Ltd, Croydon, CR0 4YY

03/10/2024

01040380-0003